Assessment of Impaired Hearing
A CRITIQUE AND A NEW METHOD

Assessment of Impaired Hearing
A CRITIQUE AND A NEW METHOD

WILLIAM G. NOBLE
Department of Psychology
The University of New England
Armidale, N.S.W., Australia

ACADEMIC PRESS New York   San Francisco   London   1978
A Subsidiary of Harcourt Brace Jovanovich, Publishers

COPYRIGHT © 1978, BY ACADEMIC PRESS, INC.
ALL RIGHTS RESERVED.
NO PART OF THIS PUBLICATION MAY BE REPRODUCED OR
TRANSMITTED IN ANY FORM OR BY ANY MEANS, ELECTRONIC
OR MECHANICAL, INCLUDING PHOTOCOPY, RECORDING, OR ANY
INFORMATION STORAGE AND RETRIEVAL SYSTEM, WITHOUT
PERMISSION IN WRITING FROM THE PUBLISHER.

ACADEMIC PRESS, INC.
111 Fifth Avenue, New York, New York 10003

United Kingdom Edition published by
ACADEMIC PRESS, INC. (LONDON) LTD.
24/28 Oval Road, London NW1 7DX

Library of Congress Cataloging in Publication Data

Noble, William G.
    The assessment of impaired hearing.

    Bibliography: p.
    Includes indexes.
    1. Audiometry.　I. Title.　[DNLM:
1. Hearing disorders--Diagnosis.　2. Hearing
tests.　WV270.3 N753a]　77-77239
ISBN 0-12-520050-1

PRINTED IN THE UNITED STATES OF AMERICA

Contents

Preface   ix
Acknowledgments   xi

PART I
EMERGENCE OF CURRENT ASSESSMENT PRACTICE

1
The Nature of Hearing, Partial Hearing, and Deafness   3

Introduction	3
The Nature of the Auditory World	4
The Functioning of the Auditory System	7
Partial Hearing and Deafness	13
Clinical Features of Hearing Impairment	19

2
The Emergence of Assessment and Tests Used in That Practice   25

The Concept of Assessment	25
Why Hearing Is Assessed	27
Tests Used in Hearing Assessment	31

3
Assessment for Compensation and the Emergence of Systems   39

The Concept of an Assessment System	39
Operational Definitions	40
Systems of Assessment	41
Historical Review of Assessment for Compensation	46
Assessment for Compensation in Various Countries	54

PART II
PROBLEMS IN ASSESSMENT OF IMPAIRED HEARING

4
Basic Assessment Concepts — 61

Reliability and Utility	61
Validity	67
Interaction of Reliability and Validity and the Concept of Generalizability	71

5
Reliability of Tests Used for Hearing Assessment — 75

Scope of Research	75
Reliability of Tonal Threshold Tests	77
Reliability of Speech Tests	99
A Note on Test Utility	108

6
Concurrent and Predictive Validity of Assessment Systems in Use — 111

Introduction	111
Tonal Threshold and Speech Reception Threshold–Speech Detection Threshold	112
Tonal Threshold and Discrimination Score	140
Discussion and Conclusions	168

7
Ancillary Problems: I. Normal Hearing — 173

The Meaning of Normal	173
Audiometric Zero	176
Normal Hearing as an Age-Related Variable	185
The "Limits of Normal"	195

8
Ancillary Problems: II. Recruitment and "Functional Hearing Loss" — 199

Introduction and Apology	199
Nature and Hypothesized Mechanism of Recruitment	200
The Measurement of Recruitment	208
Alleged Effect of Loudness Distortion on Hearing	212
"Functional Hearing Loss"	218
The "Measurement" of "Functional Hearing Loss"	224
Fakability: A Resolution of the Problem	229

Contents

PART III
A REDIRECTION IN HEARING LOSS AND HANDICAP ASSESSMENT

9
Development of Self-Report Scales for Hearing Assessment — 235

Overview of Present Practice	235
A Redirection in Hearing Assessment	237
Self-Report Questionnaires	243
The Hearing Measurement Scale	252
Appendix	264

10
Relations between Self-Report and Hearing Test Performance — 269

Purpose and Scope of Research	269
Results from Earlier Studies	270
The Hearing Measurement Scale	283

11
Advantages, Disadvantages, and Applications of Self-Report — 307

Advantages of Self-Report	307
Disadvantages of Self-Report	312
Applications of Self-Report	317

12
Future Trends — 321

References — 327
Index — 343

Preface

The assessment of impaired hearing is a large and expanding enterprise. A major cause of expansion is the increasing use throughout the world of technological procedures for the exploitation of natural resources and the manufacture of goods. Coupled with this is a growing body of statutory legislation, again worldwide, admitting compensation for impairment of hearing caused by accidental traumatic injury or by longer-term exposure to injurious levels of noise at work. In addition, war and conflict produce deafness from noise and blast, along with all the other injuries and calamities of such aggressive activity. It is impossible to estimate how many people are victims of one-time or ongoing noise exposure, but on a world scale, the impression is that these should be counted in at least hundreds of thousands.

The principal aims of this book are to review the theory and practice of current hearing assessment and to give the basis for a quite different approach to the issues. Existing practice and theory, existing interdependently, are founded on the mechanical testing of aspects of hearing function. This approach is essentially physical. The method I advocate is more psychological in style because it depends on people's own experiences and appraisals of their hearing and their difficulties in hearing.

As a consequence of this new style of approach to assessment of impaired hearing there is a transformation of attitude to the person being assessed. The individual's experience becomes the arena in which measurement is made, and his interest acquires greater prominence. The prevailing mechanical approach, in ignoring the individual's experience, also ignores his political and economic interest. Perhaps unwittingly, but very often concomitantly, the political and economic interests of the institution—industry, clinic, or the armed services—are usually the ones being served by current practice.

The focus of interest within this book is primarily on assessment of impaired hearing in *adults*. Assessment of adult hearing impairment has not received attention to nearly the same extent as hearing impairment in infants and young children. Indeed, an early motivating influence for this book's preparation stemmed from reading a recent encyclopedic work edited by Mittler (1970), *The Psychological Assessment of Mental and Physical Handicaps*. While it has space given over to visual perceptual problems of adults, the only treatment of hearing difficulty is Reed's chapter in the section on children. I think the gap in Mittler's text is best explained by the fact that prior to the appearance of the present book, there has been no extensive, highly visible source of material on adult hearing assessment.

In this book I not only assert that hearing assessment *does* go on among adults, but furthermore attempt the task of defining and articulating this large sector of the audiological world. Its major purpose is to describe issues and problems in adult hearing assessment and to argue for the reorientation of approach mentioned in the opening paragraph. The work is divided into three parts: Part I describes the emergence of the status quo in hearing assessment, with particular reference to assessment for compensation; Part II is an extensive review of problematic features of tests and systems and represents the bulk of the book; Part III describes a radical alternative to the status quo, which it is hoped may resolve many of the problems identified herein.

An important aspect of the content should be highlighted. While most of the text is addressed to purely technical and theoretical problems, there are occasional polemical passages in connection with the politics of certain aspects of this area of study. This element relates to a point I made at the opening of this preface. Assessment of impaired hearing is a social activity, having political and economic consequences, as well as a technical practice having scientific consequences (and vice versa). Unless there is acknowledgment of the first aspect, assertions may be uttered as though concerned only with the second aspect and allowed to masquerade as scientific statements. It is my view that social science, in particular, hobbles its own enterprise if it fails to take account of the larger political and economic milieux within which it is carried on.

Although the book will be of primary concern to audiologists and otologists, much of its content bears upon the endeavors of all researchers concerned with the assessment of hearing and impaired hearing for some purpose or other. Furthermore, although the text is pitched at the research level, there are short introductory passages and there is little or no unexplained jargon, so that qualified graduate students may come at the thing without fear.

Acknowledgments

It is difficult to say in what ways an intellectual career is influenced, and the best I can do is to identify two people whose professional and personal society have assuredly affected some of the ways I see problems like the ones discussed in this book. Gordon Atherley, my friend, colleague, and adviser, has such an expansive and stylish outlook that it is impossible to be narrowly constrained in one's thinking when trying to unravel problems in his company. Though we are at loggerheads over many aspects of this and other slices of the contemporary world, our mutual respect for the absurd allows disagreement to develop without calumny. And Bronwyn Davies, my closest friend and colleague, has introduced me in recent years to features of social science that I consider provide this work with much of whatever originality lies in its approach.
At a more concrete level, I wish to acknowledge two institutions in this country. The first is my own university, whose liberal policy, on this score at least, permitted me to spend the major proportion of a year's study leave at my home writing this book. The second is the Central Laboratory of the National Acoustic Laboratories in Sydney, whose director and staff, particularly of the library, allowed me to take up their time and resources in unearthing material. Without these two features, this work could not have been completed in so brief a time.
Finally my thanks to Sue Nano who produced such handsome typescripts from my disfigured drafts.
In regard to figures and tables reproduced or adapted here, specific acknowledgments of publishers' and authors' permissions are given in the text. For permission to quote from Beasley (1940b), I acknowledge the American Institute of Physics (*Journal of the Acoustical Society of America*) and the author; and I acknowledge *The Laryngoscope* for permission to quote from Fowler (1941) and from Quiggle et al. (1957).

PART I

EMERGENCE OF CURRENT ASSESSMENT PRACTICE

In this section (Chapters 1–3), two background themes are introduced. The first of these is a discourse on the nature of hearing and not-hearing. It differs from the usual accounts of both these features of human experience by virtue of a phenomenalist style of approach interleaved with descriptions of some recent technical and theoretical advances in the field. The second theme concerns the historical development of hearing assessment, first as a purely technical issue, thence as an issue embedded in a particular social and historical process. Through this approach, it is made clear from the outset that hearing, partial hearing, deafness, and the assessment of these qualities are all social phenomena as well as technical performances.

1

The Nature of Hearing, Partial Hearing, and Deafness

INTRODUCTION

Many different approaches can be made to hearing and its impairment. Since this book is concerned with assessment of hearing in adults, the approach that most naturally offers itself is to examine how people go about functioning in the performance of auditory acts vis-à-vis the audible world. This approach contrasts with one which begins with pictures of an ear and a description of how it works as a mechanism. We will from time to time be concerned with mechanical function, but that is not an appropriate primary orientation.

The performance of auditory acts is a phrase I use to describe purposive engagement in the business of attending to some feature or set of events within the audible world. This style of description, while ultimately psychological, springs partly from a sociological and partly from an ecological base. In the past decade or so, a theoretical redirection has occurred within the psychology of perception leading to a focus on perceptual systems and their functions for people living in environmental–social systems of various kinds. This theoretical change in turn has led to a change in technical experimental investigations of sensory psychology. We will, as I said, refer to the mechanics of the auditory system from time to time, but the important initial task is to describe the process of hearing from a social ecological viewpoint.

Perceiving, generally, has had a difficult intellectual history, perhaps because of its obviousness. Because perception is usually effortless and tends to be taken for granted, it is hard to step back from one's perceiving self and witness the process as an independent phenomenon. Consequently, because early attempts in our culture to analyze perceiving were carried out by contemplative scholars, theories of perceiving described a process in which the mind of the perceiver was the principal element. Although auditory perception was given considerably less attention than visual or tactile perception, constructs developed in explanation of these more apparently impressive systems were transferred nonetheless to the auditory system. For example, classical research into auditory skill looks to the discriminatory ability of the system at the level of bare acoustic quality: pitch and loudness of sinusoidal waveforms varying in periodicity and magnitude or acoustic quality embellished by such "musical" features as timbre and volume. Because the ear, like the eye, was thought of purely as a receiving system, the telephone became the ear's model just as the camera was the eye's. The function of the ear, conceived as a receiver, is to transduce complexes of waves into trains of discrete electrical impulses to be decoded and made meaningful again by the brain. In the field of auditory spatial perception, the model was much akin to the "local signs" concept of visual space. Discrete spatial positions (once again of sinusoidal waveforms) were mapped according to the temporal–intensive discrepancies between two ears with which they were associated.

It will be evident that this tradition continues to affect the way in which hearing is conceptualized, for nothing in what has been said so far will appear unusual or outdated—especially for the clinically oriented reader. Our clinical practices are based on tests which use discrete signals, be they generated by tuning forks or complicated electronic gear.

It is now time to look at the theoretical developments I mentioned and produce concepts for hearing which bear on that activity as it goes on in the social–physical environment. The foremost contemporary theoretician to adopt the ecological approach is Gibson (1950, and more particularly 1966). While I do not concur with all of his observations, I do acknowledge the worth of his theoretical attack and specifically the insights he has provided about how to construct an "ecological acoustics." I have adopted a Gibsonian approach to hearing and to the auditory world; indeed, I have borrowed some of Gibson's own insights on these matters. The reader is referred to Gibson (1966) for an exposition of that author's views.

THE NATURE OF THE AUDITORY WORLD

The task of a Gibsonian model of sense perception is to replace the classical concept, in which stimuli impinge as sensations on a receptor surface to be translated into meaningful perceptions by the brain, with one of an interlocking set of perceptual systems which actively seek out information preexisting in the sensible world. In such a model, *physically* identifiable attributes of sensible occurrences (events which are potentially detectible by sense) are for the most part incidental and usually irrelevant for a *perceptual* system. What constitutes information for an electronic analyser in no way coincides with what is informative to a human perceptual system. The pitch and loudness of sinusoidal waveforms may be discriminable by the human auditory system, but such signals are meaningless for they lack information. They have no ecological counterparts. Rather, modulations, modulation rates, and recurrence rates are the sorts of dimensions of stimuli to which an auditory system is attentive. These temporal, that is, relational, occurrences may be witnessed in physics as a series of discrete states, but they are witnessed by the auditory system as unitary events in the world.

Hearing versus Listening

It is customary, from both classical theoretical and current clinical perspectives, to consider hearing for speech separately from hearing for other types of sound. This distinction bows to a stimulus difference implied by these perspectives in the first place: pure tones on the one hand; speech sounds on the other. When we attempt to operate within the ecological acoustical perspective, it becomes more difficult to make this sort of distinction, whereas other, previously unthought-of distinctions start to emerge. One of these is the distinction between hearing and listening. As I sit at my desk, I occasionally hear the sound of my clock ticking or the sound of someone typing in a distant office. Amid this I am alerted to certain sounds potentially bearing more information—approaching footsteps or voices in conversation—and I stop to listen to that pattern, picking out from rhythm and cadence the likely identity of the parties. The distinction between hearing and listening then is the distinction between casual reception and close attentiveness to aspects of the auditory world.

The process of listening involves systematic "focusing" on critical events. These may be human speech, an animal call, footsteps, or typing. Any of these specifies a source of potential social contact, potential need for action, or potential risk, depending on its context. More than detection is involved. Identification of the specified source emerges from attention to pattern (as of footsteps). Tracking of locational change—approach, retreat, tangential movement—specifies the likely relation of the identified source to one's own self.

From a stimulus point of view, the variables within the waveforms broadcast from various fixed or changing locations, to which the auditory system may be alerted, should not be specified within the classical terms of intensity and frequency. Either the envelope shape of transients and their recurrence rate or the direction and rate of modulations of nontransients are the critical features specifying the identity of different sources. We distinguish the whine of a power saw from the grind of a truck from the roar of an aircraft from the buzz of a fly. And presumably we do this on the basis of attention not only to differences in vibration pattern, spectral shape, and the like but also to the characteristic ways in which these patterns begin, proceed, and finish as auditory events. A sound may begin as specifying "some mobile machine," but proceed in a way that narrows the category to turbine aircraft, truck, or motorcycle. Not only the change in characteristic sound as a function of internal characteristics of the source but also the specified pathway and rate of movement allow identity to be pinpointed. In the case of moving sources, these two audible qualities interlock. For instance, flying aircraft is uniquely specified as something we hear proceeding at a higher altitude and more swiftly than any other mobile machine.

Communicating versus Listening

A further distinction suggests itself: that between listening and communicating. Usually, though by no means exclusively, communication occurs between one person and another. In merely listening to some other person, one's auditory action consists of detecting and following the message in the wave train. This is specified both by modulations uniquely characteristic of different phonemes and syllables and by expression. The whole gamut of musical expression marks can apply equally to discourse—pauses, slowings, speedings, softenings, loudenings, drawlings, and staccatos. In communicating, one adds the effect of one's own self, and here one provides information vocally or visually (and in intimate situations kinesthetically and tactually) to the other person. Hence there is a dual-cuing process going on in addition to the speaking–listening process. The momentary listener cues the momentary speaker, by movement or sound or touch, about his or her ongoing reaction to what is spoken. The momentary speaker cues the momentary listener to pick up the conversation at points specified by expression, syntax, gesture, or eye contact. In this way, participants in a conversation switch smoothly from speaker to listener roles. Although such switching can be very rapid, it is usually well timed. Indeed, the high-level and multifarious interaction typically associated with communication makes that process virtually a unitary system in its own right. So much of the performance of each party is modified by the performances of the other that the event cannot be said to exist except as a changing relational structure between them.

Detailed observation by Duncan (1975) of speaker–listener interaction patterns bears out the construction of communication as a unitary system. This and other studies have pinpointed the elaborate linguistic, paralinguistic (expressive), and nonvocal code sustained by both parties to permit a smooth conversational flow.

Human communication does not occur exclusively between people.

Members of other species get roped into the human communication system, often to a degree remarkably akin to the closest of contact between people (Maxwell, 1963); and communication is involved to some extent between man and implement. The violinist, for instance, or the motor mechanic engages in a communication process when he simultaneously adjusts and listens to the note of his violin or the throb of his engine while tuning it up. The critical variables in these forms of machine work and others are once more not purely loudness and pitch. The timbre or harmonic content of the sought-for sound is as critical as the periodicity, and the relational harmony of one string or one aspect of the machine to another is also important. In woodworking, the changing shape of transient sounds bears information specifying when one item is fully malleted into another; the modulation of the rasping whine of a saw blade specifies the approaching end of a cut.

If the reader wonders why so many examples are being produced here, let me explain that this whole approach to auditory perception is fairly unfamiliar. The traditional attributes and concepts would remain paramount if ample space were not made for description of ecological audition. It should also be noted that in effect we must produce a somewhat new language to describe the acoustics of these events. Because we are talking about information for an auditory system rather than sensations in an ear, we must abandon the frequency–intensity paradigm and adopt one that more appropriately fits the variables actually encountered in the real world. It should be noted that one cannot rely on documented demonstrations of the critical nature of features such as envelope shape, recurrence rate, or modulation rate: Experiments on specifying the identity of everyday sounds have barely begun. What follows is a review of recent studies that have tried to unearth the working properties of systems in regard not only to vocalized language and other significant sounds but also to spatial location.

THE FUNCTIONING OF THE AUDITORY SYSTEM

Vocalized Language and Other Significant Sounds

In keeping with the initial orientation, the task in this subsection and the next is to consider what is thought to be involved in the pickup of linguistic and other significant acoustic information patterns and in the pickup of spatial information. It is not the task of the section to explain the physical and physiological working of the peripheral receptor system. In the first place, at least a rudimentary understanding of this is assumed for the moment. Second, far better descriptions of the peripheral system than I could succinctly produce are readily available

(Davis, 1970a; Wever & Lawrence, 1954). Third, such a description is inappropriate to the present purpose. How the auditory system functions in picking up meaningful stimuli, not how its components operate mechanically in allowing the system to do that job, is the object of present concern.

A report of considerable significance to the present endeavor is that of a Neurosciences Research Program work session, edited by Worden and Galambos (1972). These authors introduce the report by acknowledging that the informational approach to audition has only lately become the object of research concern. Their remark that "the central nervous system did not evolve to process clicks and tones [p. 8]" is a pertinent echo of the point I seek to put across here. They go on to observe that the use of isolated tones and clicks is not to be derogated, inasmuch as considerable knowledge of peripheral mechanics can be obtained using discrete stimuli. But it is significant that in the use of such signals less and less can be understood the more central the mechanism being observed.

Studies of the male cricket frog mentioned in the report have allowed synthetic patterns to be produced that mimic the recurring pattern of clicks characteristic of that animal's mating call. Gravid females of the species respond appropriately to this synthetic call, but they will not respond if the internal temporal relations of the click bursts are modified—even though the acoustic features of the clicks themselves remain intact. Hence the auditory system of this animal is attuned to a specific pattern of sound, not merely to internal qualities such as pitch and loudness. Though there may be sensitivity to variation of such qualities, ecologically the system is responsive to a higher-order variable.

This kind of observation substantiates the argument that when we consider the process of "hearing in the world" we must examine the system's operation at the level of the everyday world to discover its potential. Studies in animals with observably more elaborate vocal codes—certain types of monkeys, for example—reveal much more complex acoustic patterns and hence presumably more complex auditory nervous systems to deal with the variety of modulations in frequency, intensity, pulse rate, and duration evident in the spectrographs of various types of call.

The vocal–auditory systems of these animals are obviously closest in structure, and probably in function, to the human system. Several interesting observations have been made, particularly among macaque monkeys, whose language is more *acoustically graded* than that of other species of primates; that is, variations in modulation patterns are relatively continuous rather than discrete. Human speech is graded in this same way, and macaque monkeys show vocal behavior observably similar to that of humans. Green (1975) has reported that within a particular type of utterance produced by this species there are spectrographically distinguishable differences of a very subtle nature. These different forms of the utterance, varying in frequency modulation, are not perceptible to a human listener, but Green found that seven different varieties could reliably be categorized on the basis of spectrographic analysis. Correlating each variety of the utterance with its observed context, he later discovered that certain varieties are almost exclusively associated with certain types of encounter or social state. Thus the monkey's auditory system can detect very fine gradations of frequency modulation so that appropriate utterance varieties are made and received in different social settings. This observation is analogous to the human circumstance where a word like "please" will be uttered differently in the contexts of command, request, or supplication.

Such observations contrast with those made among less linguistically varied animal species whose utterances show, in their vocal differences, distinctly different acoustical patterns. The macaques' language patterns are acoustically closer to those of the human species. In man, spectrographically similar (though not identical) patterns are heard as distinctively different utterances. The work of Liberman, Cooper, Shankweiler, and Studdert-Kennedy (1967) on synthetic speech production has demonstrated that differentiation of certain kinds of consonants in human speech is signaled by quite subtle acoustical differences. Critical to this demonstration is the observation that stepwise changes in synthesized spectrograms are not heard as gradually changing sounds. Listeners continue to hear a given modulation as the same phoneme, despite gradual change; but at a critical point they hear the modulation as a different phoneme and go on so hearing it despite further stepwise changes in its structure. The human auditory system, like that of the macaque monkey, is constructed, or has developed, in such a way as to respond invariantly to variable patterns within certain critical ranges. This condition obviously has adaptive value since varieties of articulatory style, like varieties of graphic style, are usually equally comprehensible. It is only when letters, like phonemes, come too close to critical feature boundaries, that they become ambiguous.

A current view of the perception of human speech favors a model based on critical features and critical transitions. In their model, Cole and Scott (1974) give primacy to relatively invariant acoustical features produced by different articulatory action of the oral–laryngeal system. These features uniquely signal various consonants. Critical transitions—which are principally modulations of frequency—have been thought to provide the information to identify consonants in different syllable "environments." The place of articulation of certain consonants, |d|, |k|, |g| particularly, is governed by the vowel that follows them. Production of [di] requires an articulatory organization different from that required for production of [du]. How we recognize the consonant |d| despite this articulatory difference in its production has been the subject of much speculation. Liberman, Delattre, and Cooper (1952) showed that an invariant burst of sound centered at 1.8 kHz did not provide invariant consonantal perception when succeeded by different vowels. Thus, the sound was heard as |p| or |k| depending on the vowel that succeeded it. The corollary is the observation that certain consonants, though remaining invariantly identified in different syllable environments, display different acoustical properties in each environment. The latter obviously follows from the point made above about different articulation of these consonants. The puzzle thrown out was how the auditory system could invariantly identify consonants despite considerable changes in their spectral structure and modulation and at the same time do the opposite job of distinguishing such differences in other contexts. The transition from consonant to vowel became the supposed key to the mystery.

Cole and Scott (1974), after reviewing the evidence from a variety of different sources, put together an integrated model of the speech perceiving process that incorporates transitions and critical features in a different way. Cole and Scott's theory is not to be taken as the only way of characterizing the speech perception process. I use it simply as a current and fairly plausible account within our present understanding.

First of all, it is clear that the great majority of consonantal speech sounds, in English at least, are uniquely characterized by invariant, even if graded, features. These features are governed by the articulatory system and are invariant in that the same acoustical event occurs irrespective of the syllabic environment within which the consonant is embedded. In addition to the features that typify phonemes, there are modulation patterns that typify certain phoneme conjunctions. Thus a pattern with a markedly rising second formant uniquely specifies [bi] whereas a pattern with a slightly rising second formant specifies [di] and one with a markedly falling second formant specifies [gi]. This suggests that in some instances the auditory system analyzes information at the syllabic level rather than the phonemic. Massaro's work (1974) using a masking technique showed that the optimal duration for processing of an auditory speech signal was around 250 msec. This period is equivalent to the average syllable duration. The problem of variable consonant features can be accommodated, then, in a model that looks to the whole modulation pattern as a *syllabic* feature rather than a group of *phonemic* features.

Transitions appear to play a different role in the speech wave train. Bregman and Campbell (1971) investigated the phenomenon they labeled "primary auditory stream segregation." A sequence of tones alternating between higher and lower pitch is heard under some temporal conditions as two independent tonal lines rather than as an alternating single series. These authors point out that composers of music have exploited this phenomenon in a style sometimes called "implied polyphony." The interesting feature is that these tonal series are segregated and remain so—indeed all counterpoint in music relies upon the segregation effect to achieve the feeling of harmony. Yet speech, which is also made up of trains of frequency-separated bands of sound, does not break up in this fashion but sounds like a single continuous wave train. The reason seems to be that transitions, which are of course rapid frequency modulations, bind the formant bands together. In a further study, Bregman and Dannenbring (1973) showed that segregation is inhibited by use of gliding rather than unmodulated tones.

Cole and Scott (1974) show further that envelope modulation provides temporal and transitional information for speech discrimination, not only at the part-word but also at the whole-word and phrase level. Finally, amplitude modulation is an important transitional quality allowing discrimination between phonemes with different attack characteristics (e.g., *ch* [tʃ] and *sh* [ʃ]).

I mention earlier that it is artificial to separate speech from other audible signals. Clearly the model of speech discrimination described in the preceding paragraphs can apply to discrimination of nonspeech sounds of the kind described at the beginning of this chapter. As I also indicate there, experimental work has not yet illuminated the features permitting the discrimination of everyday sounds. Such work is beginning, and a study by Cutting and Rosner (1974) shows that a similar amplitude modulation to that which allows phonemic discrimination also allows discrimination between a "bowed" and a "plucked" musical note. Within the frequency–amplitude–time domain, the human auditory system is sensitive to features characteristic not only of speech sounds but of other sounds as well.

Indeed, it has also been found that modulations of this sort serve as aids in the location of sounds in space. This work, coming from our own laboratory, is a new departure from traditional understanding.

Spatial Location

It has traditionally been assumed that the ability to locate sounds in space is wholly provided by the lateral placement of the ears on the head. Discrepancies between the two ears in the amplitude, arrival time, and ongoing phase of a sound and the extent and direction of these discrepancies specify the whereabouts of the source relative to the listener. Information available in this way is enhanced by the ability to rotate one's head and so modulate the interaural discrepancies. Discrepancies are nullified, for example, at the point where the head is frontal to the sound source. In this way, we can literally zero-in on a source. In an authoritative review, Mills (1972) restates this classical model and goes on to remark, in connection with suggesting a possible role for the pinna in localization, that "it should not be possible to localize an unfamiliar sound, even approximately, by monaural listening without moving the head [p. 333]." A role for the pinnae is allowed insofar as they cast an acoustic "shadow" for high frequency sounds and thus aid the discrimination of frontward sources from rearward.

Usually overlooked in the classical approach to human spatial location of sound is the dynamic and ubiquitous quality of the audible world. Also overlooked are the variety and complexity of naturally occurring sounds. I try to give an idea of such variety and ubiquity in the opening section of this chapter. In need of emphasis in the current context is the functional importance for the human auditory system of all this changing, moving, universal sound. What surely takes place is a process of perceptual learning, whereby the invariant features of positional change are gradually abstracted from qualities which vary simply because of different kinds of source. In the classical view, static sources, usually sinusoids, generate information interaurally to specify their location in space, and two moving ears enable ambiguities inherent in the two-ear system to be resolved; but the view I espouse asserts that the auditory world is not composed in this way. Sources of sound move and in moving produce changes in the acoustic array to which one ear as well as two is sensitive. Just as closing one eye has little effect on the visible spatial world, so closing one ear does not negate auditory space. Despite an obvious loss of hemispheric information in monaural listening (sounds all seem to emanate from the unoccluded side) there is little other change in the structure or quality of the auditory spatial world. Recent work in our laboratory (Noble & Russell, 1972; Russell, 1975) suggests that one pinna alone and both pinnae together provide an additional system for detecting invariances of both static and dynamic location. It seems further that the nature of this additional system is high frequency transitions: As sounding objects move around the listener, invariant transformations occur in their spectral character because of the absorption and reflection characteristics of various parts of the outer ear; invariant discrepancies in spectral character are also generated between the two ears. Once the auditory system is tuned to differentiate these monaural and interaural transformations, then in Gibsonian terms it is educated to locate any moving source, no matter what its novelty. Mills is right in his assertion about a stationary ear and an unfamiliar source, but he forgets to account for the vast world of moving objects.

Of more critical interest, however, is the nature of the information to which an educated auditory system seems to attend, namely changes in frequency spectra. Given that the auditory system is especially sensitive to such transforms, as witness the evidence from perception of speech and musical signals, then it becomes more plausible to accept the idea that frequency transforms can act as important clues in auditory spatial perception. Of course, interaural differences of the kind described in classical theory are not to be discounted; they obviously have a vital role in spatial location. But it is important to emphasize other features of auditory spatial perception and even more important to retrieve the nature of the auditory spatial world lest it be construed as a static (and sinusoidal) universe.

PARTIAL HEARING AND DEAFNESS

The Meaning of Partial Hearing and Deafness

The author of this work is a hearing person, as opposed to a deaf or partially deaf (partially hearing) person. I use these three major distinctions in this section and elsewhere in this book whenever discussion turns to the phenomenal worlds of hearing and deafness or their partial state. Elsewhere I use terms like *impairment* and *hearing loss* in the context of the assessment of partial hearing. Because the author hears, the phenomenology of hearing can readily be described. The phenomenology of partial hearing is less easily captured, and that of deafness almost impossible to describe.

This book is primarily about partial hearing. Deaf people are obviously not subject to elaborate assessment procedures to establish extent of handicap. Nonetheless it is useful here to try to consider all three groups—the hearing, the deaf, and the partially hearing—to try to grasp essential qualities of the world of the last-named group. In the assessment of impaired hearing, it is always assumed that the closer it approximates deafness the greater the degree of handicap to the individual. While I think there is an argument in support of this view, there are some important implications deriving from such an attitude. Fundamentally it helps to sustain the view of *deafness* as a highly handicapping condition, such that any departure from deafness toward hearing is for the good and any departure from hearing toward deafness is for the bad. While it may be that for most hearing adults to become deaf is to become handicapped, there are without doubt cases of people who, on becoming deaf in adulthood and not suffering added problems such as tinnitus, are not handicapped by deafness. Indeed, some people find deafness useful in aiding concentration and providing peace.

Nevertheless, deafness acquired in adulthood is handicapping for most people who suffer it, and as a general rule the handicap of acquired partial deafness increases with greater impairment. We should not assume, however, that adventitious partial deafness is akin to partial deafness experienced throughout life, and we should certainly not assume that deafness acquired in adulthood is anything like deafness from birth or early childhood. It is highly probable, in fact, that lifelong deafness is less burdensome than lifelong partial deafness. We must elaborate further on all these assertions.

The Worlds of Partial and Total Deafness

People born deaf develop signing, if permitted, as a natural language. If they learn to vocalize, communication in that way is presumably a visual–kinesthetic experience—the meaning of produced language is associated not with sound but with muscular and vibratory states and changes. A concept embodied in a particular acoustic waveform for hearing people, is embodied in fluctuations of the musculature involved in vocal speech production for the deaf. These states and changes are in turn associated with visual forms of words and syllables in much the same way that words have an appearance for hearing people that matches how they sound.

But deaf people have more than the written, symbolic visual forms of words. Among other deaf people, they also have visible signs. Hearing people have, as a rule, only the visible written forms. The signs used by hearing people are more expressive of emotional states and symbolically are concrete and nonspecific. Deaf people's signs are the equivalents in all respects of hearing people's vocalized symbols, although the conceptual structure and grammatical rules of many sign systems are quite alien to the vocal and written form of a language. Signing is therefore akin to a fully developed minority dialect.

Just as signing is an alien linguistic device from a hearing person's viewpoint, so vocalized language is an alien linguistic device from a deaf person's viewpoint. As indicated in the preceding paragraph, for the deaf spoken language is presumably a kinesthetic experience. Hearing people are rarely sensitive to how words feel in the mouth, larynx, or diaphragm. Professional singers develop this sensitivity during training; another way of acquiring the experience is to practice vocalizing at a normal conversational level in noise loud enough to mask the utterance and hence nullify auditory feedback. In this fashion, one can get an experience something like that of vocalizing when deaf.

This treatment of deaf communication is presented to show that it is a system quite different from but no less evolved than the communication system of hearing people. The handicap of deafness in our kind of culture is attributable not to absence or inferiority of communication within the deaf subculture but to the barrier between the natural communication modes of the deaf and those of the hearing. Nor is that a handicap in itself, it becomes handicapping only because the deaf are a minority group. Hodgson (1953) puts it that "for the deaf themselves the real problem, of course, is not deafness but the fact of living in a hearing world. If all were deaf, then deafness would be no handicap. Theirs is a minority problem [p. 347]."

The problem of minorities is lack of power. A feature of lack of power for deaf people is that they cannot oblige hearing people to learn their language, whereas many of them are obliged to learn hearing people's language. If hearing had the minority prevalence and attendant minority status in our culture that deafness has, there would be a redefinition of handicap. It would be normative for the hearing minority to pity their own clumsy signing ability. Vocal language would be more natural for them and—presuming beneficence on the part of (deaf) educational administrators not to prohibit its use—would be developed in preference to manual signing. Hearing people would be pitied by the majority for the further handicaps of constant "noise pain" in the ears and the general lack of intelligence associated with ill-developed somosthetic sensibility. Furthermore, in a society where the majority were deaf, certain features of culture that are taken for granted would disappear. The need for acoustic privacy as well as visual would no longer exist; walls between rooms could be paper thin; motor vehicles could be unsilenced; and noisy industrial processes and the overhead flight of aircraft could continue unabated at all hours of day and night.

H. G. Wells (1904), with typical brilliance, captured this reversal of power and hence of definition in "The Country of the Blind." In this short story, a sighted protagonist, far from becoming the "one-eyed man as king" in a blind culture, gradually realizes his powerlessness and *as a result* his handicap. The antithetical nature of this realization is what is important. People who are deaf or blind are not powerless because they are handicapped; they are handicapped because they are powerless.

I construe the world of deafness, in its fully realized state, as one quite different from but no less viable than the world of hearing. For this reason, I regard deafness not as necessarily the final stage of handicapping hearing loss but rather as a different form of existence. I qualify this assertion once again by stating that adventitious deafness, for reasons yet to be examined, may be the ultimate level of hearing handicap; but fully realized, lifelong deaf "being" is merely an alternative kind of existence. Let me elaborate upon the concept of *realization*. Current societal attitudes make it almost impossible for the realization of deaf "being"; the only liberating path for the deaf leads to mimicry of the hearing lifestyle. To be in the majority society requires denial of deaf modes of being and assumption of hearing modes. The realization of deaf being will begin to occur when deaf people, *as a matter of orthodox practice*, take it that deaf modes are viable ways of being-in-society. This has started to occur and doubtless will gain increasing practical expression. In the meantime, deaf being is not realized; and as a consequence, deafness is yet another form of *deviance* (using that term in its technical sociological sense) from society's norms. Being deaf is like being black.

Just as important, being partially deaf is like being partially black. It is opportune now to turn to the world of partial hearing and to begin by pushing this parallel a little further. Partially deaf people have certain problems in common with part-Aboriginal people in Australia and no doubt with part-black and part-Indian people in many parts of North America. In Australia, most part-Aboriginal people belong to neither the traditional indigenous nor to the European immigrant society, yet they live among the whites and confront white culture through education in white schools and employment (if at all) in white firms. They are thus expected (and themselves expect) to partake of white culture, yet they are discriminated against on the basis of their mixed racial backgrounds. Partially deaf people, by analogy, belong neither to the hearing group nor to the deaf, yet they are expected (and themselves expect) to partake of hearing culture. They cannot partake of deaf culture, for their upbringing is in the culture of hearing. They do not sign. Many do not lip-read. They adopt aids to hearing in order to participate in a hearing life style. Yet they are discriminated against on the basis of their partial deafness.

The crux of my point is that being partially deaf (partially hearing) can be a more anomic state than being deaf, because faced with the expectation of hearing people that one will operate as a hearing person, one will often fail in the attempt to maintain that posture and status. The parallel between partially deaf and part-Aboriginal people is probably only meaningful in consideration of people born partially deaf or acquiring partial deafness in early childhood. These people's critical socialization experiences vis-à-vis parents, siblings, and school firmly embed them in the world of the partially hearing. The whole socialization process is geared to the remediation of their "handicap" so that they can partake of hearing culture. The socialization of urban-dwelling part-Aboriginal people has likewise been geared (at least until very recent times) to the remediation of their "cultural handicap" so as to embed them in the white culture. Lest these words sound critical, let me emphasize that the actions of the majority culture have been motivated by supposedly liberal and beneficent beliefs. Believing that partially deaf or partially black people cannot sustain a viable living if uncared for (and previous experience had borne out such a view), the majority institutions have sought to habilitate these disadvantaged peoples in the only cultural style that they knew, to provide optimal opportunity. It is only as consciousness has gradually changed, especially regarding the viability of part-Aboriginal culture, that doubts have been voiced about wholesale socialization of such people away from their own background and realization has come that help may be better directed in other ways.

A common critical feature I detect between partial deafness and partial blackness lies in the differences in language between these groups and the hearing white group. Deaf children, if permitted, will learn signing as a first language. Partially deaf children would presumably learn signing or a modified signing–vocalizing language if a partially deaf culture were allowed to develop; but partially deaf children are strongly encouraged to learn a vocal form of language, and of course they are successful in producing vocal language because their residual hearing, once amplified, allows acoustic feedback. Not all deaf children can learn to vocalize or lip-read well enough to rely solely on vocal speech for communication, and many use signing as an alternative or complementary form. The recent change in consciousness that permits deafness as a viable alternative life style has also liberated deaf communication so that children in many schools for the deaf can sign without fear of disapproval. The one-time drive to teach all deaf children to speak is giving way, though not without powerful resistance, to an attitude of encouraging deaf children to communicate by whichever means they find most natural. Signing has achieved the status in *hearing* culture of a language comparable with any other. Of course, it always had that status, albeit clandestinely, within deaf culture.

In much the same way, the nonstandard English used by part-Aborigines has come to be seen merely as a different not as an inferior language, significant of and for that culture. It has come to be realized that insistence on the use of standard English by culturally different groups represents interference with an important cultural feature of such groups. The time is a long way off (and perhaps may never come) when partially hearing people develop their own linguistic form. Technological development has allowed and will continue to allow the partially hearing to partake of the language of hearing people. To me, this is a crucial mechanism whereby the partially hearing, even from birth, identify with hearing culture. The parallel between partial hearing and part-Aboriginal origin is still real, however, because the viability of part-Aboriginal language is by no means realized. Standard English is still a major apparent goal to be achieved by such people.

Partial deafness acquired in adulthood represents a form of hearing loss different from lifelong partial deafness. A person who has lived in a hearing culture has never experienced conflict of expectation. It is probably among members of this group more than any other that the increase in severity of hearing loss genuinely represents increase in handicap. The life experience of a hearing person contains taken-for-granted features of communication, detection, and location based on the auditory system or on that system in conjunction with the visual system. At no stage has such a person been at a loss in relation to the auditory world, and when he experiences a partial impairment of hearing, the handicap is necessarily the greater the more removed from hearing—the closer to deafness—he becomes. The cultural matrix which has sustained such a person becomes less and less accessible, and there is no easy transition from one culture to another. When one is "hard of hearing," or "a little deaf," one suffers minor inconveniences, akin almost to the experiences this author has in trying to understand the Australian dialect, requiring strangers to repeat their utterances and speak more slowly. But as vocal communication becomes more restricted and as the auditory world becomes more imperceptible, feelings of occasional frustration give way to the feeling of helplessness and panic. One has become a stranger in what was once the world to be taken for granted. Deaf people may suffer in our society through their powerlessness to modify the environment to suit their needs, but their taken-for-granted world has always been stable. People who acquire deafness inevitably lose such stability, for the new world has no meaning for them, they are powerless both within this world and in regard to the world in which they once operated.

We can get a glimpse of such a process in reverse. Gregory and Wallace (1963) documented the history of a man virtually blind from early childhood whose sight was restored when he was 52 following an operation for the removal of cataracts. While it was evident that his visual skill improved over subsequent months, he nonetheless preferred to act as a blind person, showed signs of disturbance at this new world thrust upon him, because increasingly depressed, and died 2 years after the operation. Considering the positive value of a move from blindness to sightedness compared with the reverse process, it is testament to the power of the cultural milieu that any radical alteration in taken-for-granted reality can produce devastating effects. If one considers then the negative value attached to a change from hearing to deafness, one can begin to appreciate how much more devastating such a change can be.

The acquisition of partial deafness in adulthood can be particularly traumatic for an individual in an otherwise hearing social network. No preparation has been made for such a transition, and the solitary nature of the occurrence leaves the individual with a feeling of bereavement. Heaton (1968) has made a similar observation in regard to sighted people who become increasingly blind. Even in a sympathetic social environment, the person who, through disease or injury, sustains a hearing loss is largely alone in this new partially deaf world. The acquisition of partial deafness caused by cellular deterioration with advancing age or prolonged exposure to occupational noise should probably be distinguished from the solitary case. With increasing age, more and more people acquire hearing loss, and it is normative to make the transition, which is also very gradual, given that many of one's peers are going deaf too. Old people have declared to me, following interviews in which it is clear to both of us that they are partially deaf, that their hearing is "normal for their age." Such knowledge protects them from much of the alienating experience of acquired partial deafness. More than that, the aged peer group provides a society that shares understanding. One is not making this passage to a different world alone, hence there is less feeling of being a stranger.

A similar situation may obtain among people deafened by occupational noise. Once again, in interviews it is not uncommon for such people to be unperturbed by hearing loss because "everyone at work is a bit deaf." When one's social network is largely confined to the occupational peer group, there is likely to be a less marked feeling of alienation. Because this book is largely concerned with adults partially deafened by noise, I elaborate in detail on features of that group in later chapters. The main point to emerge from the present discussion is that the handicap which may result from hearing impairment is critically a function of the meaning of that impairment to the individual and to the culture in which that individual is embedded. That meaning is partly given by general cultural values (it is better to hear than not) and partly by the social situation within which the hearing impairment occurs (childhood, adulthood, old age, occupation).

CLINICAL FEATURES OF IMPAIRED HEARING

Effects on Speech Hearing

Notwithstanding social factors that define handicap, there are features intrinsic to auditory disorder, description of whose effects on the process of hearing can be undertaken rather more independently. That is to say, a person's auditory system will be disordered in such-and-such a way by such-and-such disease or injury irrespective of the social milieu of that person. Differentiating the effects of various types of auditory disorder is primarily of concern to the diagnostician, for these effects are labeled symptoms, and aid in pinpointing the nature and hence the treatment of the problem.

It is still of concern in assessment to know the sort of disorder in question and its specific disturbing effects, as well as the extent of loss of hearing. Indeed, as I argue later, it was because specific effects of noise-induced hearing disorder were largely ignored that invalid systems of assessment of that disorder have been adopted.

The classic definition of auditory disorder differentiates between that of conductive and that of sensorineural origin. In a purely conductive disorder, only the mechanical transformer subsystem of the auditory system is affected: Rupture of the eardrum, sclerosis, or mechanical breakdown of the middle-ear ossicular chain are typical examples. Pure sensorineural disorder is typified by degenerative disease affecting cells in the cochlea, the labyrinthine system, and the auditory nerve. One major difference between pure conductive and pure sensorineural disorder is that loss of hearing caused by the former is often remediable by direct surgical intervention, whereas no surgical cure is yet feasible for sensorineural disorder. Another difference between the two is that amplification of sound is often sufficient to overcome hearing loss in conductive disorder, whereas amplification is often unhelpful to people with sensorineural disorder. Pure sensorineural disorder is potentially a greater handicap because so much less can usefully be done to remediate the impairment of hearing.

There is probably more than one reason why sensorineural disorder produces such intractable disturbance and loss of hearing. The major disturbing sign is reduced ability to discriminate speech sounds. Discrimination difficulty, however it may arise, is manifest even when the speech energy level is increased. There is no great increase in intelligibility with increasing signal level. For a normally hearing listener, or for a listener with partial deafness of purely conductive origin, a speech signal becomes increasingly intelligible, virtually in a linear progression with logarithmic increase in the energy of the soundwave carrying the signal. For a listener with partial deafness of sensorineural origin, no such relationship necessarily obtains—logarithmic increase in sound energy may produce a slight increase in intelligibility with an asymptote well below the maximum possible, or there may even be a decline in intelligibility beyond a certain energy level. The situation in the first case can be likened to increasing the amplitude of a badly tuned radio—it has the effect of making things a bit clearer, but only up to a point; further increases only produce a noisier but no more intelligible signal. In the second case, the parallel might be that of an overdriven loudspeaker whose output becomes increasingly garbled as more energy is fed into it. One hesitates to draw such parallels, for the effects experienced by our hypothetical listeners may bear no resemblance to what I have just described; but these are the only analogies available to hearing people, and at least they permit some insight into a major problem of sensorineural hearing disorder. In later chapters, I consider in more detail the findings of researchers into possible mechanisms of sensorineural speech discrimination difficulty. Significant for this discussion is that such phenomena critically differentiate most sensorineural disorders from most conductive disorders and necessarily have implications for the assessment of hearing in people with each type.

Effects on Spatial Location

Less is known about the differential effects of different types of auditory disorder on auditory space perception: Until recently, the clinical significance of the disruption of auditory spatial perception was unrealized. Even now, no attention is paid in *assessment* of hearing loss to disturbance of this function. Diagnosticians have begun to explore auditory directional perception as a tool in differentiation of disorder. In particular, the work of Tonning (1975) represents a thorough analysis of this possibility. But Tonning's investigations do not (and are not intended to) provide a measure of the extent of spatial perceptual disturbance insofar as he has not yet related his laboratory observations to spatial perceptual difficulty in the day-to-day world. The work of Bienvenue and Siegenthaler (1974) is more relevant to the problem in that these authors have recognized the importance of trying to evaluate auditory spatial impairment for its own sake. Their research to date, however, is limited in scope because the test they devised has been used only in normally hearing listeners with simulated unilateral partial deafness. Bienvenue and Siegenthaler assume that only unilateral disorder will be associated with spatial disturbance. Although this assumption is well founded in classical theory, it is in fact erroneous.

A study of real-world auditory spatial ability was conducted by this author (Noble, 1969). It involved 29 listeners with various degrees of bilateral impairment caused by occupational noise and compared their self-reported ability to locate sources of sound with performance on a free-field test of directional location in the horizontal plane. The latter test was part of an investigation into directional location in open- and closed-ear listening conditions (Atherley & Noble, 1970). Self-reported disruption of auditory direction perception correlated positively, though not closely, with performance on the directional hearing test.

This research, which has been briefly described in previous publications (Noble, 1975a; Noble & Atherley, 1970) is discussed in more detail in Chapter 10. It is worth noting in passing that self-reported spatial ability seems to be reliable. It could fairly be assumed that people cannot report upon a relatively obscure aspect of everyday auditory experience, but these results suggest that they can. The reason is probably that as spatial ability deteriorates the individual becomes increasingly conscious of instances of failure to locate critical sources in the everyday world. And there is no question that directional ability is impaired as hearing loss (assessed by the tonal threshold test) increases (Atherley & Noble, 1970). Elevation of higher frequency tonal threshold is linked, though not closely, with reduced directional ability. And these data are from people with bilateral hearing disorders.

The fact that auditory spatial perception is threatened by injurious noise needs to be highlighted. Decreased ability to tell the whereabouts of unseen sources of sound could be gravely problematic for the individual in daily life. As important as the obvious difficulty this could present for safe orientation in an environment well filled by mobile machinery is the likely disruptive effect on perception of speech in acoustically competitive situations. Knowing where a novel speech signal is coming from in those famous "cocktail parties" frequented by English psychologists (Broadbent, 1958) is critical at least in initially distinguishing the signal from competing ones. If there is confusion about source, this could add to the problem of unintelligibility of speech. It has always been assumed that the speech discrimination problem experienced by people with bilateral sensorineural hearing disorder is a direct function of speech signal–receptor interaction. The possibility now needs to be considered that in day-to-day situations the problem might be partly a function of deteriorating spatial skill. The traditional assumption that auditory spatial perception is necessarily and sufficiently dependent on two ears has led to the conclusion that only unilateral hearing losses should present localization problems. Having suggested earlier in this chapter that auditory space is grasped in more than one way, I find it more plausible to accept that other patterns of hearing loss can disturb the spatial perceptual process.

Additional Dysfunction

It is clear from preceding description that partial deafness is not exhaustively described as "difficulty in hearing." That phrase suggests merely that it is hard to detect certain signals, and, of course partial deafness does entail that problem. In addition, it may entail difficulty in discriminating spoken speech, even when the speech is quite loud enough to be heard; it may entail difficulty in differentiating sources of sound. Added to these problems are effects such as tinnitus. Tinnitus may take a multitude of forms, from a single tone to broad-band noise, it may be experienced as continuous or pulsing, it may vary in intensity, and so on. From the present point of view, the critical nature of tinnitus is its disruptive emotional effect. It is bad enough to experience difficulty in hearing what one may wish to without continually being subjected to inescapable spontaneous and often unpleasant noises that distract attention and mask incoming signals.

This last feature is surely the most distressful and most in need of emphasis. Gibson (1966), whose theoretical work I mentioned earlier, has pointed out an important distinction in perceiving—that between obtained and imposed stimulation. For the most part, people actively seek information from the world to enable continuity of operation within it. In so doing, we manipulate the environment so as to highlight only those features of interest at the moment. That is to say, people exercise control by avoidance and reorientation over what they will and will not attend to.

Freedom to do this is not always complete. In my present circumstance, I can move to obtain improved musical stimulation by adjusting the volume of sound from the stereo. I can move further to reduce extraneous interference from noise outside by closing windows and doors. But occasional buzzing insects invade the house and impose their sound on my auditory system, thus interfering with concentration on work and with the pleasure of listening to music. This sudden and unwanted buzzing noise is analogous to the experience of tinnitus, but tinnitus has an additional and uncontrollable quality that makes its presence much more irritating: The buzzing insect can be dealt with, benignly or otherwise depending on one's mood and at slight cost to oneself; tinnitus is, in many cases, not susceptible to treatment.

It is worth citing, in this connection, the work of Glass and Singer (1972) on the effects of distracting noise on poststimulatory performance. They showed that when participants found that they could neither directly nor indirectly control such noise, the stress aftereffect was considerable. They attributed this result to the feeling of helplessness which reduces the person's competence to cope with the interference (Seligman, 1975). It was the meaning for the person as much as the physical presence of the distracting stimulus that these authors considered critical in producing a stress reaction. Thus the uncontrollable quality of tinnitus rather than its physical presence is probably instrumental in inducing stress. Such a postulate might help solve the puzzle of why the subjective loudness of tinnitus bears little resemblance to its measurable characteristics (Hempstock & Atherley, 1971).

Many other dysfunctions can accompany disorder of hearing. These are usually of diagnostic significance rather than aspects of assessment, and it is beyond the present purpose to examine them. Tinnitus is ubiquitous and is often found in disorders sustained by people whose hearing is assessed for some purpose or other. Our task now, having witnessed both social and clinical features of partial deafness, is to trace the development of hearing assessment and the tests and systems used in that endeavor.

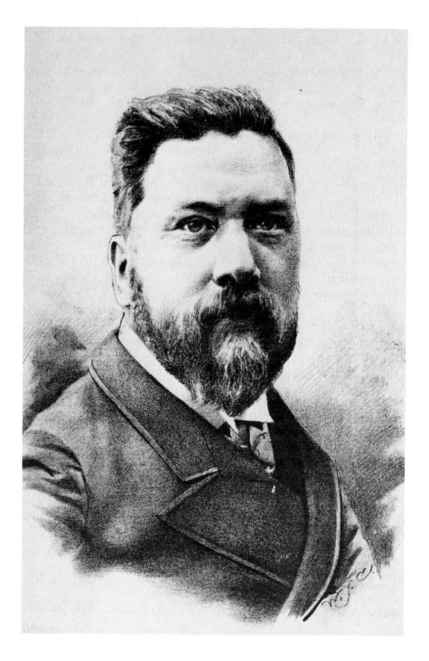

Figure 2.1 Thomas Barr (1846–1916), the Glascow otologist whose studies of hearing in children (1889) and in noise-exposed workmen (1886) mark the beginning of hearing assessment as an autonomous scientific practice. This portrait from *The Bailie* cartoon supplement of May 14, 1890 shows Barr at about the time he was publishing these reports.

2

The Emergence of Assessment and Tests Used in That Practice

THE CONCEPT OF ASSESSMENT

The first purpose of this chapter is to discuss the various contexts in which hearing assessment (as opposed to diagnosis) occurs and to define the principal area of present concern within the general field of hearing assessment. The second purpose of the chapter is to describe the major tests currently used in the hearing assessment of adults.

It might be thought unnecessary to consider the concept of "hearing loss assessment"—the idea behind this term being fairly self-evident and requiring no explanation. Although that observation is true, it is also true that the testing of hearing is a relatively recent practice, and it is valuable to reconstruct the emergence of hearing testing as a part of our everyday taken-for-granted consciousness. People occasionally ask me to test their hearing because they believe they may be a bit deaf. When I suggest that I simply interview them to find out more about the sort of difficulties they experience, their reaction is typically askance. It seems to them that their difficulties can only be "really" detected by a mechanical assessment procedure; can indeed be "realized" only from the results of such a test. Their own self-appraisals are insufficient as guides to the extent of suspected hearing difficulty.

In a way, this attitude makes sense: A mechanical test, being more standardized, can provide comparative information without the need to assemble a representative sample of people with whom to contrast the person seeking the test. The sample's responses are already built into the test's calibration. I will show by the time we reach the other end of this book that an interview can enjoy this same feature and that present dubiousness about self-report springs simply from the novelty of and hence unfamiliarity with that approach. There is at present a relative lack of standardization data using self-report methods.

Be that as it may, the assessment of hearing by means of mechanical tests is an accepted aspect of our cultural landscape. Just as we no longer rummage through piles of spectacles on a bazaar stall to find something that helps failing eyesight, so we do not go directly to the hearing aid shop for a device that may assist with auditory problems. Yet it is only in relatively recent times that the intermediate step of specialist testing has emerged in both of these areas. Consciousness regarding assessment, then, is a historical phenomenon, and as far as hearing assessment is concerned, the origin of that history can be pinpointed, I believe, in the activities of one man.

Thomas Barr (1846–1916, see portrait on p. 24) was an otologist of remarkable insight who also displayed a considerable breadth of interest in all matters pertaining to hearing. Aside from publishing a manual of diseases of the ear in 1884, a work which became a standard text in Britain and the United States, Barr showed a concern for the more public health and preventive aspects of aural disease and injury. This interest is partly explicable in the fact that Barr studied at the University of Glasgow as an undergraduate medical student at a time when Joseph Lister was initiating the principles and practice of antiseptic surgery. This effort, which originated in Glasgow, naturally had ramifications in problems of public sanitation and health. When Barr returned to Glasgow from the University of Vienna where he had studied with Politzer and others, he took up a job as honorary otologist to the children's hospital as well as a teaching post in Anderson's College Medical School. The latter establishment was later incorporated, and Barr with it, into the university. It was perhaps the children's hospital job, along with his earlier background, that provided him with the stimulus to inquire into the incidence and variety of aural disease in a large group of school children from different social districts of Glasgow. That report (1889) is probably the first public health inquiry conducted on epidemiological principles of young people's hearing. In terms of our present interest, an earlier epidemiological study by Barr (1886) established not only the principle of hearing assessment for its own sake but also the occupational origin of noise-induced hearing disorder.

Sporadic early reports of hearing loss in people pursuing noisy occupations have been cited. Kylin (1960) refers to a thesis submitted by Skragge to the University of Uppsala in Sweden in 1765 which describes the hearing impairment suffered by blacksmiths and coppersmiths; and Bryan and Tempest (1971) mention that Ramazzini, in his famous treatise of 1713 on occupational disease, noted similar cases. A more substantial study, conducted in the United States by Holt (1882), gives evidence of deafness among boilermakers in the shipyards of Portland, Maine. But Barr's (1886) study is the first to establish the causal link between the degree of noisiness of the occupation and the extent of resulting injury. Furthermore, Barr's attribution of the disorder to overstimulation of the cochlear receptor cells is the first published diagnostic statement that also happens to be correct.

Many points of detail in Barr's report reveal the penetration and breadth of his inquiries. He notes that even after a lifetime of working, there is yet a slight tendency for recovery following retirement, a point substantiated in 1965 by Taylor, Pearson, Mair, and Burns. Barr noted that about three-quarters of the boilermakers he examined found it difficult or quite impossible to hear at public meetings, a problem exacerbated, in his view, by the then current fashion for bushy beards that obscured a speaker's lips. We can see from his portrait that Barr himself subscribed to this style. He conducted the first environmental survey of boilermaker noise by recording the sounds of caulking and riveting on his own phonograph and comparing the depth of indentation on the wax cylinder with the depth typically produced by an ordinary conversational voice. He noted that loss of sensitivity was most marked for tones at higher frequencies, a substantiation of the sensorineural nature of the disorder.

But the observation of greatest potency is Barr's study comparing the hearing of 100 boilermakers with that of 100 ironmolders and 100 letter carriers (mailmen). Details of the results of that study are given in the introduction to Chapter 7. The point of present interest is that the hearing of these different groups was assessed simply for the purpose of establishing that the noise of certain occupations is injurious to hearing. This procedure, in my view, marks the beginning of hearing assessment practice as an activity independent of usual clinical inquiry. It is also fitting that Barr's study was concerned with an issue that currently occupies a major position in the assessment of hearing impairment in adults.

WHY HEARING IS ASSESSED

The three main sectors of contemporary hearing assessment practice are (a) screening of young children for early detection of hearing disorder; (b) pre- and posttreatment evaluation of hearing in clinical and rehabilitative contexts (with an analogous function in the conservation of hearing in industry); and (c) evaluation of the degree of hearing impairment and handicap in compensation cases. It is the third of these varieties with which this work is principally concerned. It follows of necessity, however, that analyses and conclusions made in regard to the technical adequacy of tests and systems used in *handicap* assessment bear upon assessment in at least the second of the above sectors and possibly in the first as well. The same tests and systems are used in both the second and third contexts, and there are some tests in common between the first and the other two contexts.

Screening in Young Children

Screening young children is not germane to the present endeavor because this book is concerned with adult hearing assessment. Certain principles attending the testing of children figure in the discussion of test utility in Chapter 5, however, and insofar as we have an overall interest in deafness and partial deafness, it is worthwhile noting why hearing is assessed in very young people. The rationale behind this practice is the wish for early detection of hearing disorder so that deaf or partially deaf children may be provided with appropriate remediation, aids, or treatment. It is reasoned that these children, especially if they are from hearing families, will be disadvantaged unless their hearing can be sufficiently restored or appropriate speech training initiated to habilitate them in the hearing world. The history of deafness is a chronicle of gradually changing attitudes. The recognition, on the part of some, of the equivalency of the deaf and the hearing in terms of functioning in society at large has eventuated in a minority educational–social posture that struggles with an older but still prevailing attitude that sees the deaf as intellectually and psychologically inferior. The struggle by the minority has produced movement toward habilitation in education and social intervention generally as the only apparent way at present to reconcile the prejudices of society at large with the knowledge of that equivalency. If the deaf can be trained to function "normally"—that is, in the hearing world—it is hoped that the prejudice against them will diminish.

Although some tests used in adult assessment are also used in the testing of younger people's hearing, the trend in recent times has been to develop specialist techniques appropriate to the population in question. The present author pretends no familiarity with this sector of the hearing assessment industry, nor has he had experience in that field. It would be simply a reiteration of what is available in the published writings of persons specializing in this sector to attempt any review of paedoaudiology. But as is mentioned earlier, certain present analyses may bear upon the hearing assessment of young people, hence there is no wish to invoke a strict line of demarcation between the problems of adult hearing assessment and those relating to children.

Evaluation of Treatment and Conservation Programs

In evaluation of treatment programs, assessment has a seemingly straightforward role. In order to judge the efficacy of some treatments, surgical operations, or rehabilitative procedures, pre-, per-, and posttreatment testing is a necessary guide. But assessment here gets into a tricky area right away when used to help therapists in their initial judgments about whether clients' complaints are sufficiently serious to warrant costly, and sometimes perilous treatments by surgery or with drugs. We will not explore this issue too deeply except to point out that the tests used in initial assessment must be proven as valid indexes of degree of impairment if their results are to provide useful guidance; and conclusions drawn in this book regarding test validity and reliability bear upon this problem. When it comes to judgments about whether a treatment or rehabilitation program has succeeded, the reliance placed on hearing tests is even more critical, and the technical quality of the tests needs that much more scrutiny.

There is an important contrary circumstance where change for the worse (or the lack of it) in performance on hearing tests is used in a monitoring way. In so-called conservation of hearing programs, routine testing is often used as a way of checking whether conditions in an industrial or military setting are adversely affecting hearing. We touch on this use of assessment when considering test reliability.

It is worth highlighting here that there is increasing interest in the problems of older people whose hearing may deteriorate with advancing age. The special problems faced by aging people as regards acceptance of aids to hearing and programs to improve their ability to cope with this difficulty are receiving considerable attention throughout the world. It may prove that as with very young people a new specialism is needed to allow valid assessment of both the degree of difficulty experienced and the extent of amelioration possible following a program of training or treatment. Indications to this author suggest that self-report methods of assessment may be particularly useful in this emerging practice. Details of studies of the above kind are given in Chapter 10, and there is further discussion of the issue in Chapter 11.

Assessment for Compensation

This sector of the hearing assessment industry is, as I indicated, the one that concerns us most closely in the present work. For it is from this context that tests themselves have often been developed, and it is in connection with this practice that most research in adult hearing assessment has been undertaken. The reason for this is quite plain. When a person lays legal claim for damages in connection with a loss of hearing, assessment of the degree of loss is used to gauge the likely handicap that person has sustained in daily life. Cash awards or pension payments are made in amounts dictated by the judged handicap. Because of this baldly economic factor, hearing assessment in legal settings has a vitally sensitive role. Interest in test validity and reliability is shown not only by scientists and medical specialists but also by plaintiffs and defendants. This is true whether the defendant is an individual or an institution. These very proper interests by all concerned nevertheless make the scientist's job harder because so much is at stake for the parties to the dispute.

It is not the scientist's task to declare what levels of handicap are such as to merit this or that amount of award. Nor is it the scientist's task to become enmeshed in the remedial and judicial functions of the courts. The scientist's task in this as in all other assessment settings is to make sure that the assessments being used by others to make these judgments are valid and reliable enough for the job. In this endeavor, the interest of scientists is partly dictated by the constructs of society at large, which enable them to know what is sought from an assessment procedure. The interest of scientists, however, is primarily dictated by evidence that bears upon society's constructs. This evidence almost inevitably will show that these constructs are inadequately served by existing tests and systems. The inevitability of this outcome arises because of the extra-scientific interests that help form the test basis in compensation settings. Tests and systems will be used as tools in the service of one or other economic interest. A realization of this fact is vital to the production of valid inquiry by scientists involved in this field.

Most important, in addition to the technical role of science, there is an innovative role induced by scientific scrutiny of the very constructs to be assessed. Evidence may emerge through disinterested investigation that reveals the inadequacy of prevailing constructs. The two major instances discussed in this treatise of each of these two scientific roles are (*a*) the inadequacy of certain tonal threshold averages in the assessment of hearing for speech; and (*b*) the insufficiency of "hearing for speech" as the construct underlying assessment of everyday hearing handicap.

The scientist in this field is therefore part technician and part radical. Scientists in their technician guise try to serve prevailing interests as best they can. In their radical guise, they undermine, oppose, and (it is hoped) improve these prevailing interests.

A word needs to be said about the special relationship that occurs, because of the *medicolegal* context, between scientists and medical practitioners. People in medicine, being entrepreneurs of their own special skills rather than students of some aspect of the natural world, are perched somewhere away from the scientists in this particular area (as I am sure they are in all areas of medicolegal assessment). The verity of this fact is not, however, sufficiently acknowledged by all participants in the medicolegal assessment game. The division between medical and scientific persons is blurred, with the result that questions of a purely scientific nature often times become clouded by medical judgment and vice versa. There is no special problem here, provided the occasions are earmarked when opinion and ideology, emanating from the scientific or medical arenas, interact with relatively more disinterested inquiry.

TESTS USED IN HEARING ASSESSMENT

It is useful to separate, as much as reasonably possible, discourse on hearing tests and their rationales from discourse on the use to which some of these tests are put in systems of assessment. A test is a procedure, involving an instrument, to gauge some aspect of function. A "system of assessment" is more abstract in that the results of a test or tests are used to calculate the degree of "functional loss" according to a scale, the basis of which is independently determined. In considering systems of assessment, one must also clarify the nomenclature ("hearing loss," "handicap," etc.) that people have devised to handle test data. This issue is of less concern in discussing a test itself where understanding what it purports to test, how it is administered, what advantages it offers over other tests, and how it relates to other tests is of most concern. Not all these features are handled in detail in this chapter, but the broader descriptions are given simply to familiarize the reader with various kinds of tests so that when we turn to assessment systems and to a more detailed study of test reliability and validity, shorthand labels can serve to inform the reader about which test is involved.

We should understand from the outset that some tests have been devised specifically with assessment in mind. Others have been appropriated by the assessment industry from the diagnostic field and elsewhere. Certain tests are used solely for diagnostic purposes (various tuning-fork procedures), others for both diagnostic and assessment purposes at the same time (estimation of levels at threshold by air conduction and by air as against bone conduction). Still others, such as speech reception threshold, have only assessment functions. We are concerned to discuss only those tests that have assessment functions and to consider procedures of testing for assessment purposes. Thus, for example, the self-recording tonal test (von Békésy, 1947) has an assessment aspect— level at threshold—and a diagnostic aspect—the Békésy "types" (Jerger, 1960). In the latter mode, test procedure is somewhat different from procedure in the former mode. Hence only the former procedure concerns us here.

A major appropriation by the assessment industry has been taken from communications research, especially following World War II. Tests using speech were devised then (and earlier in connection with telephonics research) to assess the adequacy of communications systems, especially in competing noise. The use of these tests in the context of hearing assessment was a later development. In a somewhat similar way, tests devised to assess hearing-aid performance have been used on occasion to assess hearing. It is only in recent times that tests using speech have been devised specifically to assess hearing, and it is important to keep this point in mind when considering the rationales of various types of test.

Nonverbal Tests

These tests have always been preferred over verbal tests in hearing assessment simply because once the instruction is understood the listener responds to signals without any confounding involving meaning, familiarity, or other externalities.

Various noisemakers, of which the pocket watch was perhaps the most popular, were used by clinicians in the nineteenth century. The hefty timepieces whose chains we see suspended across the sometimes equally hefty stomachs of our forebears, emitted ticks quite audible at 1 and even 2 meters from the untroubled ear. And it was a matter of measuring the distance at which the watch's tick could just be heard to gauge whether the degree of partial deafness was slight or considerable.

Politzer's *Hörmesser* (described by Barr, 1884) represented in its original manufacture a standardized mechanical noisemaker whose value Barr fully grasped when compared to the highly variable performance within and between pocket watches. Unfortunately, according to Barr, different manufacturers did not stick to the original specifications, and so *Hörmessers* of varying design, and hence of output, were used by different clinicians—thus spoiling the aim of standardization.

Bunch (1941) has described in detail the early development of the audiometer as an instrument for the delivery of pure sinusoidal wave trains through telephone receivers. It would be superfluous merely to summarize what is already a compact historical record, and the reader is referred to Bunch for further information. Most typically, audiometers are designed to produce tones in the range .125 to 12 kHz, either discretely at octaves to 8 kHz plus octaves from 1.5 kHz, or continuously throughout this range. For screening purposes, tones at octaves from .5 to 4 or 8 kHz are typically used. These octave intervals and interpolated octaves derive largely from tuning-fork frequencies, which in turn are derived from musical octaves. The older notation, namely 256 (Hz), 512, 1024, etc., is based on Helmholtz's musical notation (where middle C = $C' \equiv 256$ Hz, $C'' \equiv 512$ Hz, and so on). This scheme is approximately the same as 250 (Hz) 500, 1000, etc. I have assumed licence throughout this work to "transform" older notation to current, as this allows expression in terms of kilohertz (.25, .5, 1 kHz, etc.). I am fully aware that use of the term *octave* to describe doublings and halvings of frequency does not coincide altogether with the term as it is used in the context of musical pitch (Ward, 1970). These are different, though obviously related qualities. However, it is quite legitimate to talk of an octave in reference to doubling of frequency provided it is recognized that this is not identical with a *pitch* difference of one octave.

Various procedures have been devised for using the tonal audiometer as an instrument to determine the intensity level at the threshold of audibility. Typically, tones are presented for brief intervals at various intensities, and the level at which a tone is detectable on 50% of instances is taken as the level at threshold. In self-recording tonal audiometry, excursions back and forth across this threshold are made continuously, and the calculated average midpoint of these excursions is taken as the level at threshold. Self-recording threshold determination is made using both fixed, discrete frequencies and continuously changing frequencies (a "sweep frequency" audiogram). Another variant of the sweep frequency test, which I have observed only in laboratories in the Netherlands, involves holding intensity constant and observing excursions above and below the frequency which is just audible.

The purpose of the tonal threshold test is partly the same as that of the watch-tick test—namely, to gauge the degree of partial deafness—and partly to observe the contour of the threshold as a function of frequency. The latter feature, especially when threshold is determined by both air and bone conduction, is an aid in the diagnosis of disorder. This procedure also has an assessment function, in that a lower intensity level at threshold by bone conduction indicates that the degree of partial deafness is to some extent caused by disorder prior to the inner ear receptors, and hence more useful remediation is possible than it is when both air and bone conduction thresholds are elevated to the same degree.

One shortcoming of tonal audiometry as a means of assessment is that it examines only the level at threshold. Suprathreshold effects, distortions of various kinds, may be contributing, however, to a disturbance of hearing. Here and elsewhere, incidentally, I use the term *disorder* to mean a pathological condition of the auditory system and the term *disturbance* to mean the effect on an individual's auditory experience of one or more disorders.

Suprathreshold tonal tests are used by clinicians as aids to diagnosis but rarely as aids to assessment—despite the foregoing assertion. This is because there is little evidence of a direct link between suprathreshold distortion for nonverbal signals and hearing disturbance. This observation is examined in more detail in Chapters 6 and 8.

Another shortcoming is, of course, the very virtue of the tonal test—namely its meaninglessness. The question here concerns what has been learned with regard to someone's state of reduced hearing from a test using signals that are nonrepresentative of the everyday auditory world. This is a problem that all clinicians and researchers recognize, and it is the reason why such strenuous and extensive efforts have been made to relate results using tones to results using speech. We grapple with this massive issue in Chapter 6.

One thing long recognized is that the suprathreshold ability to discriminate speech sounds may or may not be reflected in the tonal threshold trace. For this reason, some medicolegal assessment systems are based on response to both tonal and speech signals. By and large, however, as we see in the following chapter, agencies have been content to put together assessment systems that rely solely on calculations from the air conduction tonal audiogram.

Verbal Tests

Tests using speech have been used in assessment for as long as any other procedure. Indeed, prior to introduction of the audiometer, speech testing was probably the major assessment tool. It was understood very early in clinical practice that whispered spoken speech permitted a more controlled method of presentation and allowed a better balance between vowels and consonants. Barr and Barr (1909) cite studies by Wolf on the distance required for detection of different phonemes from which it is clear that vowels have much more acoustic power than even voiced consonants.

In those times, the speech material usually consisted of unconnected, everyday words of various syllable lengths. Thus listeners would be familiar with all the words spoken but could not rely on guesswork, as they might have had sentences been presented. Words were presented to each ear separately (the other ear occluded), and vision was also masked to prevent any confounding from that source. The measure of speech hearing ability was the maximum distance at which the words could be correctly identified.

Bell Telephone Lists

Standardized word lists became available in English when Fletcher and Steinberg (1929) published their report on methods for measuring articulation. Two types of material were devised: monosyllables and sentences. The monosyllables were constructed in lists of 50—each list containing all the phonemes of English in relatively similar interlist proportions. No control was made for meaning; some syllables corresponded with actual words, some were "nonsense" words. The specification of these lists was on the basis of acoustic representativeness, the lists being intended for evaluation of different transmission systems (telephones, hearing aids, radio transmitters). In addition, lists of sentences requiring free answers by the listener were drawn up to test the overall intelligibility of meaningful speech trains through different communication systems. The key words in each sentence list also covered the range of the phonemic content of English. It is not surprising that the sentences showed far greater resistance to unintelligibility under distortion conditions because of the transition probabilities within their structure.

A test using numerals was also devised by the Bell Telephone research team and marketed on a phonograph recording which presented the numerals at decreasing levels over a range of about 30 dB. According to Hudgins, Hawkins, Karlin, and Stevens (1947) the numerals used were one, two, three, four, five, six, and eight. The test, therefore, was designed to provide maximum discriminability of signals by making them as different from one another as possible and drawing them from a very small parent population. Miller, Heise, and Lichten (1951) showed that samples of words from different-sized populations of words varied in intelligibility simply because they varied in recognizability. There being only 28 words in the English language lexicon that generate all the vocalized numerals from 1 to 999, intelligibility of 7 items from that very small lexicon is bound to be optimal. Hudgins *et al.* (1947) point out too that identification of the particular numerals of the Bell Telephone test list can successfully be made on the basis of the vowel sounds alone. Failure to discriminate or even detect the consonants would not necessarily prohibit discrimination of the items.

While the recorded numerals enjoyed considerable use as a screening test of hearing in schools, the other tests were used mainly in the technical applications for which they were originally devised, only rarely were they used in assessment of hearing. The important feature of the Bell Telephone test material is that it set the style for future and still current speech tests.

Psycho-Acoustic Laboratory Lists

Work at Harvard University's Psycho-Acoustic Laboratory (PAL) during and immediately following the war of 1939–1945 resulted in the development of several speech hearing tests for both communications and clinical application. Hudgins *et al.* (1947) reported the development of the PAL disyllable and sentence tests. The first of these used equally stressed, two-syllable words (*spondees*) recorded, like the older numerals test, in groups, each group decreasing in intensity.

The use of spondaic words rather than numerals permitted the feature of phonemic representation to be built into the test simply because there are more of such words available than number words. As in the numerals test, lists were designed to comprise readily distinguishable items, and the equal-stress quality allowed recording of each word at a relatively uniform loudness because the vowel element is uppermost in the production of equal syllabic stress. The test was intended to measure the level at threshold for the reception of speech and was not intended to include any discriminatory element. At that time, discrimination of speech sounds and the speech reception threshold were considered two separate functions requiring separate assessment. In the disyllable test, to further minimize the discriminatory element, the minimal population principle was employed. Listeners were familiarized with the test material beforehand (two lists of 42 words in six scramblings each) so that recognizability was optimized. We can see, therefore, that the disyllable test is a more extensive form of the numerals test designed along similar lines for similar purposes.

The sentence test developed at PAL (Hudgins *et al.*, 1947) was designed on a similar principle to that of the earlier Bell Telephone sentence lists. However, while the older lists required quite specific local knowledge on the listener's part to answer the questions, the PAL lists are less parochial—relying on simple everyday content ("What day comes after Monday?"). The sentence lists were also intended for the measurement of speech reception threshold using more structured and realistic material. But of course, because of that structuring, nonauditory factors come into play in the listener's grasp of the content, hence the sentence lists are less closely tied in with pure auditory sensitivity. It may be for this reason or because of the greater amount of time required for administration that the PAL sentences have rarely been used in any proving research or clinical context; the disyllable test has had extensive use, however, and is a standard assessment tool.

In 1948, Egan published a report of the PAL research and development of monosyllable lists. These lists, like the Bell Telephone Laboratory monosyllables, were devised more strictly for communication testing purposes. However, they represent a different type of content and employ actual words rather than merely syllabic sounds. In their finally revised form, there were 20 lists, each of 50 monosyllabic words, and Egan (1948) reports that the lists were constructed to be as nearly equal as possible in average intelligibility and range of difficulty. An important content development of these lists is that like the older lists they not only contain all the phonemes of English but are structured to approximate a proportional representation of the phonetic composition of English based on Dewey's (1923) statistical sampling of English speech sounds. For this reason, the PAL lists are generally known as "phonetically balanced" (PB). These lists were recorded at the Central Institute for the Deaf (CID) in Missouri, spoken by Rush-Hughes.

Revision of the PAL Lists at the Central Institute for the Deaf

In 1952, Hirsh, Davis, Silverman, Reynolds, Eldert, and Benson of the Central Institute for the Deaf (CID) reported a revision of both the disyllable and PB monosyllable material. The revised version of the first test involved reducing the original list of 84 words to a group of 36 more familiar and equally intelligible words (as observed from judges' ratings and listeners' responses). These words were recorded on tape and six scramblings produced by splicing and dubbing onto other tapes. The test was produced in two forms: at a constant intensity level (CID test W-1) and, like the original PAL test, at decreasing intensity levels (test W-2).

The revised monosyllable list involved a massive reduction of material from 1000 items in 20 lists of 50 to 200 items in 4 lists of 50. Only 120 of the 200 items came from the original PAL list, the other 80 were drawn from various other sources. Stricter criteria of familiarity and of phonetic balance were employed. The first entailed judges' ratings of item familiarity followed by a check of selected items against Thorndike's (1932) list of the most common English words in children's books and texts. All but 1 of the 200 items finally selected for high familiarity were found in Thorndike's list, and 190 of the items were in the 4000 most common words in children's English. Phonetic balance was achieved in the same way as in the original PAL lists but was undertaken more strictly in accordance with the statistical sampling of the frequency of different phonetic occurrences (Dewey, 1923; French, Carter, & Koenig, 1930). The final lists (test W-22) were recorded by Hirsh. As with the original tests, disyllables were pronounced with equal stress and effort on each syllable to give virtual identity of loudness, whereas the monosyllables were presented with more natural cadence.

The CID W-1 and W-22 lists have become standard speech test material used extensively in clinical and research settings. Although other lists of monosyllables have been devised and other monosyllable test procedures developed, as described briefly in the next subsection, the CID revisions of the PAL material continue as standard tests in themselves and as models for tests developed in different local and linguistic conditions for hearing assessment purposes.

Other Types of List

Davis and Silverman (1970, pp. 481–495) provide the best contemporary source of both bibliographic reference to and exemplars of speech tests in English developed in the United States. Probably the most important test developments since the work of Hirsh *et al.* (1952) are lists devised to test phonemic differentiation and more everyday speech-hearing ability. Tests of phonemic differentiation (rhyme tests) employ the device of presenting alternative items on a checklist, and the listener has to identify which of the alternatives he heard. By this means, a more accurate assessment of confusions between phonemes can be made. Only occasionally has the rhyme test approach been used in the assessment context, however. A more critical development is the devising of sentences of an everyday colloquial kind specifically intended for use in the assessment of "hearing handicap" (Davis & Silverman, 1970, pp. 492–495; Silverman & Hirsh, 1955). These sentences are in 10 lists of 10 sentences each, and there are 50 key words in each list. The composition of the lists takes account of phonetic balancing and also of the semantic and syntactical structure of English. Because they have only recently become available in complete form, little research has been done using them. Previously unpublished, results from the National Acoustic Laboratories in Australia using these sentences in comparison with self-reported hearing ability are presented in Chapter 10.

3

Assessment for Compensation and the Emergence of Systems

THE CONCEPT OF AN ASSESSMENT SYSTEM

Not all the tests described in Chapter 2 have been used in the various systems of assessment devised over the years. All of those tests have been used in assessment contexts of one sort or another, but only the more universally used tests form the basis of assessment according to a more abstract principle. As stated in Chapter 2, an assessment system is characterized by a set of rules whereby test results are taken as raw data and calculations are made upon them to arrive at a score or percentage. Such an exercise is vitally necessary for the purpose of making medicolegal judgments.

In discussing tests and test results, one can avoid evaluative statements by using phrases such as "higher or lower level at threshold," that refer to a physical quantity which coincides with a person's response. A common way that writers express test results, however, is to refer to such and such amount of "hearing loss." In my view, this begs the question as to both the meaning of the phrase (What is "hearing loss"?) and the validity of a test result in revealing amounts of so-called "hearing loss." I have tried throughout this book to avoid such usage except as a convenient shorthand.

As soon as we confront assessment systems, however, we are immediately faced with evaluative phrases simply because these systems purport to gauge the actual hearing experiences of individuals. I do not concur with definitional exercises that have been made over the years, and for that reason I challenge the test basis on which systems, and hence definitions applying to systems, rest. Although the main thrust of my challenge must wait until the evidence has been scrutinized, for present purposes it is necessary to be familiar with prevailing definitions within the assessment scene so that we can be clear about what is meant by terms like "hearing handicap," "disability," and so forth.

OPERATIONAL DEFINITIONS

In earlier times, the phrase that did most of the work was "hearing loss." As Davis (1970b) points out, the phrase meant not only the level at threshold but also the *shift* in that level as a result of injury, as well as the condition of partial disturbance or inability to hear. Older systems used the phrases "hearing loss for speech" and "percentage hearing loss for speech," the first referring to level at SRT (50%) and the second to a calculated figure based on some tonal threshold average. Because a level at threshold higher than audiometric zero may yet be within the range of "normal" hearing, however, it has been considered misleading to use the term "hearing loss" in reference to level at threshold. Davis (1970b) proposes that "hearing-threshold level" be used instead and that "hearing loss" be confined to descriptive diagnostic phrases such as "conductive hearing loss" and so on.

I avoid this sort of terminology simply because "hearing loss" begs the question. It assumes that a given disorder brings about a decrement in the "amount of hearing" a person possesses, and this may be an inaccurate conception of certain hearing disorders. I prefer the terms *disorder* in the diagnostic context and *disturbance* in reference to an experienced effect arising from disorder.

Davis (1970b) wishes to eschew the phrases "partial deafness" and "partial hearing." I concur with this view in the context of tests and assessment systems, but as in Chapter 1 these phrases have utility when we discuss social and psychological issues relating to hearing, partial hearing, and deafness.

In regard to assessment systems, the three main terms that have become relatively standard are *hearing impairment, hearing handicap*, and *disability*. *Hearing impairment* embodies something of both my terms *disorder* and *disturbance* in referring to a "change for the worse" in structure *or* function. *Hearing handicap* refers to the effect of impairment on everyday life—but refers very narrowly, in fact, to "hearing loss for speech" as calculated from the tonal audiogram. *Disability,* a term which has been used loosely by authors (including the present one) in reference to "handicap," has actually a distinct legal meaning, namely lessened ability to remain employed or employed at full earnings.

These are the terms encountered most of the time in discussion of assessment systems. I assume license to translate other terms into these if it is clear that authors have the same meaning in mind. Otherwise I give the terms authors themselves present as we go along.

In the following section, I describe the purpose and nature of the assessment systems developed and used in the United States. After that, I show by reference to the historical social background the way in which the most widely used system actually emerged. In the final section, I describe the assessment systems used throughout the world. The reason for this latter division is that hearing assessment systems were initially developed in the United States and what has been done there has powerfully influenced practice in other countries.

SYSTEMS OF ASSESSMENT

Fletcher's ".8 rule"

From integrated spectrographic analysis of speech samples, researchers at the Bell Telephone Laboratories concluded that the bulk of speech energy lies in the .5 to 2 kHz region. Filtering experiments confirmed this observation by demonstrating that the majority of speech elements showed significant degradation only when the filter extended upward or downward into that audio-frequency range (Fletcher, 1929). From a study comparing tonal threshold average at .5, 1, and 2 kHz with performance using numerals as speech material, Fletcher observed that multiplying the tonal average by .83 accurately predicted the speech threshold. This proposal became known as the "Fletcher .8 rule" and had some use in clinical and medicolegal assessment. We examine Fletcher's (1929) study in more detail in Chapter 6.

Fowler's and Sabine's Systems

In 1938, a committee of the Council on Physical Therapy of the American Medical Association resolved to determine a system for assessment of hearing loss that could be applied uniformly by otologists in medicolegal cases. Two influential members of that committee were Fowler and Sabine, each of whom derived his own system (Fowler, 1941, 1942; Sabine, 1942). AMA Council on Physical Therapy (1942) adopted a hybrid that owed much to Sabine's (1942) system, but Fowler's (1941, 1942) system was adopted by other agencies, principally the armed forces, for the purpose of acceptance, disability rating, and discharge of personnel.

Fowler's 1941 system was a little more complex than Fletcher's (1929) in that differential weights were applicable to levels at tonal threshold depending on frequency. Furthermore, he extended the range of audio frequencies to include 3 and 4 kHz as well .5, 1, and 2 kHz. The weights applicable to thresholds at these frequencies were

Frequency (kHz)	.5	1	2	3	4
Percentage weight	15	25	30	25	5

The tables drawn up by Fowler (1941) allowed translation of the weighted average thresholds in each ear into an overall percentage loss of capacity for hearing speech. Whereas total bilateral deafness on this scale was 100% loss of capacity, total unilateral deafness was only 10% loss of capacity—though the influence of unilateral deafness increased slightly with increasing loss of sensitivity in the other ear. The curve of weighted threshold against percentage loss of capacity was sigmoid in shape, supposedly to take account of the sigmoid shape of the articulation function (Fletcher, 1929; Steinberg & Gardner, 1940). That relationship of course depends on an assumption that loss of sensitivity for tones means the same as loss of intensity of signals to be discriminated. Fowler (1941) considered that this is true except in cases of people with sensorineural disorder, in whom loudness "recruitment" will be manifest, but he believed that this effect is beneficial in people with minor degrees of sensorineural disorder and becomes nonbeneficial with more severe impairment. Hence a minor differential correction to the weighted threshold average was included for cases of pure sensorineural disorder. The evidence in support of Fowler's (1941) system was provided by calculations on the audiograms of 20 people with various types and degrees of disorder and comparison of these calculations with the observed speech thresholds (distance for reception of normal conversational voice). In 1942, Fowler presented a simplified system based on the following weighted frequency values.

Frequency (kHz)	.5	1	2	4
Percentage weight	15	30	40	15

All other features remained as before—and the evidence in this case was taken from results in seven people with various degrees and types of disorder. We take a closer look at the evidence Fowler adduces in support of his 1941 and 1942 systems in Chapter 6.

Sabine's (1942) system was founded on quite a different precept from Fowler's, though they share certain features. Sabine based his system on Fletcher's charted calculations (1929, p. 158) of the coefficients of differential sensitivity for pitch and loudness as a function of frequency and intensity. Arguing that the perception of speech is dependent on the capacity to discriminate loudness and pitch differences, one can further argue that reduction in auditory sensitivity means a loss of the proportion of discriminable acoustic elements. We can see immediately that this hypothesis springs directly from classical psychophysics in which discrimination at the level of bare acoustic quality is taken as the fundamental function of the auditory system. Reduction in the number of discriminable tonal elements means reduction in the ear's capability to distinguish higher-order variables, which are conceived as conglomerations of these elements. Note that Sabine makes no claim for a reduction in differential sensitivity per se, merely that as threshold level is raised an increasing proportion of the total number of discriminable tones within the audible spectrum is lost.

It would indeed have been an interesting exercise had Sabine pursued this hypothesis to its limit and tried to show a relation between the number of differentiable tones and speech hearing ability. But he stopped short of that and compromised his system in two ways: first by limiting the frequency range to be considered in assessment to the .125 to 4 kHz band and second by acknowledging the principle of "the most important speech frequencies," namely .5 to 2 kHz. Hence the weight to be given in that region was arbitrarily increased and proportionately decreased in surrounding regions. Furthermore, acknowledging that even a 10 dB reduction in speech signal level from its point of maximum intelligibility has a negligible effect (i.e., the asymptotic character of the articulation function), Sabine admitted no percentage reduction in hearing capacity until at least 10 dB re: audiometric zero was reached.

In these expedients, Sabine's system has features in common with Fowler's (1941, 1942). A final feature that also aligns it with Fowler's is the assignment of an 8:1 ratio between "better" and "poorer" ears in the calculation of the binaural "percentage loss of useful hearing." The feature that distinguishes the two systems is the differential weighting for intensity in Sabine's system that owes its origin to the differential sensitivity principle from which the system emerged. Sabine (1942) presents no empirical evidence to support his system, but his principle was nevertheless incorporated into the AMA guidelines for hearing loss evaluation (AMA Council on Physical Therapy, 1942). Modifications introduced by the committee of that council were (a) reduction of the frequency range to be considered for assessment from .125 to 4 kHz to .25 to 4 kHz; (b) assignment of more weight to the .5 to 4 kHz range than is assigned in Sabine's (1942) system; and (c) a somewhat more sigmoid threshold–percentage relation. These modifications obviously bow in Fowler's direction. The main feature retained from Sabine's system is the differential intensity weighting. The better ear–poorer ear ratio was also made slightly more generous in the 1942 AMA scheme with a 7:1 weighting between values obtained on two differently affected ears

This system has in fact become known as the Fowler–Sabine formula, presumably because its structure is a hybrid of both these people's ideas. According to Davis (1971), the AMA (1942) scheme never enjoyed much popularity, the thing being apparently too complicated for acceptance by otologists. They preferred the simple Fletcher .8 formula.

The AMA Council on Physical Medicine (as it was now called) tried to respond to this problem by producing a more simplified scheme (1947) prepared by Fowler and Sabine. According to Harris, Haines, and Myers (1956), the new formula is even more in the direction of Fowler's (1942) scheme; so it is perhaps fitting to label AMA (1942) the Sabine–Fowler formula and AMA (1947) the Fowler–Sabine formula. Certainly the plot of threshold over the .5 to 4 kHz range against percentage loss used in the 1947 scheme shows an even greater sigmoid shape than the 1942 scheme. This feature therefore conforms with Fowler's (1942). And the differential intensity weightings are quite negligibly variant from one intensity level to the next. Finally, the proportional weight applicable to each frequency is, on average 15.3, 30.1, 39.6, and 15%—virtually identical with Fowler's (1942) weights of 15, 30, 40, and 15% at .5, 1, 2, and 4 kHz, respectively.

The 7:1 better–poorer ear ratio was retained in AMA (1947), and Fowler (1947) voiced his objection to this, saying that a fixed ratio of better–poorer ear did not do justice to the varying importance of better–poorer ear relations depending on the levels of hearing loss in each. In Fowler (1941, 1942), there was allowance for precisely this sort of changing relationship.

In 1955, the AMA Council on Physical Medicine and Rehabilitation (yet another restyled committee, but speaking now for both the AMA and the American Academy of Ophthalmology and Otolaryngology—AAOO) produced a statement of principle regarding hearing loss evaluation. In essence, this statement declared that the existing AMA (1947) system was not satisfactory for people with sensorineural disorder and that studies were needed to find out more precisely what the relationship was between the tonal audiogram and the ability to hear speech in heterogeneous groups. Another principle held that the statistical limit of normal on the audiometer is about 15 dB (ASA) so that beginning hearing handicap should be taken as levels at threshold in excess of that value. From the style of the statement, it is clear that direct assessment of speech hearing ability is preferable to exclusive reliance upon tonal threshold. However, the development since the time of that statement has been even more firmly in the direction of the tonal test; and it is now unlikely, if present practice continues, that this test will be superseded. The model provided by the United States medical groups has influenced most legislation in that country and in most other industrialized countries, as we see in the final section of this chapter.

The American Academy of Ophthalmology and Otolarynology Formula

The most important change to occur in the 1950s was the insistent assertion that the average threshold levels at .5, 1, and 2 kHz best represented hearing impairment for speech. The rejection of any measurement beyond 2 kHz has been firm and complete. The evidential basis for using only .5 to 2 kHz tonal threshold is obscure. We examine most of the research that purports to validate its use in Chapter 6. Some of it should be commented upon here, however, and a general appraisal of the problem is also in order.

The agency most responsible for promoting use of the .5 to 2 kHz average in assessing hearing impairment for compensation and other purposes is the AAOO. The deliberations of its Committee on Conservation of Hearing (1959) in turn affected the AMA Committee on Medical Rating of Physical Impairment (the latest name), so that in 1961 that committee adopted the AAOO formula and rating scale as far as hearing impairment is concerned. The two bodies have concurred on the .5 to 2 kHz issue ever since.

It should be clear from the outset that the rating of impairment has its major purpose in medicolegal deliberations. As far as rating of hearing is concerned, that context will largely be inhabited by persons claiming injury caused by noise. There are other functions of handicap rating: clinical appraisal or judgment about the success of a therapeutic measure. These are important and legitimate assessment occasions, but the assessment for compensation, largely of people with a specific kind of hearing disorder, is the primary purpose of the systems described here. That being the case, it should have been the aim of interested agencies such as the AMA, the AAOO, and the Veterans Administration to seek explicit information on tonal threshold–speech hearing relationships in that group, as well as in the general population of people with impaired hearing, but this has never been undertaken.

Davis (1970b) refers not only to heterogeneous population studies in the context of .5 to 2 kHz–speech hearing interrelations but also to the research that led to his own assessment system—the Social Adequacy Index (Davis, 1948). With respect to the population study evidence, discussion is better postponed until Chapter 10 because these studies involved the use of self-report scales. The Social Adequacy Index, however, can be dealt with here. It is my contention that reference to the Social Adequacy Index in the context of assessment of hearing for compensation is misleading. This index was derived from measures of speech hearing ability in various groups of people, and its purpose was to establish a matrix through which, from measurement of speech reception threshold and maximum discrimination score, a person's social hearing adequacy could be pinpointed. The validation of the index from self-reports by persons who underwent the fenestration operation was never well established. The critical point is that tonal threshold was not involved as a predictor of social adequacy in the development of this scheme: Not only is the index uncertain as to its internal criteria of "social adequacy," it has not been related subsequently to tonal threshold measurement in people with other than pure or predominantly conductive disorders.

The actual evidence underlying the .5 to 2 kHz tonal threshold as a valid speech hearing predictor is in fact very specific. Threshold levels in that region relate very well to the highly restricted speech tests using numerals or disyllables, but these materials are arguably far removed from everyday speech. Furthermore, in the specific population of primary assessment concern, people with noise-induced disorder, there is no evidence that even these speech test results relate closely to .5 to 2 kHz tonal threshold. To detail these assertions further is to anticipate the extensive analysis and review of this issue in Chapter 6. But the point needs stressing here that the .5 to 2 kHz formula rests on very shaky foundations. In the next section, I give the reasons I perceive why there has been such insistence on using this average in assessment for compensation.

Other Formulas

The AAOO–AMA formula has not received universal assent or official acceptance. Authors such as Kryter (1973) and Harris (1965) have argued the better validity of an average over 1, 2, and 3 kHz or even 2, 3, and 4 kHz, and in some states of the United States and at the federal level, systems along these lines have been adopted; but the great majority of states that use an averaging formula have adopted the AAOO–AMA guide. The pattern of choice of formulas outside the United States is similar.

Systems of assessment other than these described here have been devised from time to time, but they have never gained acceptance. A concise review of these is included in Harris *et al.* (1956). Precise details of the AAOO–AMA formula are given by Davis (1970b). The following section traces some of the important historical moments in the medicolegal assessment context principally to show the social milieu in which the AAOO–AMA system emerged and was used. The final section details the kinds of system presently in operation in various states and countries throughout the world.

HISTORICAL REVIEW OF ASSESSMENT FOR COMPENSATION

Presumably the assessment of hearing from a medicolegal point of view began when the first cases in which a disorder of hearing was claimed to have arisen from someone else's negligence were brought to court. Early cases of successful common-law suits of this kind are rare. The more usual remedy has been sought under Workmen's Compensation law, in which negligence is not the point at issue.

Workmen's Compensation first emerged in technological society in Germany in 1884 (Nelson, 1957). Its purpose was to compensate the victims of industrial accidents during the periods when they were laid up and hence unable to earn. Previously, accident victims had to rely on charitable handouts to survive. The German philosophy held that accidents to people, being an inevitable feature of the industrial process, should be covered by compensation simply as one of the costs of that process. In other words, part of the price of producing goods includes the necessary cost of insurance to compensate the victims of industrial accidents. This purely economic view of industrial hazards has prevailed, especially in the United States. Because of its solidly economic base, compensation for a long time was seen only as a means of making up for lost earnings and reduced ability to earn in the future. The fact that people were harmed, sometimes severely and permanently, was not in itself seen as problematic.

The Workmen's Compensation Act of 1906 in the United Kingdom embodied principles similar to those of the German act but provided for the inclusion of certain scheduled diseases arising out of specific occupations. In 1907, the British Committee on Compensation for Industrial Disease heard evidence relating to "Boilermakers' Deafness" with a view to its inclusion in the schedule. It was well known in 1907 that boilermakers and similar tradesmen, mainly employed in the shipbuilding regions of the United Kingdom went deaf as a result of their noisy occupations. Barr's (1886) study had demonstrated beyond doubt that this was the case. But there was, of course, no evidence that the gradual loss of hearing experienced by these people prevented their continuation in their jobs. There was no case for inclusion, therefore, because there was no loss of earnings: "Then they do not mind the deafness?" "No; it does not inconvenience them beyond that they do not hear [Minutes of evidence of Dr. A. Mechan to the Committee, 1907, p. 163]." When the British law was changed in 1946 by introduction of the National Insurance (Industrial Injuries) Act, the loss of wages condition was dropped from the statute, but surprisingly noise deafness was not included in the schedule of diseases prescribed as compensable. One says "surprisingly," but perhaps compensation for deafness following combat in the 1939–1945 war helped mop up prewar industrial cases so that there was no pressing need to write noise deafness into the statute. This was certainly considered to be what happened in the United States (see pages 52–53). Not until 1975 in fact was legislation introduced in the

United Kingdom allowing claims for noise-induced deafness under the revised National Insurance (Industrial Injuries) Act. Prior to 1975 a few successful claims were made at common law (Coles, 1975; Grime, 1975; Hinchcliffe & Hinchcliffe, 1974).

The real medicolegal history of occupational noise deafness assessment occurred in the United States. Events in that country have shaped the pattern of compensation systems for noise deafness in most other parts of the technological world, because the whole issue got off the ground there years before other industrial societies began to take the matter seriously.

The first American Employees' Compensation Act was a federal statute introduced in 1908 that covered traumatic (sudden) deafness caused by accident and included a loss-of-earnings feature built into its terms. In 1917, the Federal Employers Liability Act was introduced in the United States, and Keck (1955) reports a "Catch-22" case which was heard that same year in Florida. A railroad fireman sued his employer under common law for traumatic hearing injury resulting from the blast of a train whistle let off while he was close to it, but on appeal to the Florida Supreme Court, this decision was reversed. The plaintiff was informed that his exclusive legal remedy was under the new 1917 act. However, because there was a 2-year limiting statute under that act and presumably the injury had occurred more than 2 years before, the action was barred!

Keck (1955) reports other cases from various parts of the United States from as early as 1918 in which damages were awarded for traumatic deafness and even, in the case of a boilermaker, for blast-induced tinnitus. That incident occurred in Oklahoma in 1931.

The Case of *Slawinski* v. *J. H. Williams and Co.*, New York

The classic case, however, is that of *Slawinski* v. *J. H. Williams and Co.*, heard in 1948 by the New York Court of Appeals. Workmen's Compensation in New York began in 1910 with an act akin to the federal statute covering accidental injury that resulted in loss or reduction of earnings (Symons, 1955). The concept of injury as an inevitable part, and hence cost of industrial production was clearly expressed in the revision of that act in 1914. It was not until 1920 that disease arising out of the industrial process, as opposed to injury from accident, was included in the statute and a schedule of prescribed disorders drawn up. In 1935, the act was amended to cover any and all diseases, provided occupational cause could be established. Loss of earnings was still a feature of the law, however. Traumatic injury to hearing was specifically included in the

Workmen's Compensation Act of 1922, and in 1938 a case was brought and an award made for "partial loss of use" of hearing, presumably following an accidental trauma.

Matthew Slawinski, however, a drop-forger, claimed compensation for "occupational hearing loss" as an industrial *disease,* not as the result of accidental injury. This case was heard in 1948, and the claim was controverted by the defendant on the grounds that "occupational hearing loss" was not a disease within the meaning of the act and that in any case no loss of earnings was involved. The referee nonetheless awarded compensation.

According to Williams (1957) this was the first time, in New York State at any rate, that compensation was paid without demonstrated loss of earnings. The decision was appealed in various further hearings, but the original judgment was upheld. A spate of claims followed the Slawinski case, and employers and their insurance carriers had to operate swiftly to reduce the impact of unforeseen costs. The first stopgap measure was to persuade the legislature to rule that claims could not be dealt with until the claimant had been away from exposure to the injurious noise for a 6-month period. In effect, this meant that most claimants would have retired before a claim could be brought, and since there was also built in a "presbycusis" correction, then claims by retired persons would necessarily be that much reduced. New York adopted the Fletcher .8 system at that time in assessing claims. The 6-month rule was ostensibly recommended by an advisory medical committee on the grounds that noise-induced disorder is an impermanent condition, so assessment should not take place until well after removal from noise. Since there was not a scrap of quantitative or substantiated evidence at that time to support this notion, it is fairly clear that the medical opinion was simply a way of disguising a maneuver to give insurance companies and industrial management time to build up funds to meet the claims. Later a more open admission about the 6-month rule was made. That rule remains the law in New York State.

One very nice point, according to Symons (1958), is that whereas the original rule said 6 months after the end of *exposure* to the injurious noise, the final agreement was 6 months after the end of *employment* in the noisy workplace. One reason for this change was that were employers to reduce the noise by engineering means—which they were genuinely anxious to do—then 6 months later they would have faced compensation claims under an exposure concept. Through the employment concept, noise reduction measures would not result in having to pay compensation immediately. Subsequent changes in New York law include abandonment of the presbycusis correction and adoption of the AAOO formula.

The Case of *Wojcik* v. *The Green Bay Co.*, Wisconsin

Wisconsin was the scene of the second case of compensation despite no loss of earnings, but the ramifications of that battle have spread throughout the entire world. Yet another migrant worker, Albert Wojcik, and also a drop-forge operator, sued the Green Bay Company through the Wisconsin Industrial Commission. On appeal, a circuit court judge reversed the commission's decision on the no-loss-of-earnings argument, but in 1953, 2 years after the case began, the Supreme Court of Wisconsin restored the original judgment, ruling that loss of earnings was not a demonstrable requirement in the case of disorder induced by occupational noise. The AMA (1947) system was used in the Wojcik case to assess the percentage loss of hearing. As in New York, a flood of claims emerged in Wisconsin (Nelson, 1957). The response of management was to invoke the 6 month waiting period and to engage the services of medical consultants to investigate the assessment system and the extent of the problem they were likely to face. The result was a series of recommendations: (*a*) that .5 to 2 kHz tonal threshold average should replace the AMA (1947) system; (*b*) that there should be a "low fence" of 15 dB (ASA); and (*c*) that a population survey of the highly industrial Milwaukee region of Wisconsin should be undertaken as part of the state fair in 1954. The results of that survey, as is well known, have subsequently been used for a variety of purposes. One of these of course has been to suggest that in the United States population hearing level as a function of age shows quite massive deterioration, so one should not overemphasize the degree of industrially caused loss of hearing (Symons, 1958). Such an argument is, of course, absurd, precisely because the highly self-selected group of people who participated in the survey would undoubtedly have contained a high proportion of people from heavy industry and even more likely would have come from the very industries involved in the litigation going on at the time. The interest among such people to check out their own hearing would be greater at that time than it would in the population at large.

While the 1954 Wisconsin State Fair survey has ramified in various unfortunate ways over the years, it is now largely recognized as a source of unreliable and unrepresentative data. What is not perhaps realized is the purpose of the survey in the first place, namely to find out the extent of hearing loss in that part of the state so that insurance companies could make some sort of prediction regarding the likely rate of claims over subsequent years (Fox, 1957).

Much more important, the recommendation for use of the .5 to 2 kHz tonal threshold is one many agencies and legislatures have embraced; it received the endorsement of the AAOO and then of the AMA. We scrutinize the .5 to 2 kHz average later; a revealing remark about it is given by Sharrah (1966). After discussing the fact that occupational noise had become less of a major issue at the time of his writing, Sharrah goes on to say that this could lead people concerned with the problem to feel that it had been successfully overcome. But the apparent reduction in the problem's magnitude was caused by "two basic safeguards which have kept claims experience in the noise field at a fairly low rate. The two safeguards are: (a) The six-month waiting period; (b) The hearing measurement formula recommended by the American Academy of Ophthalmology and Otolaryngology and the American Medical Association [Sharrah, 1966, p. 276]."

Here then is open acknowledgment that the .5 to 2 kHz formula is a money-saving device, simply because so little threshold change is typically observable at these audio frequencies in people with noise deafness. Sharrah (1966) goes on to observe that were 3 kHz threshold included in the averaging system, compensation costs would rise by 25%, and were 1 to 3 kHz rather than .5 to 2 kHz used, as some authorities recommended, claim costs would double.

It is rare indeed to find an admission by those professionally involved in this field of the bald economic forces underlying the rules of the assessment game. Medical researchers in particular have perpetually stressed the "scientific" basis of the AAOO–AMA formula. As I indicated earlier, in Chapter 6 we observe the evidence that "sustains" the .5 to 2 kHz system.

Despite pressure from unions and from less interested observers, the .5 to 2 kHz system has gained wide (though by no means universal) acceptance both in and beyond the United States. Union pressure has been sufficient in California, for example, to have 3 kHz included in the averaging formula in that state, and the federal system uses 1 to 3 kHz as its formula. Lest it be taken that I simply favor formulas that cost more money, let me make the following points. Sharrah's (1966) assertion that use of 1 to 3 kHz would double compensation claims is only true if the payout rate remains the same as at present. Further, it is not part of the present author's interest how unions and management battle over compensation claims. It is in the nature of their struggle to engage in such activity.

Two features of the problem do concern me though: As an ordinary citizen, I join the rest of society in paying compensation costs in the price I pay for goods produced under dangerous conditions. Frankly, I would prefer to pay the cost of making these conditions nondangerous. As a scientist, if I am nonetheless faced with the fact of compensation, then my concern is that it be fair in terms of relative assessments, that is to say valid and reliable. This book is, as I said in the preface, partly technical, partly polemical. My reason for making it so is that there is no value in doing social science without reference to the political structure of that aspect of the world one is doing one's social science to. If there is no such reference, then one's social science is naive at best, and most typically wrong. Writing and practice in this field predominantly pay lip-service to the political outlook of management. This situation is both naive and wrong and leads to naive and wrong science. So the polemical ingredient of this work is more than the mere airing of my (fairly ordinary) political views; it is in fact vitally tied in with the science I am attempting to do in a field of inquiry that has suffered from unspoken interest in only one facet of the political structure that surrounds and interacts with this feature, as with all features, of social being. In other words, as a scientist, I attempt to abstain from identification with any of the interested parties to the dispute and to concentrate my effort on scrutinizing the means used to gauge the degree of damage to a person's hearing as a result of occupational exposure to injurious noise.

The Role of the Veterans Administration

The historical timing of the first American industrial compensation claims is worthy of note. Prior to World War II, there had been claims against industry in the United States under both common and statute law for traumatic injury following blast or other accidental episodes. But the first allowable claim for deafness of a more chronic nature did not occur until after the war. I think one can locate the reason for this change in actions taken following the war. Veterans in many countries were compensated for deafness resulting from combat, be it traumatic or insidious. This very likely acted as the precedent, in the United States at least, for nonaccident industrial claims. This point has backing from a couple of unrelated sources. In a report by the International Association of Industrial Accident Boards and Commissions (1961), a largely American body, the observation is made that surprisingly few industrial claims for deafness were heard prior to World War II. It is further observed that the Veterans Administration no doubt mopped up a large number of prewar industrial injuries in their postwar compensation program.

This point has force, in view of the contrast between the way the Veterans Administration assessed the hearing of servicemen at induction and the way it was assessed at discharge. According to Johnson (1957), the law concerning veterans' compensation at that time specified that unless a hearing disorder was specifically identified on enlistment any disorder detected at discharge must be assumed to be service connected. Up to the time of Johnson's (1957) article, at enlistment the only hearing test used was the spoken live-voice test, whereas both that test and tonal threshold testing were administered on discharge. One can very well picture the administrative mind, anxious for recruits, allowing a fairly lax assessment of hearing at induction; and one can further speculate that the more careful discharge assessment was in fact deliberately designed to pick up all cases of disorder, no matter what their origins. Given the close bureaucratic links that have ever existed between industry and the armed services in the United States (Galbraith, 1974), it requires no great leap of the imagination to picture the sort of understanding that prevailed between industry and government regarding the function of postwar veterans awards within the larger political and economic structure. However, the effect of veterans awards would have been to mobilize efforts among people whose ages or occupations prevented their enlistment during the war. Presumably drop-forging was a vital industry in wartime, hence many workers in that industry would not have seen service. Yet they would very well realize that many of the people receiving "service-connected" pensions for hearing loss had in fact acquired some at least of that loss in industry.

It is I think for this reason that the courts allowed claims such as those of Slawinski and Wojcik at the period in history in which they were filed. It is also for this reason that the first major claims emerged from the large metalworking industries of New York, Wisconsin, and New Jersey.

The Present Picture of Assessment in the United States

The pattern of compensation for noise-induced hearing disorder developing in the United States since the 1950s can only be sketched in the present text. Specific legislation was drawn up first in New York and Wisconsin, then in Missouri and California. Fox (1965) reported a survey by himself and R.E. Gintz of provisions existing to 1963 in various states. While all but one of the 50 states and the District of Columbia covered deafness caused by accident, only 31 had statutes covering nonaccidental noise-induced disorder. Fourteen of these states used the AAOO (.5 to 2 kHz) system; two used the AMA (1947) system; California, as mentioned, used .5 to 3 kHz; and the remaining 14 states used "medical evaluation," namely unstated and perhaps unstandardized systems based on otologists' opinions and assessments.

In 1975, an article in *The Machinist,* the periodical of the International Association of Machinists and Aerospace Workers, gave the more recent picture in the 50 states and the District of Columbia. Forty-two of these now covered occupational nonaccidental loss of hearing; and of these 28 used the AAOO system. As is evident, the proportion of states adopting the AAOO method has increased in recent times, the exceptions (apart from "medical evaluation" which still operates in some states) being only California and the District of Columbia.

The Veterans Adminstration, according to Suter and von Gierke (1975), uses a system based on tonal threshold at octaves from .25 to 4 kHz and on SRT and monosyllable discrimination score (DS). From personal communication between myself and the Veterans Administration it emerges that low fences of 26 dB (ISO) and 92% correct identification apply, respectively, to SRT and monosyllable DS. In addition, a low fence applies to tonal threshold, namely, that if levels at each of the 5 octaves from .25 to 4 kHz are less than 40 dB (ISO) and if levels at any 4 of these 5 frequencies are less than 25 dB (ISO), no compensable impairment is judged to exist. All three of the audiometric tests must show results within the fence criteria described for an assessment of "normal" hearing to be made. The precise rating of handicap, once one or more of the fences is surmounted, is not described in the material made available to me, but a remark appears in the draft of the revised Professional Manual of the agency that, in regard to service-connected hearing impairment, audiological assessment is made for the purpose of finding the "disability rating" and this in turn relates to the Social Adequacy Index.

As shown in pages 45–46 of this chapter, the Social Adequacy Index is an assessment device whose reliability and generalizability are quite uncertain.

ASSESSMENT FOR COMPENSATION IN VARIOUS COUNTRIES

Information about industrial countries other than the United States is more patchy. From a variety of sources, some kind of a picture can be built up, but the information available to the present author is undoubtedly incomplete.

In the United Kingdom, average tonal threshold in the "better ear" at 1, 2, and 3 kHz is used as the basis for calculation, but with a low fence of 50 dB (ISO). Furthermore, claims are allowable only from people employed in metalworking industries, and only after they have been employed for at least 20 years in such industries. This highly restricted provision is frankly dictated by budgetary constraints. There is presently a review to find ways of making the provision somewhat more liberal.

In other countries of the European Economic Community, according to Claass and Jolivet (1975), compensation systems vary considerably. No specific system is used or publicised in West Germany, but compensation is payable according to medical evaluation of persons exposed to excessive noise. In Belgium, a system like that used in the United Kindgom has operated since 1974, namely better-ear average threshold at 1, 2, and 3 kHz—with a low fence of 55 dB (ISO). In Denmark, it appears that the AAOO system is used—with a low fence of 60 dB (ISO).

In France, a modified AAOO system is used, namely twice the threshold level at 1 kHz, plus levels at .5 and 2 kHz, the sum divided by 4, and a low fence of 35 dB (ISO). Better-ear values only are used in the calculation. While a list of occupations most likely to be injurious to hearing is published in the French system, it is not, according to Claass and Jolivet (1975), a restrictive one as in the United Kingdom.

No provision as yet exists in the Republic of Ireland, though that situation will obviously change in future years with increasing industrialization. In the Netherlands, social security legislation since 1967 has made no distinction between occupational and nonoccupational accidents and diseases. Compensation is payable to victims of disease or injury whatever their origins. No specific system is given for calculating handicaps from hearing disorders. This approach to disease and injury reparation has also recently been adopted in New Zealand. An interesting development in New Zealand is adoption of the Australian National Acoustic Laboratories system (described on p. 56) to provide a percentage estimate of loss of function. This is elaborated, however, by use of the Hearing Measurement Scale (Noble, 1969) and various speech and lip-reading tests, to obtain a more direct gauge of actual everyday experience and disadvantage. Adoption of the Hearing Measurement Scale is an important sign that self-report is beginning to find application in assessment for compensation.

No system as yet exists in Luxembourg, but the problem is presently under review. In Italy, the official system, according to Claass and Jolivet, uses the average at frequencies from .5 to 4 kHz with a low fence of 20 dB (ISO). In a paper by Mazzella di Bosco (1975), that system is attributed to Finulli and to Bocca and Pellegrini, who suggest weightings of 25, 30, 40, and 5% to be attached to levels at threshold at .5, 1, 2, and 4 kHz, respectively. Other systems are used or at least recommended by other authorities in Italy, including the AAOO and one using thresholds from .25 to 4 kHz, with weightings akin to those of Fowler (1941).

In Japan, according to Yamamoto (1971), a modified AAOO system like that in France is used—but with a low fence of 60 dB (ASA). A report by Westerman (1975) contains a list of systems used in certain countries of the world. According to that source, the AAOO system plus medical evaluation is used in Austria, but with a loss-of-earnings provision included in the statute. In Taiwan, only virtually total deafness for speech is compensable. In Israel, the AAOO system is used with a 40 dB (ISO) low fence; the AAOO system is also used in Brazil and Iran, in the latter country a loss-of-earnings principle also operates. No stated procedures are given for South Africa, Sweden, Switzerland, the Soviet Union, East Germany, Hungary, Egypt, or Turkey, but compensation is payable in all these countries. There is no compensation cover for occupational noise disorder in India or Peru, and in the Phillipines spoken live-voice testing is still the method of assessment used. Westerman (1975) also reports that various Canadian provinces operate different systems. Basically, the AAOO system is favored, but apparently in Nova Scotia, and possibly in Ontario and Saskatchewan, a .5 to 3 kHz average is used. According to other sources (Cordell, 1972; International Association of Industrial Accident Boards and Commissions, 1961), as of 1961 Canadian authorities generally adopted the AAOO system with certain modifications. It may be that only federal Canadian boards use the AAOO system as a standard, while provincial boards have various modified forms. Whatever the finer detail, the AAOO system is the most widely used in that country overall.

Castelo-Branco (1971) reports that a .5 to 2 kHz tonal threshold average is used in Portugal but the system of assessment of degree of handicap does not follow that of the AAOO. Instead, the role of each ear is more evenly balanced, according to a table that Castelo-Branco presents in his paper.

Finally, in Australia a return has been made to a system that owes something to both the Sabine–Fowler (AMA, 1942) and Fowler–Sabine (AMA, 1947) methods. The system, recommended by the National Acoustic Laboratories (1974) and used by federal though not necessarily as yet by state agencies is based in part on the work of MacRae and Brigden (1973). From their study applying the articulation index (AI) principle to tonal threshold levels and comparing AI values with everyday speech hearing ability, it was shown that virtually the whole central frequency spectrum is important in prediction of speech hearing ability. We consider that research in detail in Chapter 6.

While the AI is unfortunately not the system actually adopted federally in Australia, the compromise system now being used involves thresholds in each ear at .5, 1, 1.5, 2, 3, and 4 kHz with variable interaural balancing, though typically in a 6 : 1 better–poorer ear ratio. *Better* and *poorer* ears are defined as the lower and higher levels at threshold at each tested frequency rather than average over all frequencies, and the "percent loss of hearing" varies in curvilinear fashion with rising threshold at each frequency. This is because the AI–everyday speech hearing function was found by MacRae and Brigden (1973) also to be curvilinear—a vindication of the old Fowler–Sabine rule. The maximum weights attaching to threshold at each frequency are

Frequency (kHz)	.5	1	1.5	2	3	4
Percentage weight	20	25	20	15	10	10

and a low fence of 15 dB (ISO) operates at each frequency. MacRae (1975–1976) has shown not only that the new Australian system accords better than the AAOO system with experienced difficulty in handling everyday speech but also (1977) that the system is as reliable as that of the AAOO.

Given the much more powerful data base on which the new Australian system rests in comparison with the data base for the AAOO, it seems evident to me that the former must eventually supersede the latter in assessment for compensation. Only bureaucratic intransigence coupled with naked economic interest will prevent that development. What is likely is that schedules of compensation will be rewritten so that no markedly greater cost is involved in the use of this system. Even if that occurs, the advantage of the new system will remain: namely, that it provides a fairer relative assessment than the most popular system in present use. It more accurately rates the difficulties experienced by people with noise-induced disorder.

The foregoing survey is not intended as an exhaustive study of assessment systems in use. Its function has been to highlight the fact that the AAOO system was born in response to a sudden upsurge of claims against American industry and designed to minimize the cost of these claims and that this feature alone is what makes it attractive to governmental and commercial institutions. I show in Chapter 6 that evidence in its support is virtually nonexistent.

Before we reach that stage in the present work, other technical aspects of tests in current use must be examined. An introduction to the theoretical constructs we will be adopting for this examination forms the content of the next chapter.

PART II

PROBLEMS IN ASSESSMENT OF IMPAIRED HEARING

This central section of the book (Chapters 4–8) is the largest, technically the most detailed, and theoretically the most complex. This cannot really be avoided, for the section represents analysis and criticism of a large but scattered volume of research, only occasional and isolated parts of which have been brought together by previous authors. In general terms, it should be seen as a series of reviews of basic features and some ancillary features of current hearing tests and assessment systems. It should also be taken as a necessary preliminary step in the presentation of arguments for radically revising adult assessment practice. That is the task of the final section.

This part begins (Chapter 4) with a brief methodological scheme which is designed to orient the reader to the framework of inquiry in the subsequent two chapters. Chapter 5 examines most aspects of test reliability. Chapter 6 is pivotal to the whole work, for its lays bare the main evidential prop of current assessment systems. Chapters 7 and 8 examine certain important ancillary issues, and the attempt there is to present a critique of certain taken-for-granted concepts. The surprise rate in these two chapters was not inconsiderable to this author in their preparation.

4

Basic Assessment Concepts

RELIABILITY AND UTILITY

A major function of this work is to examine the technical and theoretical adequacy of procedures used in hearing assessment. A necessary first step in that examination is to describe its method. The two principal concepts in assessment are reliability and validity. Various features of measurement and meaning are contained in these concepts. Although readers will be familiar with the terms, they may not be familiar with all their ramifications. A distinction of special importance is that between concurrent–predictive validity and content–construct validity. Tests and procedures can be examined separately in connection with each of these forms, so it is important to establish their distinctive realms of concern.

The Meaning of Reliability

In the Pavillon de Breteuil at Sèvres, near Paris, lies a metal bar inscribed with two microscopic marks 1 meter apart. A person using this bar as a ruler would be fairly well guaranteed that within certain tolerances the distance between the marks indeed measures 1 meter, for the bar is made of platinum–iridium and was manufactured precisely to serve as a standard against which other measuring sticks could be judged. The concept of a *meter* is arbitrary, although its invention was an attempt to gain rational universality. The meter was originally defined as one ten-millionth of an earth meridian from the North Pole to the Equator (Danloux-Dumesnils, 1969). Enormous care went into the manufacture of this standard prototype, and it officially served the metric world from 1889 until 1960. A new standard was then officially adopted based on the wavelength of light corresponding to a specific energy transition of the atom krypton-86.

One reason for replacing the old standard was that accurate as it may be its *reliability* was less than tolerable for an increasingly molecular scientific physics. That is to say, imperceptible fluctuations of its length caused by equally imperceptible changes in temperature and pressure were nevertheless enough to make it an uncertain gauge. The new standard suffers a similar problem but to a lesser extent. Fluctuations are of the order of only 5 to 10 Ångströms (1 Ångström = 10^{-10} m).

For people working in a clinical research field, such a problem may seem laughably unreal. If we generate measuring devices with a reliability of 90%, we consider the job very well done. But I did not choose the example of the meter as a fanciful way to undermine human research aspirations. It serves rather as a neat and concrete model to illustrate the meaning of the word *reliability*.

If an assessment tool is to be reliable, it has to be *stable* in use from one occasion to another. Alternatively, a reliable assessment tool should come up with a measurement *consistent* with one derived independently but according to the same specifications. To illustrate the stability concept: The platinum–iridium bar, if stable, should provide similar measures from one occasion of use to another. To illustrate the consistency concept: The original meter, geodetically defined and derived from an actual survey of part of the earth's surface should be, if consistent, the same length as a meter derived from the wavelength of krypton-86.

Of course, there is a problem in all measurement, a problem that affects metal bars as much as it affects tests of human capacity. To judge the consistency or stability of systems requires reference to a further system—that which is being measured. The problem is how do we know whether fluctuations in measurement result from the unreliability of the instrument or from a fluctuation in the thing being measured?

The answer to this question faces us with the larger issue of the interaction between reliability and validity which will be considered later on. For the moment, confining attention to the purely technical problem, the answer to the question is, in a sense, contained in the question. The only practicable way to try to discover to what the variability is attributable lies in repeated measurement by various methods of the property in question. If we can assume that the different measurement methods assess the same thing, then certain conclusions follow from repeated assessments using them. If the methods produce inconsistent results between themselves from one test occasion to the next, this variability can be put down to the inherent unreliability of the methods themselves. The method or procedure that provides the greatest fluctuations relative to others from one occasion to the next would presumably be the least reliable.

If, however, different measurement methods produce results which though varying from one occasion to another are more interconsistent, on average, in that variation, this result can be put down to change in the system or quality being assessed. These two sets of events are schematized in Figure 4.1 (page 64).

As regards the everyday measurement of some simple quality such as length, we can be highly confident about the reliability of assessment. Within the tolerances required by a cabinetmaker or even by an engineer, measuring instruments will remain stable enough from one occasion to another. Furthermore, the structures or systems which need to be measured for length usually remain stable and accessible so that the measuring device can provide identical data and be applied in identical fashion time and again (i.e., the interface between system and measuring method is constant). With respect to the measurement of various qualities of people, the apparent unreliability of assessment reflects the dynamic character of the system being assessed and the interface between assessment tool and system as much as it reflects the inherent unreliability of the measuring device itself. A physical ruler can be brought into contact with a structure in almost exactly the same way from one occasion to another. A psychometric scale (for instance, a personality questionnaire) applied to a person on one occasion and reapplied on another will provide different outcomes because the person changes through intervening experience and the meaning of the questions correspondingly changes. Hence both the system being assessed and the interface between system and assessment scale are variable.

We can see the analogy of this example even at the level of psychoacoustical assessment. The threshold of audibility of a tone for an individual listener varies from one occasion to another, even though the energy output of the audiometer may be highly consistent over time. Not only does the physiological and psychological state of the person change—resulting in a changed response; but if a contra-aural earphone is used, variations in the placement of that device from one test to the next will result in a variable interface and hence the energy in the listener's ear will vary.

We should mention the concept of "sensitivity" in this connection. A test susceptible to minute inter- and intraindividual differences in the dynamics of the quality being assessed can be considered *sensitive*. To the extent that it also reflects changes attributable to irrelevant features of the person (irrelevant, that is, to the assessment task in hand), it becomes unreliable. The contrary situation is a test of high reliability but low sensitivity, that is to say a test so crude that though its consistency is guaranteed, its discriminative capacity is negligible. We are back once again to the interaction of reliability and validity. A test sensitive to irrelevant features of the system being assessed can be said to be both less valid and less reliable than one which has similar properties but concentrates its measurement only on relevant features. This critical fact of interaction is discussed later.

To sum up at this point: The concept of reliability refers to the reliance one can place on a measuring device; the certainty one has that its character is consistent with that of other devices constructed to measure the same quality; the stability of the device itself from one occasion of use to another; and the sensitivity of the device to changes in the quality being assessed.

While I have stressed the incomplete independence of reliability and validity, there is nevertheless room to examine purely technical issues in the estimation of test reliability; and an argument can be made at a theoretical level for maintaining some separation of the two concepts. As a purely coincidental fact, within the field of hearing assessment, reliability and validity have always been tackled separately by research workers. There is therefore some present value in maintaining that separation, conceptually at least, for the time being.

Measurement of Reliability

Consistency

Ideally, to assess consistency of a measure in relation to other measures of the same quality, two or more independent studies would be initiated, each with the same task specification. This might be, say, to devise a mechanical means of estimating the absolute threshold of hearing. The measuring devices independently designed to meet that specification would then be compared in various samples of people. The schematic illustration in Figure 4.1 (A) can be seen in this context as the variance model for results obtained by three tests (A, B, and C) from

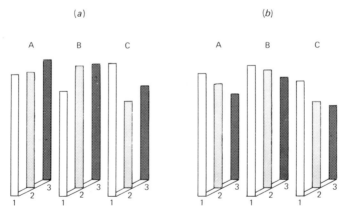

Figure 4.1 Schema for a general variance model of test reliability, also applicable to the concepts of consistency, stability, and content validity. (a) Three tests (A, B, and C; y-axis) applied on three occasions (1, 2, and 3; z-axis) give inter- and intrainconsistent results (x-axis). Variations are assumed to be within the tests themselves. Test A looks like the most reliable (least variable). (b) The same set-up, but this time all three tests show interconsistent results. Variations are assumed to be within the quality measured. See text for details of the general and specific applications of the model.

three similar samples (1, 2, and 3). The similarity of the samples would have been independently specified. The scheme in Figure 4.1 (B) can stand as the variance model for results obtained in three dissimilar samples (again, dissimilarity is independently specified).

In practice, tests are not produced with such foresight and planning. They are more usually the result of an individual researcher's attempt to wrestle with a specific assessment problem. Only afterwards is comparison made by others, using similar devices they have constructed for a somewhat similar purpose. Given the different orientations and theoretical preferences of different investigators, specifications of tests devised for "somewhat similar" purposes will in fact be rather different in content. Direct comparability for the sole purpose of measuring test consistency is thus usually rather difficult.

More typical of actual measurement of test consistency is the construction of parallel forms of a single test. The performance of these forms is then compared in a sample or series of samples. The objective is to observe the degree of agreement between each form and the degree of agreement between changes in response to each form from one sample to another. In this way, the relative reliability of each subtest in the set of parallel forms can be observed. A simpler procedure still is to assign items in a single test (say a questionnaire or performance test of some kind) at random to two equal subgroups and treat these split-halves as parallel forms. This technique can be extended indefinitely to examine the consistency–reliability of smaller and smaller groups of items, down to single items. In this way the *internal consistency* of the test—the agreement between its elements and the thing as a whole—can be estimated.

The theoretical drawback in the parallel forms or split-halves procedure is the lack of true independence of content of each test. Because the same theoretical structure informs the design of each subtest, the outcome is bound to show a consistency whose generality remains unknown. The analogy here would be the construction of several platinum–iridium bars that perform interconsistently yet all turn out to be unreliable when compared with a method developed for the same purpose but along quite different lines.

Stability

This technique can be extended to provide an indication of the consistency of measurement provided by a test reapplied to the same population after an interval of days, weeks, or months. The scheme in Figure 4.1(A) shows this variance model, 1, 2, and 3 representing reapplications in time of each test on the same population. The final outcome of a consistency study is to permit a stability study using parallel forms of known similar characteristics in reapplication. This avoids the problem that people being retested may grow familiar with the content of a given subtest.

Tonal threshold testing has been the particular subject of stability study, because the tonal audiogram is the major tool used in long-term monitoring of hearing capacity in both clinical and industrial settings. The internal consistency of pure tone audiometry has also been examined but for the specific aim of finding short forms of the test for screening purposes. This issue can appropriately be used as one example of the following concept.

Utility

The utility issue is an application in clinical settings of the economic concept of cost-effectiveness. The concept in simplified form involves balancing one cost—that entailed in gaining information to make a decision, for example—with the consequent cost of not seeking that information and so avoiding the first cost. Consider, for example, the development of a weather forecast system. A cost-effective analysis would seek to balance the price involved in producing the most effective system currently possible (say, satellite monitoring) against the cost, using weather balloons, of not knowing with any real certainty what changes are on the way. This second option entails the costs of whatever greater misfortunes are likely to occur to people and material in the absence of better warning.

In personnel selection, to bring discussion closer to present interest, the costs involved in misselection of an airline pilot are enormous (and deadly). Misselection of a steward will have a less calamitous consequent cost. Thus the effort and expense involved in the first task are extensive, and those in the second are comparatively small.

Within the context of hearing assessment, Bench and Mentz (1975) and Bench, Collyer, Mentz, and Wilson (1976) have investigated the effectiveness of screening in babies up to 6 months old for signs of hearing loss. They concluded that the cost involved is unwarranted because the chance of correctly diagnosing hearing difficulty is so low. The consequent cost of waiting until a baby is older than 6 months is negligible.

Among older age groups, the cost of instituting a complete clinical audiometric system, in a school or health center, for instance, may be unwarranted whereas installing a less expensive screening system might provide an effective routine service for early detection of children with some form of hearing loss. As regards both infant hearing testing and this sort of solution, the important question is whether the screening device is reliable enough to produce low "false-alarm" and "miss" rates.

These terms are borrowed from the signal-detectability field and refer to the sensitivity of a system to signals broadcast in its vicinity. A highly sensitive system will not only pick up "genuine" signals but also respond to "noise" (random occurrences which at times achieve signal-like dimensions). These are false alarms—instances of nonsignals categorized as signals. An insensitive system will display the opposite characteristic and miss genuine signals of low strength. Clearly, a screening device will be costly in its consequences if it displays either characteristic too grossly. *Sensitivity* in this context has the same meaning as it does in the reliability context considered earlier.

Thus the representative quality of a screening device is its all-important characteristic. By this I mean simply enough that the most critical function of the full-scale system must be represented in the screening system. If, for instance, we adopt the (disputed) notion that average threshold level for tones at .5 to 2 kHz can reliably indicate the general state of someone's hearing, then an audiometric screening system should allow *reliable* testing at these particular frequencies.

Clearly, to design the optimal specification for a screening device requires extensive study of the internal consistency of the full-scale test. By this means, the most representative elements (those parts which correlate most closely with the test as a whole) can be abstracted for screening purposes so as to provide the best approximation to the more complete picture. The implications in the foregoing concept of *representativeness* bear on the concept of *generalizability* discussed later in the chapter.

This section points to the question of the economics of instituting some system of measurement as opposed to the economics of failure so to do; it also points to the utility of adopting a screening or shorthand system of assessment as an alternative to either the full-blown system or nothing much at all.

VALIDITY

The essential characteristic of validity is the question of what the measuring device actually does assess. In most circumstances, we can assume that a straight metal bar 1 meter in length will truly measure the shortest distance between two points on the earth's surface which are close enough to be connected by it. Consider, however, a straight metal bar 10,000 km in length. Can it be regarded as a valid instrument for measuring the shortest distance between two points 10,000 km apart on the earth's surface? Presumably not, for over such a distance the earth's curvature would increasingly invalidate that particular measurement.

All tests obviously measure something, but not all tests measure what is claimed for them. Traditionally, there are two major aspects (each with two subaspects) to the estimation of the validity of a test: (*a*) its concurrent and predictive validity; and (b) its theoretical construct and content validity. I have lumped *concurrent* and *predictive* together and *construct* and *content* together because in my understanding the grouped concepts have at least a certain commonality of meaning.

Concurrent and Predictive Validity

If I claim to assess someone's everyday capacity to hear on the basis of a test of speech, the validity of my assessment can be judged by its degree of concurrence with other test results recorded for that person. The reader will immediately note that this seems merely like a restatement of reliability. And in many instances it is; as I foreshadowed, reliability and validity are interrelated. But there is surplus meaning in the validity concept; for if my speech test accurately reflects general hearing capacity, then results using it should concur with those from quite different forms of assessment—direct observation, a clinical interview, or peer rating—which supposedly do truly assess everyday hearing capacity. In other words, in claiming such validity I go beyond the demand that the instrument used be reliable to make a claim about the character of its informativeness. In producing a reliable test, I need make no particular claim about its character beyond its stability over time or its consistency with *similar* tests. Note also that I need make no claim about *what it actually is* that the test measures, merely that the result it produces is consistent with results otherwise obtained. But in treating validity I must claim a certain quality for the test beyond consistency.

Predictive validity may amount to the same thing, namely that I can predict the level of the person's performance on other, perhaps quite different tests as a result of assessment using this one. In predictive validity, there is the added feature of prognostication—prediction of a given course of development in the future as a result of present capacity, plus knowledge of contingent features. Thus if one determines the average temporary change in threshold for pure tones in a group of newly recruited people following a typical working day in a noisy environment, one may claim to predict the average persistent threshold level for that group 10 years hence if they continue working under the same conditions (Glorig, Ward, & Nixon, 1961). Predictive validity is also exemplified in the work of Burns and Robinson (1970). Their results show that one can predict, on the basis of noise measurement, the incidence and distribution of persistent threshold-level values in a noise-exposed population up to 25 years in the future if conditions remain constant. Note that in both these examples the predictive validity claim is limited to the group level. Attempts to predict an individual's future fate have not had much success (Burns, 1971).

Theoretical Construct and Content Validity

This is a more fundamental and complex feature of validity, conceptually more abstract and technically more difficult to determine. A *theoretical construct* is an hypothesized quality that governs or underlies behavior. For example, psychologists have produced theoretical constructs such as introversion–extraversion (Eysenck, 1953; Jung, 1923) and motivation for achievement (McClelland, Atkinson, Clark, & Lowell, 1953). They have devised a variety of tests to assess the incidence and degree of these hypothesized qualities. Such theoretical constructs are likely to be refined or even debunked as succeeding research points up inadequacies in the original formulation.

In that a test is a scale for the assessment of the construct in question, it is then also an expression of that construct's dimensions. The content validity of the test will therefore be undermined as soon as a refinement occurs at the theoretical level in the construct of which it is an expression. The construct validity of a test, of course, may be quite negated if the "parent" construct is itself debunked.

The theoretical construct labeled *intelligence* has undergone radical transformations in the history of psychology. Around the beginning of this century, the prevailing view among many influential psychologists held that intelligence had as much to do with sensorimotor performance as with scholastic. Cattell (1890) used a "mental test" which assessed keenness of hearing and vision, hand–eye coordination, muscular strength, reaction time, and so forth as well as arithmetic skill, memory, and the like. This construction of intelligence was radically overthrown by Binet and Simon (1905) whose test concentrated on more purely cognitive capacities and was linked to the more abstract scholastic curriculum. The Binet–Simon construct was wholeheartedly embraced by most of the psychological community, and from then on a valid test of intelligence was seen to be one which assessed the ability to manipulate words, solve conundrums and arithmetic puzzles, and perceive conceptual relationships (cat is to kitten as _____ is to puppy).

Now it might at first seem hard to think of times when the theoretical construct *hearing loss* has undergone radical revision. Indeed, this does not look like a theoretical construct at all; but here the power of social definition is at work. Current understanding takes it for granted that a person who cannot detect common everyday warning signals or follow a vocal conversation is the victim of loss of hearing and presumably has always been so labeled. There are surely universally recognized signs that are automatically perceived as those of "deafness." Although this construct has perhaps become more stabilized in recent times, historical evidence demonstrates quite clearly that these signs have been labeled "crazy" or "dumb" or "mentally defective" in different cultures at different times. Hearing loss may be a more straightforward construct to put together than intelligence, but it suffers shifts in definition and taxonomy no less than the latter as a result of changes in human consciousness and ideology.

Theoretical constructs in social and human science are produced in response to observed or inferred characteristics of people, and their natures are bound to change as general views of people change. Even so, such constructs do stabilize, often for long periods. The Binet formulation of intelligence, which held sway for several decades, has been seriously undermined only in recent years (Goodnow, 1976; Riegel, 1973). While a construct is stable, we can conclude that relevant scientists are satisfied that it truly (validly) describes an aspect of the psychological or social universe. Attention then is directed to the refinement of the *content* of scales devised to measure the construct's dimensions. A vast technology has been generated to provide tools to do such a job (Wiggins, 1973). It is less germane to the present purpose to review these methods than to describe the aim of such exercises. That aim is to discover to what extent the content of a test actually reflects the construct that gave birth to it, to what extent the test measures other features, to what extent the construct is univariate or multivariate, and whether the test is sensitive to the construct's form in the population.

In regard to hearing loss, assuming that the construct has stabilized as I suggested earlier, there is nonetheless considerable variation in the content of tests devised to assess it. These variations reflect disparate views of what constitutes hearing loss. This might look like a paradoxical pair of statements. However, when I say the hearing loss construct has stabilized, I mean that although we generally take it these days to mean something other than mutism or mental deficiency, the precise nature and characteristics of the differentiated construct have yet to be agreed upon. Indeed, this book is an attempt at least to refine and extend the prevailing concept of *hearing loss* and argue the invalidity of the content of most tests in use.

We can see then that the content of a test may be taken as valid for assessment of a construct insofar as its characteristics conform to the features of the construct and do not spill over into neighboring territory; that a test of general intelligence is not merely a test of scholastic achievement (assuming the wish is to distinguish these two constructs). We can see further that a current construct (of intelligence say) may be shown to be invalid as consciousness about psychological nature changes with changing experience and knowledge. Finally, we can see that decisions regarding a test's content may rest critically on outcomes from predictive and concurrent studies. Thus if a test measures intelligence, it should relate as much to observations of problem solving in the everyday world as to performance in the classroom.

Construct validity has an historical quality. What is valid today inevitably becomes invalid tomorrow in a culture like ours which is continuously modifying its behavior and values. One main reason for this perpetual drive to modification is the presence of science as an accepted part of our world-view. Science is the system par excellence which unceasingly undermines not only the assumptions underlying its content but even the assumptions about how it actually works (Chalmers, 1976; Kuhn, 1962; Lakatos, 1970). The process of refinement which I have equated with content validation can be seen in historical terms as exemplifying Kuhn's (1962) process of "normal science." That is to say, during a period of construct stability, the task at hand is to iron out details of content within that construct viewed as a paradigm. When the construct itself is overthrown, all tests relating to the debunked paradigm are also largely negated. Their content refers to a nonacceptable theoretical structure. This is an example of "revolutionary science." That process is, as I say, increasing. Validity cannot be universal or timeless because it has to do with how the aspect of the world being assessed is perceived by people. And people's perceptions change with changes of knowledge and practice.

INTERACTION OF RELIABILITY AND VALIDITY AND THE CONCEPT OF GENERALIZABILITY

The discussion in this chapter at times has labored to maintain a distinction between reliability and validity. From a different theoretical view, no such distinction exists except, I maintain, in the exposition of theoretical construct validity.

If we turn once more to Figure 4.1, we can understand why it is that, with the exception noted, reliability and validity interact. In the model given in Figure 4.1, three tests are devised to assess the same quality in somewhat different ways. Each shows a unique pattern of variability, and if we assume that each is indeed measuring the same thing, then these inconsistent variations are attributable to the unreliability of the measurement itself. The platinum–iridium bar is less reliable than the light emission system in the measurement of length because it fluctuates to a greater degree in its length from one occasion to another. But if we view the problem from another direction, we can see that it is an issue in validity as much as one in reliability.

Within the discussion of content validity, the point made was that effort is directed to ensuring that a test measures only features relevant to the construct in question and that it is not being influenced by irrelevant features. Another way of putting this point is to say that the test is not also measuring irrelevant features. The metal bar fluctuates more than light emission because it is less controllably affected by changes in temperature and pressure. In other words, in addition to measuring length it also, though not very sensitively, measures temperature and pressure. It is thus less *valid* in its content because it is influenced by irrelevant features.

Within audiological measurement, the same model can apply. For example, if our three tests are parallel forms of a measure of speech hearing ability applied successively to the same group of people, we would conclude that the most reliable form is the one that shows the least fluctuation. But in this case we have dodged a couple of issues. In the first place from one occasion to another there may be fluctuations in the quality being measured, so that the unchanging test may simply be an insensitive one. Second, each form may be reliably tapping slightly different but equally relevant features of the quality being measured. In the assessment of human characteristics, because we cannot be so precise about the thing being tested, this more circumspect view of the matter needs to be taken. The principle is the same as the principle involved in the measurement of length, however, and the reliability problem overlaps with the question of validity. A further implication is that in the effort to make a test more consistent by excising items that fluctuate more extremely, its validity could be affected. This is true because the excluded items may be *reliably* reflecting actual moment-to-moment changes in a relevant feature of the measured quality, but it is not to say that all variability has some critical meaning for the quality being tested. There are undoubtedly features of tests whose unreliability results purely from ambiguous internal structure, so that responses of different kinds are governed as much by the "sloppiness" of meaning of the test item as by change in the subject's behavior or perception. The foregoing points must be emphasized because the qualities assessed in psychology and audiology cannot be specified with complete accuracy, and there can therefore be no certainty that unreliability is exclusively attributable to a test. The most to be expected is that genuine inconsistency will show up in areas outside of internal test inconsistency.

In an effort to clear away the confusion of reliability–validity interaction, Cronbach, Rajaratnam, and Gleser (1963) proposed the concept of *generalizability*. They point out that in regard to the outcome of any test result the question asked by the researcher is "what do I know as a result of this outcome on this test?" In other words, how far can one *generalize* on the basis of a single observation (using *single* in the sense of a single test occasion)? Three aspects of generalization can be listed. On the basis of a single observation one may be interested to

1. Infer or predict results from other tests of the person's functioning
2. Infer or predict results from other occasions of observation of the person, of the same quality

3. Infer or predict results from occasions of observation of the person in other conditions

The first type of generalization refers to the representative nature of the test result. If it is a screening test, for example, then one is concerned to estimate the chances of the screen's being accurate. If it is a full-scale test, then it is the predictive–concurrent validity of the measurement that is of concern. The second type of generalization has to do with the stability of the test or the consistency of its various forms—in other words, the classically defined reliability of the test result. The third type of generalization covers both sensitivity and content validity of the test, a most interesting juxtaposition. For the question here is whether the test can reliably reflect changes in the quality under consideration and at the same time be relatively immune to changes in extraneous factors not supposedly relevant to its content.

It seems that the reformulation of Cronbach *et al.* (1963) is a more effective way of conceptualizing most problems with regard to technical features of test construction and analysis. The major area left unaccounted for, and quite rightly, is the theoretical. This is not a technical issue but rather a social, at least within sciences concerned with human behavior. That it bears importantly on content validity (what is or is not an irrelevant tested feature?) is not to detract from the generalizability concept. It shows rather that the generalizability concept can be operated successfully only in concert with larger, nontechnical schematizations of the world's structure. It means that validity and therefore reliability are not reducible to mechanical matrices but must always relate to the changing consciousness people have of their own being.

In conclusion, I must point out that the plan of this text in the chapters to follow does not attempt to synthesize the reliability–validity problem under the umbrella of the formulation advanced by Cronbach *et al.* Certain novelties of approach do spring from an understanding of that scheme, but it is quite outside the present purpose to realign the research in this field according to the generalizability approach. It is daunting enough to try to confront the mass of research that has gone into the issues of test reliability and concurrent validity. Perhaps an interested student of the area can take the present exposition and perform the necessary intellectual acrobatics to display the research about to be reviewed in these terms. My aim in the next two chapters is merely to consider hearing assessment tests in terms of more classical technical features.

5

Reliability of Tests Used for Hearing Assessment

SCOPE OF RESEARCH

Aims and Procedures

As is emphasized in Chapter 4, the rigid separation of reliability from validity in consideration of test specifications is not possible, but for practical purposes the main technical features of each aspect can be separately reviewed if not theoretically distinguished.

In research studies to determine the reliability of tonal threshold testing, the main procedure involves repeated application to observe the stability of test results. This technique is feasible because the task for the listener involves little by way of meaning, so problems of learning and memory are not necessarily at issue. The observation of reduction in tonal threshold levels with practice is a familiarization effect. The nature of this effect is somewhat different from that of an effect arising from the listener's remembering a signal.

By contrast, some tests using speech can only be examined for consistency. Parallel forms of word or sentence lists are applied on separate occasions. Any observed differences reflect the content equivalency as well as the stability of the test. The exceptional speech tests are Speech Detection Threshold (SDT) and Speech Reception Threshold (SRT) whose respective functions are to locate the sound level required for bare detection and for 50% correct identification of material with which the listener is already familiar. In the SRT test particularly, there is control of the familiarity effect. Thus the stability of that test can be measured; but because the function of speech discrimination tests is to find the listener's capacity to distinguish unpredictable speech sounds, repeated testing with the same material is generally ruled out. By varying the order (scrambling) of items on a discrimination test, this problem can be got around to some extent.

Consistency can be a procedure in tonal testing, as, for example, when different methods of threshold determination are compared for equivalency of performance. However, the aim of studies of this kind is not so much to show consistency of tonal threshold per se, as to compare techniques of determination with respect to their stability in relation to one another.

Some studies in the field of test reliability have been conducted simply to observe how reliable or otherwise a test is. Others have attempted to explore the components of variance. We begin this review with the straightforward kind of enterprise before discussing the theoretical problems attending more elaborate investigations. Certain other distinctions need to be noted. The bulk of studies have been conducted using the conventional (operator-controlled) audiometric procedure; more recent work has used the self-recording procedure (von Békésy, 1947). Although there are some data on comparative stability of these two basic types of determination, for the most part only the broad pattern of difference between studies using exclusively one or the other can be drawn.

A distinction of some importance is the test population and conditions of testing. Some studies have used carefully selected, young, normally-hearing listeners; other have examined reliability in people with hearing disorder tested in a field situation. Some direct comparative work has been done across certain of these conditions, but again we must rely more on the overall pattern emerging from different kinds of studies.

Common Statistical Techniques

Various statistics have been used to express reliability. Most of these can be transformed at least approximately into each other's terms. The major statistics are correlation, standard deviation of differences, and standard error of measurement. The correlation coefficient (r, product–moment correlation; r_s, Spearman's rank correlation) expresses the closeness of agreement between two sets of values. In the present context, this would be the original and repeated test sets. The standard deviation of differences (σ_{diff}) is an expression in actual numerical terms of the variation in values between one test occasion and another. The standard error of measurement (σ_{meas}) is usually reserved for multiple retests since it expresses the range of deviation about the "true" scores to be expected. However it can be derived from only two sets of scores, since a value for it is computable from

$$\sigma_{\text{meas}} = \sigma_{xy}(1 - r_{xy})^{1/2} \tag{1}$$

where σ_{xy} is the standard deviation of the sets of scores and r_{xy} is the correlation between these sets of scores. The standard error of measurement is also approximately derivable from the standard deviation of differences by dividing the latter by $\sqrt{2}$.

As regards two sets of test values, correlation and σ_diff (standard deviation of differences) are the most straightforward statistics. However, the former is affected by the variance of values obtained in a test series. As can be seen from Equation (1),

$$r_{xy} = 1 - (\sigma^2_\text{meas}/\sigma^2_{xy}). \tag{2}$$

Hence, the smaller the value of σ_{xy} (the more restricted the range of values in the test series), the smaller will be the correlation coefficient. The value of σ_meas (hence of σ_diff) will be unaffected by range effects, only by the amount of agreement or disagreement between the sets of scores. These latter are therefore more useful statistics to express reliability in most circumstances. However, correlation is valuable when the reliability of two types of incommensurable tests are to be compared and where the distributions of values obtained from each test are relatively similar.

The correlation analysis bears upon the closeness of agreement between two sets of test values though it says nothing about the absolute stability of measurement. The standard deviation of differences bears upon the variability of results; and in common with all standardized expressions, it is a measure of the proportion of changes observed within plus or minus certain test values. A σ_diff of 6 dB, for example, means that about two-thirds of repeat test values lay withing ±6 dB of original values, and about 95% lay within ±12 dB of original values. The σ_meas does a different job, for it is an expression of the variance within persons. A σ_meas of 5 dB means there is a 2:1 chance that a person's score on a single test lies within ±5 dB of his "true" score; and there is a 20:1 chance ($p = .05$) that the score is within ±10 dB of the "true" score. The concept of "true" score is simply the concept of the average score a person attains over multiple repeat tests. The standard deviation of the distribution of scores about that average is the σ_meas. It can be seen that an expression of σ_meas from only a single repeat test can be only an estimate of the σ_meas not an expression of its actual value, which can only be derived from multiple testing.

The following review does not pretend to be exhaustive, but I am confident that all major studies among adults are included, so that the emergent picture is essentially complete.

RELIABILITY OF TONAL THRESHOLD TESTS

Studies in Clinical–Industrial Samples

The earliest published report among adults from a clinical population is probably that by Witting and Hughson (1940). An extensive series of repeated tests was conducted on 17 people aged 16–47 years with various sorts and degrees of conductive disorders. At least 10 threshold tests were made on each person over a period ranging from 2 to 28 months. No form of therapy was introduced during an individual's test series, and testing was avoided at times when any listener suffered a minor complaint likely to influence the typical threshold level. Thresholds were determined at octaves from .125 to 8 kHz. No details of actual test technique are given, nor is any mention made of monitoring of instrument variation during the study.

A series of repeat tests was also conducted on 7 listeners who had no auditory disorders. No details about these people or the duration of the test series are given, however. Standard deviations were calculated in each individual at each test frequency from the person's average threshold over 10 or more audiograms. The average standard deviations of the 17 partially hearing listeners were plotted, and these range from 3.28 dB at 1 kHz to 4.67 dB at 8 kHz. By comparison, the normally hearing listeners showed a range of 2.74 dB to 4.50 dB. Deviations in the former group were greater at every test frequency, and in both groups, maximum deviations were at the lower and higher ends of the audiofrequency range. One should note that average standard deviation is akin to but not identical with σ_{meas}, though it has the same function.

Among other analyses by Witting and Hughson (1940), one of practical interest was comparison of the deviation of the first test from the average of all tests. Expression of the spread of these deviations was not in the same terms as above. Rather the proportion of first test values lying within ±2.5 and ±5 dB of the average was given at each frequency. Over all frequencies, 76.7% of first test values were within ±5 dB of the average on all tests. Thus σ_{meas} could be said from these data to approach 5 dB as an overall estimate of audiogram reliability in a clinical sample. Harris (1946), on the basis of his own data and unpublished results from other investigators, confirmed Witting and Hughson's (1940) result at the frequencies .5, 1, and 2 kHz.

A highly detailed report was made by Brown (1948) of three studies using Royal Air Force personnel, examining different features of tonal threshold reliability. In the first study, listeners were retested almost immediately but by a different operator and in slightly different ambient conditions. Thirty people, 24 with various degrees and types of hearing disorder, were used in this study. Test procedure involved continuous attenuation of an audible signal with periodic interruption. Listeners had to indicate when the signal was "on" or "off." Attenuation was increased to the point where listeners no longer reliably signaled "on" and "off," then decreased until there was synchrony of listener signal and operator interruption. Threshold was taken to be this point. Testing was undertaken on both ears of listeners at octaves from .125 to 8 kHz.

The standard deviation of differences between the two measurement systems ranged from 5.97 dB at .5 kHz to 9.93 dB at 8 kHz. As in Witting and Hughson's (1940) study, greater deviations were observed at the higher and lower test frequencies.

In the second study, test conditions were identical. The outcome of this investigation therefore allowed the effect of different conditions of test on reliability to be isolated. Thirty further listeners comparable with the first group were involved in this experiment. Standard deviations of difference were somewhat reduced, ranging from 5.1 dB at .125 kHz to 6.9 dB at 8 kHz. Oddly, the frequency extremity effect was absent from these results. The final study controlled for operator effect as well as the effect of test conditions. Its outcome thus allows the isolation of the effect of interobserver difference on reliability. Yet another group of 30 listeners was involved. In this group, however, there were somewhat more people with conductive disorder and somewhat fewer with sensorineural disorder than in previous groups. Standard deviations, which were generally reduced somewhat compared with the second study's result, ranged from 4.36 dB at .5 kHz to 7.1 dB at 8 kHz.

Overall, this study demonstrated that in a heterogeneous sample, test conditions have a critical bearing on the stability of tonal threshold determination whereas, at least in the conditions of the study, the effect of different operators appears to be negligible. The raw data presented allow comparison of conductive and sensorineural cases as regards reliability. A check on the σ_{diffs} at 1 and 2 kHz in the two samples of listeners in the second of Brown's studies revealed no difference in reliability of thresholds for each diagnostic type.

High and Glorig (1962) presented results from a nonclinical sample of industrial workers. Test conditions were arranged to be similar to those typically found in an industrial audiological setting. A self-recording technique was used, and listeners numbered 79 people—factory and office workers allegedly not exposed to injurious noise (to prevent TTS effects from contaminating the results). Median age was 40.8 years. The stated aim of this study was to check the reliability of industrial audiometric operations. "The importance of industrial audiograms in legal proceedings, hearing conservation programs, and job placement makes it necessary to know more about . . . the reliability of these measurements [High & Glorig, 1962, p. 56]." It does seem to defeat this aim somewhat to use listeners who do not exhibit noise-induced disorder. At the least, a comparison of reliability in groups from similar industrial backgrounds, one of which comprised people with noise disorder, should have been undertaken to fulfill the study's purpose. The study was carried out at factory sites using a mobile audiological laboratory. Test–retest interval was 6 months. One feature of interest noted in the study was that threshold for the first tone presented (in this case 1 kHz) was always higher than threshold for the next tone. Repeat testing at 1 kHz after all frequencies had been presented in one ear generally showed a reduction in level at the 1 kHz threshold.

Reliability results were expressed in both correlation and σ_{diff}, the latter values lying between 3.65 dB (2 kHz, right ear) and 5.44 dB (6 kHz, left ear). A slight extreme frequency effect was apparent in the results. These data show much smaller test–retest variability than results from previous samples. Given the lengthy intertest interval, this result suggests perhaps that the method of testing (self-recording audiogram) may be an influential factor in tonal test stability. I mentioned that High and Glorig's (1962) sample was nonnoise exposed. Nevertheless, threshold levels at 3–6 kHz were 15–25 dB above (ASA) zero with standard deviations of 15 dB to 22 dB. Furthermore, the average level at threshold of the group rose at all but one audio frequency from the initial test to the retest 6 months later. Though the change in average threshold is not significant, the consistency of its occurrence suggests the systematic influence of some factor on the group or on the test records.

Another industrial study was reported in 1962 by Jackson, Fassett, Riley, and Sutton. There were two aspects of the research: a study of operator–instrument variability and a study of listener variability. The program is in fact akin to that of Brown (1948), though Jackson et al. are unaware of that work. The design of the first part of the study is elaborate. Listeners were multiply retested on various audiometers by various operators. There were only four listeners in the study, but each was tested 18 times in a factorial design that allowed operator and instrument variability to be independently analyzed. As in Brown's (1948) study, operator effect was negligible, but a slight interaction was found between listeners and test conditions.

To study listener variability, two audiometers were used on 30 inexperienced listeners (new employees). With half of these, the initial test was done using one audiometer, the retest using the other, and the reverse process was used with the other half of the sample. Retests were conducted 1 to 4 hours later. This counterbalanced design allowed systematic differences attributable to test order and test instrument to be accounted for. The residual ("inherent") variance was expressed as mean absolute intertest difference remaining after test-order effect ("learning") and instrument effect had been subtracted from the overall variability. These values are not comparable with σ_{diff}, but the higher and lower frequency pattern is strongly evident. Mean deviation at 4 to 8 kHz is twice as great as .5 to 3 kHz and slightly greater at .25 kHz than at .5 to 3 kHz.

Jackson et al. (1962) ascribe the reduction in retest threshold level to "learning." Such improvement, observable across the whole frequency range, was not observed by Brown (1948) in very similar test conditions.

More recent study reveals a "learning" effect, but one of a different character from that reported by Jackson *et al.* (1962). We return to this issue when considering sources of variance in threshold determination.

Jerger (1962) reported retest reliability in a clinical sample on various tests. As only tonal threshold and speech test reliability in connection with assessment are our present concerns, certain features of Jerger's report need not concern us. For the record, the tests administered in this reliability study were

1. Conventional AC tonal threshold
2. Conventional BC tonal threshold
3. Self-recording threshold; sweep frequency; continuous and interrupted tone
4. Self-recording threshold; fixed frequency (.25, 1, and 4 kHz); continuous and interrupted tone
5. Tone decay test
6. SISI test

Only the first three tests are of present concern. The inclusion of a description of results from BC threshold testing is useful. The AC–BC relationship has an assessment function as well as a diagnostic. Many decisions will be made regarding rehabilitative or therapeutic procedures, and about the degree of handicap attributable to noise, on the basis of AC–BC patterns. These decisions will be only as reliable as the test results consulted in making them.

In Jerger's (1962) study there were 27 listeners with sensorineural disorder aged 14 to 54 years (average 44 years). While people with a definite diagnosis of Ménière's disease were excluded, 10 of the listeners had a tentative diagnosis of this condition. As is well known, people suffering from Ménière's disease characteristically have fluctuating episodes of severity of disturbance. It is in fact in the service of people with this disease to obtain realistic estimates of test reliability from people with more stable types of cochlear disorder. By this means, the fluctuation which typifies Ménière's can be more readily identified rather than put down to test error.

Testing was carried out in the usual conditions of a clinical audiological examination (much in the way that High and Glorig (1962) used typical survey conditions in their study). Retesting was carried out 1 to 18 months after initial testing. Two operators were used, one of whom conducted some initial tests and all retesting. Conventional threshold determination was made by the ascending method (Carhart & Jerger, 1959). Correlation coefficients as well as σ_{meas} values were computed on the test–retest data. To compare Jerger's data more readily with those of other people, his σ_{meas} figures are expressed as σ_{diff} by multiplying them by $\sqrt{2}$; and these figures are shown in Table 5.1.

TABLE 5.1

Values of σ_{diff} in Decibels Calculated from Values of σ_{meas} Found by Jerger (1962) for Various Tonal Threshold Tests

Test	Frequency (kHz)		
	.25	1	4
Conventional AC	6.9	8.5	6.6
Conventional BC	8.5	5.9	7.1
Self-recording AC (sweep frequency; interrupted tone)	8.5	6.9	6.2
Self-recording AC (sweep frequency; continuous tone)	8.6	7.9	5.8

These values are greater than those observed by High and Glorig (1962), suggesting that in the sample studied threshold fluctuation was greater, perhaps because of the composition of the group. Two features are of interest: Conventional BC testing has a similar order of reliability to AC testing in this sample. Jerger refers to a study of BC reliability by Carhart and Hayes (1949). These authors observed σ_{diff} values for BC testing of 7.7 dB at .25 kHz, 7.65 dB at 1 kHz, and 9.4 dB at 4 kHz. Carhart and Hayes' study involved 250 people from a clinical population, with retest about 1 month later. While their values are not wholly coincident with Jerger's BC result, neither are they widely different from it.

The other feature of interest is that self-recording threshold testing provided somewhat more reliable results than the conventional procedure at 1 and 4 kHz. This outcome is in line with the possibility mentioned in relation to High and Glorig's (1962) study that the self-recording technique may show less fluctuation than conventional methods. In the sweep frequency procedure in Jerger's (1962) study, both an interrupted tone and continuous tone were used. There is little difference in reliability between the two signal types, but a consistently higher level at threshold for continuous tone was observed. This particular feature is discussed in the next section.

A long-term industrial study described by High and Gallo (1963) provides several instructive features. Six test series were conducted in a factory where employees were exposed to potentially injurious noise. These tests, made at approximately 8-month intervals, were carried out by an audiometric technician employed at the factory. The purpose of this routine testing, "was to protect the employees' hearing [p. 17]." This use of audiometry was mentioned in Chapter 2 as one of the reasons why hearing is assessed. And of course yet another reason why the reliability of the test needs to be known is to permit improbable fluctuations in threshold to be identified. The statistic chosen by High and Gallo to express reliability was Pearson's correlation coefficient. These authors also give standard deviations of test results, and an estimate of σ_{meas} between different series can therefore be computed from the formula given earlier in this chapter, and σ_{diff} can be derived by multiplying that value by $\sqrt{2}$. The standard deviations of each test series only are given, but an approximate combined standard deviation is derivable from the square root of the mean variance between each test series.

From these calculations, the σ_{diff} between the various test occasions at 5 test frequencies are estimated and shown in Table 5.2. It is clear that

TABLE 5.2

Calculated Estimates of σ_{diff} in Decibels Observed between Six Separate Test Occasions by High and Gallo (1963) on Conventional AC Tonal Threshold Tests

Between test occasions	Frequency (kHz)				
	.5	1	2	4	6
1 and 2	7.8	8.8	8.8	11.3	10.9
2 and 3	6.2	6.4	7.4	10.9	8.9
3 and 4	5.5	5.8	6.8	10.0	8.1
4 and 5	5.5	6.1	7.1	9.6	8.6
5 and 6	6.6	6.6	7.4	9.6	10.7

reliability improves after a repeat test, suggesting that the initial test may vary considerably from the "true" score. This finding conforms with that of Witting and Hughson (1940) who showed that while the first test was within ±5 dB of the "true" score in 77% of cases the average of the first three tests was within ±5 dB of the "true" score in 93% of cases. Test–retest σ_{diff} between successive tests in High and Gallo's study was in the 5–10 dB range, hence they are comparable with results from Jerger's (1962) study. Agreement dropped steadily, however, from the start to the finish of the research period, so that σ_{diff} between first and final test values were

	.5	1	2	4	6	kHz
$\sigma_{diff}(1-6)$	7.9	10.0	9.3	12.4	13.6	dB

Inspection of correlation and standard deviation values suggests that second and final tests were not much closer in agreement, but third and final tests begin to approximate successive test σ_{diff} values given in Table 5.2.

The gradual loss of agreement with increasing intertest interval would be an expected outcome. In the case of High and Gallo's study, the mechanism creating increasing variability is deterioration in hearing caused by noise. A gradual but steady increase in levels at higher frequency threshold (significant between certain test series) is observable with the passage of time, and it is clear to the authors themselves that this change is attributable to progressive injury resulting from exposure to occupational noise. Given that people are variably affected by the same noise and also show changing rates of cumulative injury (Burns & Robinson, 1970), then it is not surprising that test results started to show increased variability with the passage of time.

Of course the question remains why there should be such obvious signs of deterioration when the hearing of employees was being constantly monitored and the purpose of that monitoring "was to protect the employees' hearing [High & Gallo, 1963, p. 17]." The purpose of the monitoring was, in fact, to detect people who showed the most extreme changes (> 15 dB at any test frequency) on any occasion of test relative to the preemployment test. What became of people who did so is not stated. But one aim of the High and Gallo (1963) study was to find out the likely incidence of this sort of extremity. The fact that nonextreme but significant deterioration in threshold levels was observed throughout the survey period demonstrates that the purpose of the monitoring exercise was not to protect hearing but to protect management from nontrivial compensation claims. The only way in which hearing would be protected was, and always will be, by reducing noise to noninjurious levels. The pious disclaimers of those who advocate the monitoring of hearing as a "protection" measure in noisy industry are here shown in a different light.

A study, also reported in 1963, which bears upon the monitoring-of-hearing issue is that of Atherley and Dingwall-Fordyce. Their purpose was to estimate the inherent variability of the tonal threshold test in order to find out how much change in a person's hearing could be attributable to nonchance factors. Data were therefore presented in such a way as to show what amount of change would constitute an unlikely variation and hence more probably be caused by an extrinsic effect on the person's hearing. A very careful check was made of instrument variability to ensure that this was not a feasible source of error. The thresholds of 12 young male listeners with no apparent disorder of hearing were determined by conventional technique four times, tests being separated by intervals of a day, then a week, then another day.

Atherley and Dingwall-Fordyce (1963) express their results in a format somewhat different from usual—presenting the estimated variance of measurement across the four determinations. The square root of their presented values is thus σ_{meas}

	.5	1	2	3	4	6	8	kHz
σ_{meas}	2.9	2.7	2.6	2.4	4.1	4.4	4.8	dB

Since data are from four test series, σ_{meas} is a legitimate expression of their result. These values are in good agreement with Witting and Hughson (1940).

On the basis of these values, Atherley and Dingwall-Fordyce (1963) give the amounts of change in threshold that would have to occur in an individual before it were decided that this change is unlikely on a chance basis. They conclude that quite considerable changes would have to occur—of the order of 12 to 15 dB at higher frequencies—before such a "nonchance" decision were taken. Since these are the frequencies at which change is likely to occur among people exposed to noise, it seems clear that the tonal test could be an unreliable guide in that circumstance. If we look again at the High and Gallo (1963) report, we could conclude that the requirement for change in an individual test of at least 15 dB was a proper procedure, since such a change would be expected by chance at the higher, noise-affected frequencies.

The first flaw in such an argument as regards the High and Gallo situation is that a change in the group as a whole of only 3 or 4 dB is significant and hence provides evidence that the population has been injured by the noise to which they are exposed. The second flaw in this whole approach to what is and is not a chance fluctuation lies in the following point. In observing fluctuations of level at threshold whose direction of change is equiprobably positive or negative, we must treat any such change with a two-tailed test of significance. In that case, the .05 level of chance has to be split between each tail of the distribution of changes. But in observing possible effects of noise or some other intervening variable, we know the direction of effect beforehand. The situation is one tailed, and hence the whole of the .05 rejection region can be located at one end of the distribution. A less marked change in the expected direction is therefore needed to be considered significant. Atherley and Dingwall-Fordyce overlook this point in their calculations. And were High and Gallo's (1963) study a genuine exercise in hearing conservation, their result would illustrate the price of applying a two-tailed decision to an essentially one-tailed situation.

The detailed results of other field studies conform with those given here. More recent work in the field has addressed itself to identifying different sources of variance. We return to some of these studies when we consider the details of audiogram variability. The overall picture from field studies is that roughly within ±5 dB lie two-thirds of the variation likely to arise from repeat testing. Hence, within about ±13 dB will lie about 99% of differences. Any given clinical or survey-type audiogram has 1 chance in 100 of being ±13 dB different on a repeat test, presuming no intervening effects.

The question, now, concerns the factors that contribute to this not inconsiderable variability. Some of these may be subject to better control if their influence can be isolated.

Laboratory and Field Studies of Reliability

Establishing a Taxonomy

While most work undertaken to identify factors contributing to threshold variability has been carried out under laboratory conditions, some important work has gone on in field settings. In the foregoing review, we have already touched on such influences as learning, type of testing technique, and testing conditions as possible sources of change not accounted for by extrinsic agencies such as noise exposure. In the following review, then, we alternate between field and laboratory research.

Before we proceed, it is necessary to reiterate the theoretical construct, *reliability*. In many reports in this field, authors speak about "sources of error variance" and typically produce a tripartite scheme within which to locate these sources. Thus "physical," "physiological," and "psychological" categories are used, often with delineation of numerous subaspects of these main categories. While such an approach has technical merit, it is theoretically unacceptable. The requirement for reliability, in reference to the performance of a test, means (*a*) that the test will provide stable measurement from one occasion to another (where the stability of the thing to be measured is known or presumed); (*b*) that the test will be consistent with independent measurement systems designed to assess the same quality; and (*c*) that the test will accurately reflect actual changes in the quality being measured. These are the features of reliability, and they refer to the test itself. A test is unreliable if an erroneous or uncertain measurement occurs either because it allows irrelevant factors to influence its assessment or because its procedure permits nonidentical application from time to time.

Distinct from reliability is *variability* of the quality being measured. A test is reliable if it fulfills the third of the criteria listed in the preceding paragraph. It is *unreliable* if it does *not* respond to variability within the quality to be assessed because it is then insensitive and hence erroneous. Discussing "physiological" and "psychological" factors as components within reliability admits a confusion to the problem of test reliability. To be sure, some factors within people being tested may contribute to unreliability (faking of results, for instance), but variations in a person's threshold of audibility are independent of the reliability of the system being used to detect that threshold.

For this reason, we will not adopt the sort of schemes put forward by previous authors in this field but consider instead two major subdivisions in our taxonomy: sources of threshold test unreliability and sources of threshold variability.

Sources of Test Unreliability

CALIBRATION

Aside from the obvious unreliability introduced by variations in instrument output or earphone performance, the calibration problem relates to certainty regarding actual output to the listener when that is referred to an agreed-upon standard. National standards are based on surveys of so-called "normal" hearing, and they vary considerably. Provided the conversions applying to a set of data are reliably known, then results can be expressed according to various standards. Since the publication of International Standard R389 (International Organization for Standardization [ISO], 1964) it has been presumed that all data are reducible to a common reference—provided the appropriate conversion figures for a given earphone–coupler arrangement are used. But Delaney and Whittle (1967) have shown that these conversion figures, as given by Weissler (1968), are themselves unreliable. This means that data sets obtained from a listener on two different systems which are then expressed in terms of ISO zero will actually appear to provide different results.

Although this problem is not of practical significance in an isolated testing situation, it certainly becomes problematic when data from different systems are compared or when a standard for minimum acceptable risk or beginning hearing handicap developed in one country is adopted by agencies in another using different calibration standards and systems. In such a case, reliance on official conversion figures may lead to erroneous conclusions about the extent of injury to hearing that has been sustained.

TESTING TECHNIQUE

From the previous review, it seems fairly certain that different techniques for determining tonal threshold level are more or less similarly reliable. A possible exception is that the self-recording procedure may be more stable than conventional procedures. A study by High, Glorig, and Nixon (1961) compared multiple-repeat testing by various conventional techniques with a fixed-frequency, self-recording procedure in seven listeners. Data were analyzed using correlation coefficients only, so the actual numerical variability is unknown. However, no differences were observed between methods as revealed by the correlation analysis. Assuming homogeneity of variance between methods (unfortunately, no data are given), this result suggests—contrary to the possibility suggested by findings from other investigations—that self-recording is no more reliable than conventional procedures. No final conclusion can be drawn at this stage, therefore, regarding comparative stability of the conventional and self-recording procedures. It can at least be asserted that they are no different in outcome in this regard.

The consistency of the two procedures has been the subject of considerable study. An investigation by Robinson and Whittle (1973) is probably the most systematic in its design. Counterbalancing of order of test technique was made on initial test and on repeat test 15 months later. Even though comparative stability data were generated in this study, no details are given in the report by Robinson and Whittle (1973). Listeners were 48 people from the local population, aged 29–73 years (average on repeat test, 51 years). Elaborate data analysis was undertaken, but the outcome of present relevance is that while no appreciable difference emerged between the two procedures on the first test frequency, the self-recording technique provided lower levels at threshold than the conventional technique at subsequent test frequencies. The average difference between the two methods was about 3 dB, a finding that conformed with those of some previous studies.

Two previous studies which bear upon this result are those by Jerger (1962) and Hempstock, Bryan, and Tempest (1965). Although Robinson and Whittle (1973) do not refer to either work, a feature of these reports could explain the difference between self-recording and conventional modes observed by the latter. Robinson and Whittle used a pulsed signal (2 per second) in self-recording tests and a continuous 1- to 2-second signal in conventional tests. With respect to the Jerger (1962) study, it will be recalled that listeners provided lower levels at tonal threshold when an interrupted tone was used than when a continuous tone was used. However, slightly lower thresholds were also observed by Jerger between conventional and interrupted-tone, self-recording methods. Hence from his (1962) study it could be postulated that type of signal as well as type of technique might affect results. Because Jerger's data are taken from a clinical sample, that factor could provide a further interaction and make his observations nongeneralizable to the sample of ordinary listeners used by Robinson and Whittle (1973). Hempstock *et al.* (1965), in quite different test conditions from those of Robinson and Whittle (1973), nonetheless used normally hearing listeners, so their results perhaps bear more relevance to the Robinson and Whittle finding.

Hempstock *et al.* (1965), used both pulsed and continuous signals in *both* self-recording and conventional modes. Listeners were 10 normally hearing people aged 20–32 years, and all tests were in free-field anechoic conditions. An average difference of 3.3 dB was observed between conventional and self-recording methods when continuous tones were used (the latter method giving lower levels at threshold). But no difference was observed between the two methods when pulsed tones were used. Furthermore, no difference was observed between pulsed and continuous tone self-recorded thresholds.

This result was interpreted by Hempstock *et al.* (1965) in terms of minor adaptation effects. In the conventional mode, with a continuous tone burst the energy to the ear during the test will be greater than it is in a self-recording mode because signal level, uncontrolled by the listener, will at times be further above the listener's threshold in conventional methods than it is in self-recording methods. A pulsed tonal burst presents less total energy to the listener, even at that higher level, than a continuous tone. In addition, there may be microscopic recovery effects in the pulsed condition because of the signal's discontinuity. Hence the self-recording–conventional difference interacts with signal type, and at least in the study by Hempstock *et al.* (1965), signal type explains all of the difference between the two procedures. Whether that explanation accounts for the difference observed by Robinson and Whittle (1973) cannot be stated with certainty.

Jerger's (1962) result is at odds with that of Hempstock *et al.* (1965) as far as pulsed–continuous self-recording threshold is concerned. Once again, that difference might be attributable to differences in sample composition. The conclusion that can be drawn is that signal type seems to be a critical variable that interacts differentially with other variables to affect results. It is therefore premature to conclude that different outcomes between self-recording and the conventional mode are attributable solely to that procedural difference.

Earphone Placement

As has been noted fairly consistently, threshold stability is reduced at higher and lower audio frequencies, and the major reason for this is earphone placement (Kylin, 1960). I mention in Chapter 4 that the reapplication of a measurement device is a source of unreliability, that this problem is especially apparent in human-type assessments, and that even typical threshold determination procedures suffer from it. The problem with earphones is simply that the apposition of such a device to the ear cannot be identical from one occasion of test to another. This means that from the cavity engendered by earphone and external ear at lower frequencies there is variable leakage of sound with slight positional variation from one occasion to another. At higher frequencies, the variable cavity resulting from slight positional change itself produces changes in resonance pattern, so that energy at the tympanic membrane varies considerably.

Different kinds of studies bear out the earphone positioning effect. Hempstock, Bryan, and Webster (1966) showed that the reliability of threshold testing in free field improved at both higher and lower frequencies compared with earphone testing. The "replacement" of a sound source in free-field conditions is of course unaffected by the cavity problems attending earphone use. Hickling (1966) showed a short-term reduction in higher frequency (6 and 8 kHz) threshold variability (frequencies below 1 kHz were not tested) when earphones were left in position on the listener's head between tests rather than removed and replaced. Atherley and Lord (1965), in a more exotic design, had head masks manufactured to conform with the contours of the heads of 2 listeners. These masks contained earphones, and replacement on the head meant that the earphones were brought into almost identical apposition with the listeners' ears on each test occasion. In a carefully designed experiment, it was found that threshold variability was lower in the mask than it was in standard earphone-headband conditions.

In an effort to overcome the earphone placement effect, Atherley, Lord, and Walker (1966) designed a circumaural earphone assembly whose acoustical characteristics reduced the effect of placement variation. The reliability of tonal thresholds from the new earphone device (Atherley, Hempstock, Lord, & Walker, 1967) showed reduction in variability at 6 and 8 kHz to levels approaching free-field determination. In the 1 to 3 kHz region, performance was akin to that using the usual earphone construction.

Thus the problem of earphone placement can potentially be overcome, but no commercial development of the circumaural device has taken place. Part of the problem with circumaural earphone assemblies is the design of a reliable calibration system (Delaney, 1971). It should be mentioned finally that ordinary circumaural earphone assemblies designed to attenuate external noise are no more reliable than standard types (Coles, 1967; Delaney, 1971).

In sum, unreliability of the tonal threshold test springs from earphone placement, testing technique, and calibration variation. The second and third sources can be controlled, the first source remains a continuing problem.

Sources of Threshold Variability

ADAPTATION AND FAMILIARIZATION

It is not possible to say precisely how much variation is attributable to this or that source of threshold fluctuation, but the major source is probably contained in adaptation and familiarization. These are components of an effect that has been labeled *learning* by various authors. I hesitate to apply that term too generally since it connotes a change in a person's state, and there is no evidence that people learn to change their absolute hearing sensitivity. There is considerable evidence that with practice people learn to detect, or at least respond to, lower signal levels, but I think we are dealing in that case with the dual effect described by adaptation and familiarization.

We must begin this review with a discussion of the concept of *threshold*. It might be a fair assumption that the lowest recorded energy level acknowledged by a listener as audible should represent that person's threshold of hearing. If this construction of the term were acceptable, then the problem of reliability would diminish, for any given threshold determination might lie above "true" threshold, but it could not be below it. Measurement error would be unidirectional, and the distribution of values approximating threshold would be subject to a one-tailed rejection region.

The question begged by this approach concerns the status of observations at levels above the lowest observed level. In this model, these would presumably be erroneous values; but such a view results from a theory of the threshold as a fixed entity—a detectable locus on an energy continuum. Enough is known about the way people and their sensory systems respond to incoming signals to make such a theory unsupportable. Research into the fine structure of signal detection (Green, 1960; Swets, 1961) has provided a concept of threshold as a variable commodity because the likelihood of a listener's detecting a signal is not altogether predictable. Random fluctuations in the level of competing "noise" generated within the total transmission–reception system make signal detectability uncertain at the "threshold" region. This effect is quite independent of any systematic change that may be occurring through adaptation or familiarization.

In addition to this random variation, a more systematic change can occur in the listener's criterion of what constitutes a signal. In Chapter 4, mention was made of the "false alarm" problem in connection with auditory screening devices. This concept, which emerged from signal detectability research, is manifest in the forced-choice design of certain experiments within that paradigm. In these, the listener has to declare whether or not a low-level signal occurred within a given time interval when it is known that a signal may or may not have occurred. Variation in signal level and random distribution of signal–no-signal occurrences allows the threshold region to be plotted and listeners' criterion changes to be recorded. Listeners may commence such a task by adopting a conservative decision strategy and responding only when they are sure that a signal has occurred. In other words, signal level will usually be high before it is acknowledged. As testing proceeds, adaptational effects occur, and the listener also becomes more confident about what constitutes a signal. (Adaptation effect is discussed at length later.) Thus, whereas at the start of testing many signals will be missed, later in the test signals will be acknowledged that did not in fact occur. These are "false alarms." The rate of misses and "false alarms," varying throughout the test session, is an index of the listener's changing decision criterion. Criterion can be manipulated by varying the sanctions visited upon correct and incorrect identifications (Swets, Tanner, & Birdsall, 1961). To some extent, this effect models a motivational influence which we also discuss later. Seen from this perspective, "threshold" is clearly a statistical expression with no fixed psychophysical locus. The lowest output level cannot be designated the "true" threshold because it is an occasional station point and not a constant. Likewise, the 50% correct detection zone is not a "true" threshold for it will vary because of the kinds of effects discussed in the preceding paragraphs. There is in fact no locus that can be designated as "threshold." All that exists are agreed-upon conventions about what "threshold" will be taken to mean.

Many authors talk about more and less "reliable" threshold determinations (Jerger, 1962; Robinson, Shipton & Whittle, 1973) as though a varying threshold was less reliable and a consistent one more so. We have already dismissed the imputation of reliability to the quality being assessed. What these authors observe are more and less *variable* thresholds whose *reliable* determination (as being variable or stable) is solely a function of the sort of test conditions discussed in the previous section. The most realistic expression of "threshold" can only be in terms of the confidence interval or the standard error of measurement associated with a given result. There can never be a narrowing down of measurements to a specific point.

The constructs developed within signal detection theory can be applied to issues within threshold variability. The observed change in level at threshold associated with practice signifies change in criterion. Criterion change can be labeled *learning:* Operationally, either label refers to a process of familiarization with the task, usually leading to increased sensitivity to signals (though the opposite can occur when listeners learn to fake poorer hearing sensitivity than they have). Adaptation is the process whereby consistent changes in signal–noise relations take place: Again, operationally this usually leads to increased sensitivity, though the opposite can occur if the "threshold" sought is, for instance, the "discomfort" level.

The value of the signal detection approach is in permitting the separate conceptualizing of these two processes: familiarization ("learning") and adaptation. For researchers have confounded the two and labeled any change in level at threshold as the result of one or the other depending on the theoretical tenor of their investigations.

A classic instance is in the study by Corso and Cohen (1958). They observed a consistent reduction in level at threshold among 10 normally hearing listeners tested periodically over 50-minute sessions. They described the result as a learning effect. This explanation is difficult to sustain in view of the reversion to virtually identical initial levels of these listeners' thresholds on repeat tests a few weeks later. Actually, levels were on average .7 dB lower at the start of the retest than at the start of the initial test session, a finding that has been observed by subsequent investigators (Robinson & Whittle, 1973; Robinson et al., 1973). This effect might very well be attributable to "learning," in the sense that listeners familiar with the task on the second occasion commenced with less conservative criteria of "signal-present." To suggest that a long-term reduction in hearing sensitivity had occurred would be rather farfetched.

Explanation of the within-trials effect observed by Corso and Cohen (1958) in terms of "learning" is also difficult to sustain because the curve of reduction of level at threshold with successive trials on the second test occasion exactly paralleled the first test curve. There was, in other words, no "savings" effect of the sort classically observed in typical learning–relearning experiments.

An explanation that makes more sense of Corso and Cohen's (1958) result conceives it in terms of adaptation. Over a 50-minute listening session in quiet conditions, the auditory system of a listener would adapt in much the same way that the visual system adapts in darkened conditions. Bryan, Parbrook, and Tempest (1965a) labeled this effect "quiet threshold shift." They found an exponential reduction in level at threshold among listeners tested periodically over hour-long sessions under the infinitely low noise conditions of an anechoic chamber. It can be argued reasonably that the auditory system is conditioned to the medium-level noise environment of the day-to-day world, just as the visual system is light adapted. Removal of sound and removal of light lead respectively to quiet and dark adaptation, and entry to the noisy, lighted world leads to readaptation of both systems.

As proof that the effect is attributable to adaptation and not to familiarization, Bryan et al. (1965a) tested 7 listeners in an anechoic room then retested them according to the same schedule but with time out between tests in ordinary ambient noise conditions. No "quiet threshold shift" was observed in the latter treatment.

A refinement of this design (Bryan et al., 1965b) bears nicely upon the results obtained by Corso and Cohen (1958). Three groups of listeners were tested periodically over 1-hour sessions in an anechoic room, and between tests each group was exposed to white noise at either 30, 50, or 70 dBA during the first 30 minutes of the session. A fourth group listened throughout in the "0" dBA conditions of the anechoic room. Figure 5.1

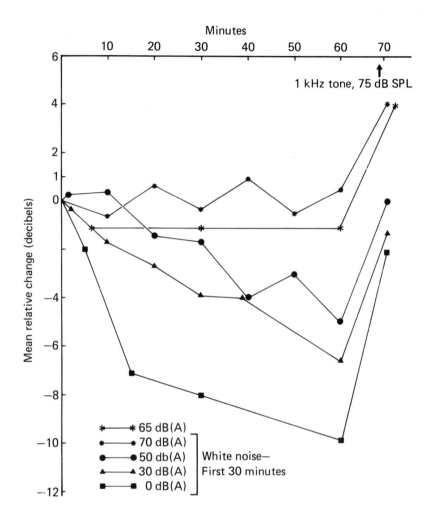

Figure 5.1. Results obtained by Bryan *et al.* (1965a, b) showing the dependence of "quiet threshold shift" on intertest ambient sound level. The plot of mean relative change in threshold labeled "65 dB(A)," from Bryan *et al.* (1965a), shows the absence of quiet threshold shift when listeners remain in ordinary ambient conditions between threshold tests. The other plots (1965b) show the variable amounts of threshold shift in the first 30 min of testing associated with intertest exposure to different amounts of white noise. The introduction of a 75 dB(SPL) 1 kHz tone (arrowed in figure) is followed by relative upward shifts in levels at threshold—extent of relative change being inversely related to degree of previous quiet threshold shift. From Bryan *et al.* (1965b); reprinted with the authors' permission.

shows the differential rates of threshold level reduction over time in the different groups. This demonstrates the dependency of quiet threshold shift on intertest ambient noise conditions.

An impressive feature of this result is the marked effect on quiet threshold shift of even very low (30 dBA) noise compared with 0 dBA conditions. A level of 30 dBA is not untypical inside standard audiometric test booths. It was inside such a booth that Corso and Cohen (1958) sat their listeners for 50 minutes and gave them 10 threshold tests at 5-minute intervals. Figure 5.2 shows the tabulated data of Corso and Cohen, graphed here in terms of relative change in mean level at threshold as a function of time, along with the data of Bryan *et al.* (1965b) from listeners exposed to 30 dBA white noise between tests during the first 30 minutes of the test sessions. The data fall on practically the same curve, suggesting an adaptation explanation for Corso and Cohen's result.

Not all listeners in the 1965b study by Bryan *et al.* showed quiet threshold shift, and the variability among subjects prompted a highly

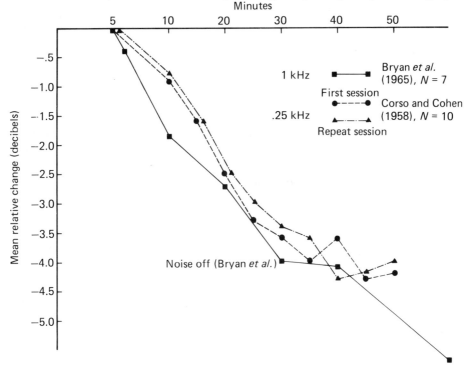

Figure 5.2. Quiet threshold shift observed by Bryan *et al.* (1965b) under intertest noise conditions of 30 dB(A) during the first 30 min of testing, compared with the mean relative change in threshold on an initial and repeat test series observed by Corso and Cohen (1958) under ordinary acoustic-booth test conditions.

illuminating though unfortunately small-scale study of longer-term threshold variability and its relation to degree of quiet threshold shift. Listeners were given weekly threshold tests in free-field conditions, thereby eliminating earphone positioning variance. Six of these listeners then underwent the 1-hour quiet threshold procedure. It was found that the extent of longer-term threshold variability at higher frequencies (6 and 10 kHz) correlated fairly positively with extent of quiet threshold shift at these same frequencies ($r = .67$ and $.75$, respectively). This result suggests that variability in threshold in the longer term, being significantly associated with auditory adaptation in the shorter term, may be partly accounted for by real changes in sensitivity resulting from variations in everyday noise exposure prior to each threshold test. Certainly such an explanation best serves to account for the increased variability of threshold over 2 hours as against a few minutes or seconds observed by Hickling (1966).

It would require a larger-scale investigation to establish whether auditory susceptibility to low-level noise is a sufficient condition governing individual threshold variability. In the meantime, the results found by Bryan et al. (1965b) underscore the point made earlier that change in threshold across audiometric tests can be a reliable indicator of real change in sensitivity, not merely a source of error.

Familiarization, as distinct from adaptation, has not been systematically studied. That is to say, very large-scale investigations, like those by Robinson et al. (1973, 1975) into the reduction of level at threshold with practice, have not isolated the adaptation effect from the familiarization effect. This situation is very unfortunate since it needs to be ascertained whether it would be more useful for listeners to have adaptation periods prior to threshold testing or to have "warm-ups" in order to gain familiarity with the task. Certainly from the studies by Robinson et al. (1973, 1975) and by Hartley, Howell, Sinclair, and Slattery (1973) it is clear that initial audiograms typically show higher levels at threshold than series of repeat tests.

PERSONAL FACTORS: STATE OF HEARING

No systematic study has been made of threshold variability as a function of degree of hearing loss or type of disorder. The picture that emerges from the opening review in this chapter is that normally hearing listeners may show less variability than some sorts of hearing-impaired listeners (Jerger, 1962; Witting & Hughson, 1940). In regard to people with noise-induced disorders, among whom test results could have critical compensation implications, there seems to be no clear result. However, Robinson et al. (1973) tested people exposed to marginally damaging noise levels. Their study was intended to tease out indicators on an initial test of likely high threshold variability. Many parameters were examined, but degree of hearing loss was not a distinguishing feature. On present evidence, it does not seem that increasing noise-induced hearing loss is associated with greater variability, whereas it may understandably be the case that certain types of hearing disorder, like Ménière's disease, are so associated. Clearly, variability will be increased in people exposed to noise if testing is not carried out with due control of recovery time from temporary threshold shift.

MOTIVATION

Two features associated with differences in variability in the study by Robinson et al. (1973) were age and status. Highly inconsistent results tended more often to come from younger and from poorer paid participants (all data were from shop and office employees in the one factory). The authors make no comment about this result, and perhaps none is to be made. It is a suggestive finding, however, with respect to differences in attitude between different groups of listeners. Younger people in low-status jobs would be relatively uncommitted to their jobs and to the factory institution generally and see little value in cooperating with government researchers. Older people, having worked in the place longer and having acquired higher status, would perhaps be more likely to respond conscientiously to a management request for cooperation in the study.

One should not press such a possibility too hard in the absence of actual information about attitudes. Nor should it be inferred that age or social class per se might generally be associated with variability of audiometric performance. It is more feasible that the features noted by Robinson et al. (1973) were peculiar to that research context. And a further finding by Robinson et al. (1975) helps back up a motivational basis for their 1973 outcome. In the later study, listeners (staff employed by an airline company) showed the expectable change in threshold on a repeat visit, but on the occasion of a third visit some listeners began to show responses quite inconsistent with previous results. The authors report that it was also evident that participants were becoming disgruntled on the third visit by having to undergo yet another (boring) threshold test. We need only postulate a greater initial degree of disenchantment among the younger, lower status employees in the 1973 study to secure an explanation for the earlier finding.

This example is a possible instance of motivational influence on test outcome. The magnitude of the effect of this influence is hard to pin down, but fairly clear instances of its operation are available both experimentally and in clinical and field surveys. It was mentioned earlier that in signal detection experiments the decision strategy of the listener can be modified by differentially rewarding, or withdrawing reward from, different sorts of response. Zwislocki, Maire, Feldman, and Rubin

(1958) observed more rapid improvement in auditory signal detection ability from one day's testing to the next's when listeners were paid to outrank their previous day's results. Here is a straightforward motivational change producing change in "threshold."

Differences of motivation are also clearly to be witnessed in cases of people who fake high levels of threshold for the purpose of gaining some reward. This, however, is a test reliability problem. Insofar as a test is susceptible to faking, then it is unreliable. But faking can also be seen as a motivational effect leading to variable results. An instance of its opposite, namely production of highly sensitive threshold levels in a natural field setting, was reported by Atherley and Noble (1967). We asked the local branch of the British Rail medical service for help in contacting men employed in the operation of rolling stock. The medical service permitted us to bring our own mobile audiological laboratory to the medical center so that threshold measurements could be requested of railwaymen when they appeared for obligatory medical examinations. The audiogram results obtained, plotted as a function of age, showed lower levels at threshold than was anticipated from the results of studies of other railwaymen. The mean level at threshold for the 20-year-old group was also lower than the levels used in determining "normal" British hearing threshold (British Standards Institution, 1954). Since that level was obtained under rigidly controlled laboratory conditions, such a finding from an initial test was surprising.

An explanation of the finding can probably be made in terms of a situational factor. The men were motivated to be in the "best of health" (medical screening is used by British Rail to weed out people considered unfit to drive locomotives, etc.). Even though the threshold test results were for our purposes only and the men were informed that our presence was fortuitous and unconnected with the overall medical examination, a generally heightened motivation (perhaps one could say high arousal) very probably carried over to the threshold test.

Personality Differences

So far we have looked at possible extrinsic influences affecting attitude, motivation, or whatever which in turn might influence an audiometric test outcome. In closing this section, we turn to the somewhat impenetrable area subsumed in psychology under the heading *individual differences* to find out whether any intrinsic features of people are associated with variability of threshold. In the discussion of the work by Bryan et al. (1965b), a possible physiological feature differing among people was identified. Psychological features might also play some part. I should point out that I am cautious about "personality" categories, not because they are unobservable but rather because their parameters are difficult to define in universally meaningful ways. Furthermore, I would not want to isolate biological features using a taxonomy that holds psychological characteristics to be exclusive aspects of the person and physiological characteristics to be exclusive but different aspects of the person. On this score, the work of Eysenck (1967) is highly relevant, for he has championed the idea that the factors he purports to identify in human personality (extraversion, neuroticism) relate in turn to certain physiological and performatory features of people. It is not my wish to enter the maze of psychophysiology. I mention the foregoing simply to establish some credentials for research that tries to relate differences in response on an Eysenck-type questionnaire to differences in threshold variability. There appears to be less test–retest variability among persons who produce high "introversion" scores on a suitable inventory than among those scoring high on "extraversion" (Stephens, 1971). Furthermore, using a signal-detection paradigm, Stephens (1969) found that while persons who score high on "extraversion" show high variance in lower threshold sensitivity, persons who score high on "neuroticism" show high variance in criterion of what constitutes a signal. It thus appears that different kinds of people produce variable thresholds in different ways, and as might be expected, the most highly variable thresholds are provided by persons scoring high on both "extraversion" and "neuroticism." In sum, variability in the quality being measured (which has, I have emphasized, nothing to do with the reliability of the test) arises from adaptation, practice, and change in attitude or motivation. Certain intrinsic features of individuals, at least as they are reflected in tests of introversion–extraversion, also lend themselves to greater or lesser variability of threshold—though such relationships may be the consequence of more direct links between psychoacoustical performance and physiological mechanisms.

RELIABILITY OF SPEECH TESTS

The problem of speech test reliability has not received the same intensive study as that of the tonal test. This is understandable because speech testing is not used to the same extent in assessment of hearing. Speech testing has an important role nonetheless, particularly in evaluation of therapeutic or rehabilitative programs. The Veterans Administration uses speech test results in evaluation of hearing for compensation purposes, but it is the only major agency, to my knowledge, which does so. For the most part, reliance is placed on the tonal test and an assumption that certain configurations of that test's results have predictive validity with respect to speech hearing ability. Chapter 6 examines the foundation for that assumption.

Speech test reliability needs to be thoroughly explored because of the predictive validity issue. If the speech test performance to be predicted by the tonal threshold test is itself highly variable or if speech tests are unreliable devices, this will add to the uncertainty about what is being predicted.

We can assume that many of the factors influencing tonal test reliability and tonal threshold variability also play roles in some kinds of speech testing—particularly tests of speech "thresholds." We can assume further, and results to be reviewed concur, that tests using speech in which factors of meaning, interpretation, and so forth play a part will be subject to a new range of influences of a kind not attending a tonal or speech-detection-type task.

Obviously, as soon as signal meaning becomes critical in the successful performance of a hearing task, then structural factors within the material must interact with human cognitive variables to influence the consistency of the test's operation. The most straightforward path into the speech test reliability problem is to begin with the simplest detection-type tests using the simplest verbal material and work our way toward meaning-laden tests, such as those using everyday sentences at comfortably audible levels.

Speech Detection–Reception Threshold Reliability

Early tests using spoken or recorded numerals were probably highly reliable although I am not aware of any study that examined this feature. From the work of Miller *et al.* (1951), mentioned in Chapter 2, one can predict that numerals, coming from a restricted verbal population in the English language, would be highly intelligible. A listener requires very little information to detect and comprehend spoken numerals because their content is so predictable. Recall that the original number test used only numerals whose vowel components were readily distinguishable from those of other numerals in the set. This feature would make the numeral test at least as reliable as a test using disyllables. The one main source of unreliability with early tests was the technique. Distance at which the spoken material could just be comprehended was the measure, and without doubt the speaker's enunciation and delivery would introduce variability to the signal from one occasion to another. Fowler (1941) mentions the extreme variability of results obtained on retest using distance for comprehension of live-voice speech material but gives no details. When prerecording or monitoring of live-voice became the routine procedure, this problem diminished.

Disyllabic material (so-called "spondees")[1] was designed to provide a

---

[1] I say "so-called spondees." Nabokov (1964, Vol. III, p. 472) points out that in English the occurrence of two-syllable, equally stressed words is virtually nonexistent (the word

better sample of speech sounds. This material was designed for use in assessing the speech detection and speech reception thresholds. The former is the level at which the listener is just able to recognize the signal as speech without necessarily comprehending it. The speech reception threshold is conventionally the level at which 50% of the items are correctly identified. In the interest of gaining good reliability and at the same time sampling more of the speech sounds of English, disyllables from a limited set are presented to the listener. These understandably show a very steep articulation function (Hirsh, 1952, p. 135). With increasing gain, their intelligibility rises very rapidly; as with numerals, listeners require not much information for full identification. The test–retest reliability for disyllables was studied by Falconer and Davis (1947) as part of their work on development of the connected discourse test as an alternative to the disyllable list. Listeners were retested during a single session, but it is not stated whether they kept earphones on their heads throughout the whole proceeding. A group of 25 young, normally hearing people was used. The σ_{meas} for PAL disyllables (PAL recording) in this group was 2.86 dB. The threshold for connected discourse gave retest σ_{meas} of 2.4 dB, and in a group of 47 listeners with largely conductive disorders a σ_{meas} of 1.95 dB. The disyllable outcome was in line with the result reported by Hudgins *et al.* (1947) using both normally hearing and impaired listeners. No details about listeners or test–retest procedure are given by these authors, however.

Both Hudgins *et al.* (1947) and Falconer and Davis (1947) found little or no familiarization–learning effect with either disyllables or connected discourse. Presumably the high intelligibility of the material is the reason for this. Hudgins *et al.* (1947) found the σ_{meas} of SRT for the PAL sentence lists to be of a similar order to those of the disyllables. This result is more interesting. The PAL disyllable lists are merely scramblings of a basic list of 84 items, hence retesting examines the stability of the items. The PAL sentence lists, however, each contain different questions (though with similar content) requiring single word answers. In any measure of their reliability, the consistency of their different content is being tested. Once again, the intelligibility of the material is high and the cognitive involvement is negligible.

The picture at this stage is therefore very clear. In assessment of thresholds using simple speech material, reliability appears to be much better than it is for tones. Test conditions, however, have been designed to be highly favorable to such an outcome.

When we turn to measurement of discrimination ability, a whole series

---

"spondee" is a rare exception). The disyllables of traditional SRT test lists are given an artificial spondaic quality, a feature they do not exhibit in everyday use.

of problems emerges because of the sort of material and measurement involved.

Speech Discrimination Reliability

Procedural Factors

Since the essence of speech discrimination testing is to determine the intelligibility of a speech signal, the mode of presentation usually adopted includes the inflections and modulations typical of everyday speech. Furthermore, material is less readily grasped since it usually consists of disconnected monosyllables. The aim has been to find out whether a person can discriminate the phonemes of these short words sufficiently well to repeat them correctly. As can be appreciated, the vocabulary of monosyllables is enormous and their predictability is low; they are therefore often sufficiently ambiguous to elicit plausible alternatives in response when a listener has not distinguished the entire word. The articulation function for monosyllables is much shallower than that for either numerals or carefully enunciated disyllables.

Indeed, enunciation is one major factor affecting discrimination score. Two aspects of this factor have been studied—intra- and intertalker variability. As regards intratalker variability, data are actually equivocal. Kreul, Bell, and Nixon (1969) observed only slight and insignificant variations in listener response with repeat testing using sets of different recordings by the same talkers. Test material was a list from the Modified Rhyme Test (House, Williams, Hecker & Kryter, 1965), and listeners were college students. Whereas different recordings by the same talker resulted in no significant variation in test results, the variation in response to lists read by two different talkers was considerable.

This result is at odds with one reported by Brandy (1966). He contrasted three repeats of a single recording with 3 separate recordings, all by the same talker, of 25 monosyllables from the CID W-22 list. The first condition he called "recorded," the second a "live-voice." Whereas 12 listeners showed no variation in response in the "recorded" condition, another sample of 12 listeners showed significant variation in response to one of the 3 "live-voice" recordings by the same talker. There appears to be confounding in Brandy's study, however, first in that the sample of the speaker's utterance used in the "recorded" condition was adjusted so as to even out fluctuations in the loudness of different words. Since no such modification was introduced in the "live-voice" condition, the advantage of "prerecording" over "live voice" in this study does not clearly emerge. The fact remains that "live-voice" testing did produce significant changes in performance. The problem is that the exact source of this variance cannot be pinpointed in Brandy's data. Another confounding feature of the data is a marked difference in mean performance between the 2 samples subjected exclusively to series of either "recorded" or "live-voice" treatments. A counterbalanced design would have helped partial out variance caused by what appear to be differences in characteristics between the two samples tested.

So, the picture remains unclear as regards live-voice presentation of test material. Intuitively, increased variance would be anticipated from use of such a mode of presentation, but evidence to date does not satisfactorily support such a notion.

On the matter of increased variability introduced by listening to different speakers, there can be no argument that such an effect is substantial. The classic instance is that between recordings by Rush-Hughes (Davis, 1948) of the original PAL monosyllables (Egan, 1948) and by Hirsh (Hirsh et al., 1952) of the modified form of these monosyllables (W-22). Tests using these two recordings produced markedly different articulation functions in both hearing and partially deaf listeners, the Rush-Hughes recording producing a much shallower gain in intelligibility with increasing signal level. Hirsh et al. (1952) postulated that the smaller size of the W-22 test (4 lists of 50 items each) compared with the original 20 lists of 50 items somehow meant that W-22 was an easier test. In a later publication (Silverman & Hirsh, 1955), this explanation, whose basis was never clear, was rejected in favor of one based on actual voice quality. Rush-Hughes spoke the monosyllables in a clipped way and with considerable modulation, Hirsh tended to enunciate them in Standard American English and more slowly. The most interesting outcome of this difference was not so much its effect on intelligibility gain functions among hearing listeners but rather in the differential effects of each recording among people with conductive or sensorineural disorders. The Rush-Hughes form distinguishes more readily between people with these different disorders than the Hirsh recording, and this outcome has interesting clinical implications. Distortion of speech is considered more fully in the next chapter.

In the present context, the importance of this difference is obvious. Different speakers cannot be used to test the reliability of parallel forms of a speech test. This point is substantiated in the study by Kreul et al. (1969) who, while finding no significant variability in listener performance with repeated live-voice presentation of lists by the same speaker, observed significant differences in performance when the same lists were presented by two different speakers.

Response mode, a variable that appears to have little effect on tonal or SRT determination, is obviously critical in discrimination testing where error of "translation" is the critical quality being assessed. Obviously, if a listener is asked to repeat words to an auditor, translation errors will be compounded. As Jerger, Speaks, and Trammell (1968) nicely point out in discussing the problem of vocal repetition of test items, "Under conditions of less than ideal electronic communications systems it is sometimes ambiguous as to whose speech discrimination is being tested, the patient's or the audiologist's [p. 319]."

Merrell and Atkinson (1965), in a somewhat tortuous investigation of this issue, had 25 hearing judges ("auditors") assess the vocal responses of one partially deaf listener and observed differences of up to 20% in the discrimination scores awarded. The auditors heard each test word—standard CID W-22 recording—followed by the listener's repetition of what *he* had heard. One interesting feature of the Merrell and Atkinson study is that the listener's written response (which was taken to be an accurate record of his discrimination ability) provided a much lower score than his vocal response. The authors comment that the auditors had a tendency to accept incorrect utterances as correct. There may be a problem here in that the labeling of a vocal response as "correct" or "incorrect" was judged on the basis of its correspondence with the written record, as though a priori the written record was a truer account. However, the listener in this study was selected on the basis of his good speaking voice and ability to spell and write. It seems plausible then that slightly aberrant vocal responses were translated as accurate by the hearing people who formed the auditor panel. Whatever may explain the vocal–written discrepancy, the outcome shows that the two forms of response provide markedly different results and that the vocal mode gives rise to considerable variability, at least between one judge and another. A more thorough examination of the problem would have usefully included intraauditor and interlistener designs to discover how the variability in scoring of vocal responses is distributed between talkers and auditors.

Interlist Consistency

Assuming that procedural issues of the sort just described can be sorted out—and there seems no reason why standardized and controlled test conditions cannot be attained—the major problem that remains in regard to speech discrimination test material is that of equivalency of content. This, as I mentioned earlier, is an issue of test consistency. The reliability of a test from this point of view lies in the similarity of measurement provided by equivalent or parallel forms of the device. We look first at some of the studies undertaken to examine consistency of the classical discrimination tests (PAL–CID monosyllables) then at more recent attempts to overcome certain sources of unreliability in these kinds of tests and at the work done using everyday sentence lists.

PAL AND CID LISTS

When Egan (1948) published the original phonetically balanced monosyllable and sentence lists (PAL lists), he noted many of the factors that govern the consistency of performance from one test list to another. The specifications of the original test were carefully worked out to try to achieve equivalency of difficulty and difficulty range. No actual data on interlist consistency were presented, but a learning curve was calculated (Egan, 1948, p. 970) from 8 days of successive test sessions in six listeners. This shows a marked increase (from 60 to 80%) in correct identifications of monosyllables. This result suggests that familiarization could have considerable influence on test consistency.

When Hirsh et al. (1952) published the revision of the original PB lists (CID tests) they showed the average articulation functions for the four lists of the new monosyllable test (W-22) to be virtually identical. However, as they themselves point out, listeners were familiarized with the test items, so the data are not generalizable to the typical test situation. Also, average data say nothing about the interlist consistency for an individual listener.

Silverman and Hirsh (1955) reported that the CID recorded revision of the PAL recorded lists was not doing the same job clinically as the older test; and from a comparison of performance on the two tests among 218 heterogeneous clinic listeners, it was found that the new recording provided much higher scores than the old and hence failed to discriminate listeners so well as the old. We have already touched on this difference in the context of talker effect on discrimination score. Silverman and Hirsh also reported that the new test was not as useful in discriminating persons with sensorineural disorder from those with conductive disorder. These findings, plus the recognition that disconnected monosyllables were hardly representative of everyday speech, led to the devising of the CID everday sentence lists. We consider the performance of these presently.

In regard to the consistency of monosyllable tests, Silverman and Hirsh (1955) report that whereas there was a .98 correlation between results from two recordings of the CID W-22 lists, the correlations between each of these and the original PAL recording were only .88 and .85. Despite the recognition by these authors that monosyllables were not altogether adequate as material for assessing everday speech hearing ability, the Veterans Administration continued to use the CID monosyllables in assessment of speech hearing ability. A study that followed up on the findings of Hirsh et al. (1952) with respect to interlist equivalency was conducted by Elpern (1960). In this study, conditions of testing were of the typical clinical kind rather than of the kind used by Hirsh et al. (1952). Using data from six Veterans Administration clinics in various parts of the United States, Elpern (1960) compared results from the four CID W-22 monosyllable lists. He found significant differences between the lists in terms of both average scores and range of difficulty. List 1 particularly gave higher discrimination scores than the others. In the original development (Hirsh et al., 1952), List 1 was found to give lower discrimination scores, and in consequence its recorded level was boosted by 2 dB. Obviously it was boosted too much. Elpern concluded that despite the observed differences in interlist performance some of the lists (2 and 3; 3 and 4) could be used interchangeably without risk of introducing serious differences in results.

Ross and Huntington (1962) assessed the reliability and equivalency of the CID recording of the W-22 monosyllables in a group of 33 listeners with sensorineural disorders. Each person listened to one scrambling (C) of all four lists, then to a different scrambling (D) of all four, after a rest period. Lists were presented at 30 dB: SRT or at a 5 dB lower level than the uncomfortable listening level if a less than 35 dB difference was noted between SRT and uncomfortable listening level. Details of diagnosis, hearing range, age, and so forth of the listeners are not given though it is mentioned that 3 listeners had levels at AC tonal threshold of at least 30 dB (ASA) at one test frequency in the .25 to 4 kHz range and the others showed at least 30 dB threshold levels at two or more frequencies in that range. The overall mean discrimination score noted by Ross and Huntington on the eight lists, was 80.6%; a somewhat lower average than was noted by Elpern (1960). The average standard deviation of the means on each test was about 13%. These results suggest a fair range of performance in Ross and Huntington's (1962) sample—given the high scores to be expected on the CID recording of W-22 (Silverman & Hirsh, 1955). Significant differences between means were found by Ross and Huntington between Lists 1 and 3, 1 and 4, and 2 and 4 on both the C and D scramblings. Significant differences were also observed between Lists 2C and 3C and 1D and 2D. Correlations between scores on each of the eight possible pairs of results ranged from .74 to .92, and standard errors of estimate (the predictability of results on one list from those on the other) ranged from 5 to 9.6%. The test–retest reliability coefficient of each list ranged from .91 to .95 and σ_{meas} ranged from 2.9 to 3.9%. Hence while the consistency (equivalency) of lists and even of scramblings of lists is not good, the stability of each list is fairly high. Ross and Huntington's (1962) result is akin to Elpern's (1960) at least in demonstrating that Lists 3 and 4 are roughly equivalent.

In 1965, Carhart showed test–retest results using the Northwestern University Test no. 4 in various samples of listeners. The statistic used was the average absolute difference in discrimination score. Carhart found that with increasing signal sensation level test–retest variability was reduced considerably. Listeners with sensorineural disorder showed the greatest variability, especially at sensation levels up to 24 dB. The expression of variability used by Carhart (1965) is not very informative as it gives no indication of the spread of variability observed.

Carhart notes that his finding in regard to sensation level is consistent with the shape of the articulation function. Because it is a sigmoid, then as Egan (1948) pointed out, greatest variability will occur in the region of the steepest slope of the curve, minor fluctuations in level being associated with major fluctuations in discrimination score. This is turn means of course that a sensitive test which also has the dynamic characteristics of W-22 will be bound to show high test–retest variability. The original PAL recording of PB lists suffers less in this respect because while it is more sensitive than the CID W-22 recording it also exhibits a shallower intelligibility–signal level slope.

Engelberg (1968) confirmed one of Carhart's (1965) results; Comparing consistency of the 4 CID W-22 lists in listeners with predominantly conductive or predominantly sensorineural disorder, he found greater σ_{diff} among the latter type. In addition, with increasing level at SRT, the σ_{diff} also tended to increase in people with sensorineural disorder, but it tended to remain fairly constant with increasing SRT level in conductive cases. The σ_{diff} range in the conductive group was 2.4 to 5.8%; in the sensorineural group it was 4.9 to 9.5%. These results on interlist consistency are similar to those obtained by Ross and Huntington (1962).

More Recent Test Lists

Paralleling these studies designed to assess the performance characteristics of classical speech discrimination tests, one observes the development of alternative test types using single words. In particular, the closed-set ("rhyme test") format has been popularized in clinical settings. Fairbanks (1958) devised the original closed-set "rhyme test." This was modified by House et al. (1965) and again by Kreul, Nixon, Kryter, Bell, Lang, and Schubert (1968). The test–retest reliability of the version by Kreul et al. (1968) was estimated by Gengel (1973) in a group of listeners with sensorineural disorder. Gengel (1973) comments that a closed-set approach ought perhaps to reduce variability by preventing cognitive variables from interacting with clinical variables. The closed-set method involves the identification from a written list of alternatives of the test item presented. In the development of such tests, list equivalency was examined with great care. Gengel's (1973) is the first study reporting clinical reliability, however. Four scramblings of the first list from the Kreul et al. (1968) Modified Rhyme Test were presented to each person on four separate test occasions. Listeners were 16 Gallaudet College students with various degrees of long-term sensorineural disorder. Variability was high across repeat sessions and is not accountable for in terms of practice effect (although some improvement is observable).

On average, there was an 11% range of differences in scores across list scramblings and test sessions. On this evidence, the closed-set technique does not seem to offer an advantage over traditional methods.

Another recent development has been the introduction of CID sentences containing everyday colloquial words the listener has to repeat, scoring being by either number of key words correctly identified or number of sentences. No systematic study of the reliability of these lists has been undertaken. The specifications for the original lists are given in Silverman and Hirsh (1955), presented by Davis and Silverman (1970), and revised and extended by Harris, Haines, Kelsey, and Clack (1961). The consistency of the original and revised CID sentence lists was examined by Giolas and Duffy (1973) who found low levels of interlist agreement and considerable differences in interlist difficulty when the lists were heard in filtered conditions by normally hearing listeners.

The foregoing review does not pretend to present an exhaustive coverage of published literature in the field of speech test development. Rather it is a representative account of the major work that has been addressed specifically to the reliability issue in clinical conditions. It seems evident that as meaning increases so does variability of listener response. This, as was asserted from the beginning, is understandable because other nonauditory factors begin to play a critical role. The practical effect of increased variability is of course decreased estimability of discrimination test results from other test data. We will see the ample evidence for that, particularly in people with sensorineural disorder in the next chapter.

A NOTE ON TEST UTILITY

The utility or cost-effectiveness of a test is very difficult to estimate. The concept is inseparable from both reliability and validity, indeed could be said to represent another way of expressing these qualities. Hence it is a concept that springs directly from generalizability (see Chapter 4). In gauging the utility of a test, one is asking about the amount of information obtainable from using it rather than another assessment form. The actual cost in economic terms is bound up with utility in the academic, information-gaining sense. Certain tests, in order to provide reliable and valid information, require elaborate procedures, conditions, and equipment and highly trained personnel. The overall equipment cost for obtaining a reliable estimate of tonal threshold is not inconsiderable. The cost of obtaining a reliable estimate of speech discrimination ability is high in terms of equipment and time. The question of the costs of these procedures in relation to each other brings in the issue of their respective generalizability; the cost-effectiveness of assessing both rather than one or the other bears upon the same issue. These aspects of measurement from an assessment point of view have rarely been investigated. In diagnosis, the question of utility is more often faced because there are fairly obvious cost differences between alternative procedures. In hearing assessment, the cost is usually ignored because assessment relies on procedures that are also usually basic to diagnosis. The utility factor is considered only in relation to short forms of tests.

The tonal test, for example, is typically carried out only at discrete frequencies in octaves from .25 or .5 kHz to 8 kHz and at 3 and 6 kHz. The choice of these test frequencies is based partly on reliability and validity estimates. Beasley (1940a), for example, used the United States Public Health Service 1935–1936 survey data to correlate tonal threshold levels at frequencies in octaves from about 62.5 Hz to 8 kHz. He showed that in that large population sample thresholds at frequencies up to .5 kHz were highly interrelated and interfrequency correlations declined from that point upward. Hence .5 kHz has become the lowest tested frequency in most screening or survey procedures.

On the assumption that .5 to 2 kHz tonal threshold is the valid frequency range for meaningful reception of speech, some portable screening devices test only in that range with the addition of 4 kHz to detect early signs of noise trauma.

In the speech testing field, occasional attempts have been made to produce short forms of discrimination test lists (for example, Elpern, 1961; Resnick, 1962). Grubb (1963a, b) has shown, however, that short forms, at least of the CID W-22 lists, do not show good stability or interconsistency because critical differences of content are generated by casting whole-list items into separate shorter forms. Campbell (1965), however, has analysed the whole-list consistency of the W-22 test in a carefully selected sample of veterans. From this analysis, he devised eight new half-lists whose content was determined from word-difficulty analysis. These new half-lists, at least within Campbell's developmental research, are closely equivalent with respect to relative level and range of difficulty.

A final word on utility anticipates a point that is emphasized in Chapter 11. The cost involved in production and administration of a self-report scale of hearing loss is negligible compared with the cost of mechanical testing. The information potentially obtainable from use of such a method is far more detailed than can be obtained from a tonal or speech test, as far as *assessment* is concerned. It remains to argue the utility in the larger sense (of generalizability) of such a device. Before entering that realm, we must first consider other technical problems attending current methods of assessment.

6

Concurrent and Predictive Validity of Assessment Systems in Use

INTRODUCTION

For a procedure to be valid, it must measure what it claims to measure. We have earlier been at pains to separate the concurrent and predictive element from the content and construct element of validity (Chapter 4). This chapter looks mainly though not exclusively at the concurrent and predictive aspect of assessment procedures and systems in use. It is largely an empirical and technical review of the evidence relating to claims that assessment of hearing by means of pure tone testing is valid for estimating degree of hearing handicap. Hearing handicap is understood, for present purposes, to mean lessened ability to hear the sounds of *everyday speech under everday conditions.* The reader will recognize that this phrase is a metaphorical construction that really means speech as it is represented in various standardized tests constructed with an eye to everyday usage and conditions (see Chapter 2). It is claimed that the actual performance of a partially hearing person listening to speech in everday life is predictable from these tests. Some agencies use speech tests as well as pure tone tests in assessment of hearing. In such cases, the concurrent and predictive validity of the latter no longer needs to be worried about. But the practice of using speech tests impresses the need to scrutinize *their* validity in gauging hearing handicap (as defined above). However, that is better done in the course of a broader review (Chapter 9) because discussion of the validity of speech tests brings in questions of content and construct validity, and I want to avoid where possible a compounded mixture of these different elements of the validity concept.

Complete separation of such elements is impossible, though; and in this chapter a certain amount of comment will be made, as required, about the content and representativeness of speech test material used by investigators in their studies of tonal threshold–speech test relationships. The subdivisions used in this chapter have been adopted solely for the purpose of organizing the published literature that I analyze and discuss. In addition, two thematic features dictate the orientation of the following review. Since my concern is to evaluate evidence relating to systems of assessment for compensation, data that bear upon various tonal-averaging techniques are of special interest, and data from listeners with sensorineural disorder, particularly noise-induced cochlear injury, are also of special importance.

In a more general review of studies in this area (Noble, 1973), I concluded that in people with sensorineural disorder disyllable SRT was to some extent predictable from tonal threshold whereas monosyllable discrimination score (DS) was not readily predictable. This was especially true among people with noise-induced disorder. Although that conclusion is basically unchanged as a result of further examination of published literature, the earlier review itself needs revising, extending and updating. In any case, the organization of the earlier work followed historical lines whereas the present approach is systematic and topical. A semihistorical approach is still inevitable, even under a different organization, because data relating to different tests of speech hearing tend to occur in rough succession rather than in parallel. Naturally enough, the invention of a new speech test or technique is sometimes a signal for abandoning an existing test or technique. However, to ignore studies using "outmoded" material is to miss essential data bases for current systems of assessment. Some demonstrated relation between an older test and tonal threshold will have been and continue to be taken as support for that test's validity. The quality of such correlational evidence needs to be examined, as does the validity of the speech material used. An excellent case in point is the very first recorded study of relations between tonal threshold and SRT in partially deaf people.

TONAL THRESHOLD AND SPEECH RECEPTION THRESHOLD–SPEECH DETECTION THRESHOLD

Numerals

In his classic work, *Speech and Hearing* (1929), Fletcher summarized the program of research carried out to that date at the laboratories of the Bell Telephone Company into various aspects of the speech transmission–discrimination process. Telephonics was of course a developing technology, and considerable resources were put into finding effective transmitter–receiver systems at least cost. Analysis of speech spectra was a vital part of such effort, and transmission of spoken numerals a key feature of any telephone research in those operator-connected times.

Fletcher showed that the bulk of speech energy is to be found in the .5 to 2 kHz region, and he therefore suggested that people's ability to detect speech sounds will presumably be related to their average threshold for tones in that same region. To bear out this point, 10 people, 9 of whom had various degrees of partial deafness, were tested using both live-voice and recorded voiced numerals. The distance and intensity at which the numerals just failed to be identified were then compared with their levels at tonal threshold in the .5 to 2 kHz region.

It should be noted that the phrase "just failed to be identified" refers to a speech threshold concept that is more akin to SDT than to SRT. It is for this reason that "SRT–SDT" is the phrase used in this subsection's heading. Although the concept of SRT as the level required for 50% correct identification of material did not emerge until later, there is a theoretical point to be made in this connection, and we will return to it later.

From comparison of speech–tonal threshold results, Fletcher concluded that the two measures were closely related. Harris (1946) in fact calculated a correlation of .95 between the data sets presented by Fletcher (1929). Fletcher gave no details about diagnosis or age of the 10 people involved in his study, but he did reproduce their tonal audiograms (1929, p. 217). Inspection of these shows that the bulk of listeners had relatively uniform threshold elevations as a function of audio frequency, and only one or two had traces characteristic of noise-induced disorder. The generalizability of Fletcher's proposal about .5 to 2 kHz tonal threshold and speech hearing ability is uncertain in view of the unknown nature of the disorders suffered by his listeners, and of course the small number in the sample. It is apparently on this data base nonetheless that Fletcher advanced the percentage of hearing loss scale calculated from .8 times the average tonal threshold values at .5, 1, and 2 kHz.

In contrast to Fletcher, McFarlan (1940) reported data from 22 clinic listeners using recorded numerals and average .5, 1, and 2 kHz tonal threshold. No details are given about the listeners as regards diagnosis, age, and the like nor about test procedures. McFarlan simply noted a poor correspondence between the two test outcomes. Harris (1946) calculated a correlation of only .65 on McFarlan's data.

A report by Curry (1949) appears to be another approximate replication of Fletcher's study. Live-voice whispered and voiced numerals were used, and distance at which they were just identifiable (as opposed to just not identifiable—a minor variation) was the measure of speech hearing performance. Of various tonal threshold averages, that for .5, 1, and 2 kHz correlated best with the test using *voiced* numerals. Curry described his sample of listeners as having sensorineural disorder. Their ages range from 14 to 56 years, but their number is unstated. However, the confidence levels associated with the reported product–moment correlations allow one to surmise that there could only have been 13 or 14 people in the group.

Not quite 20 years after Curry's (1949) report came a study by Meyer zum Gottesberge and Plath (1967) reporting relations between distance for "full discrimination" of live-voice whispered and voiced numerals and average tonal threshold at octaves from .25 to 8 kHz plus 3 and 6 kHz. Relations were also calculated between voiced and whispered numerals and tonal threshold at 4 kHz alone. Unfortunately, there is no report of relations between each frequency or .5, 1, and 2 kHz average and the speech test, so no direct comparison with the earlier studies is possible. The authors state that their data are taken from 227 men with noise-induced hearing disorder. Correlation between whispered speech hearing ability and average tonal threshold was .780, and it was .642 between tonal threshold average and voiced speech in a group of 251 "ears" classified as having a definite dip in the audiogram trace. Correlations of .719 and .709 were reported for the respective comparison in a group of 203 "ears" classified as having a gradual threshold elevation with rising audio frequency.

In regard to relations between tonal threshold and speech hearing ability for *numerals*, to my knowledge, these four reports represent the only detailed data available. Harris (1946) reports en passant a correlation of .69 between threshold (distance) for live-voice whispered numerals and .5 to 2 kHz tonal threshold in 335 "ears." No other details are given. Other speech testing procedures viva voce have included numerals in the presented material, but no reports are known to me other than those already mentioned which have investigated relations between tonal threshold and ability to hear numerals exclusively.

As was noted, this subsection has been headed *SRT–SDT* because no percentage-correct procedure was used in any of the studies described. It seems that the speech thresholds obtained by the procedures described were relatively all-or-none "points" in space where the numerals could or could not (all) be correctly identified. The original application by Fletcher (1929) in the context of telephonics provides some content validity for the use of numerals. As a test for general speech hearing ability, numerals are nonrepresentative. The major arguments about them have already been given in Chapters 2 and 5 and can only be underlined here. Listeners are very likely engaged in a pure detection task when numerals are used—the number of possible stimulus alternatives is small, the number of potential confusions between stimuli smaller still. Redundancy in such a circumstance is obviously much higher than it is even in everyday colloquial conversation. Thus, once a minor proportion of available energy is detectable, the content of the transmitted message can be fully worked out.

In the voiced condition, energy will of course be in the .5 to 2 kHz region, whereas in the whispered condition there will be a more equal representation of energy across the audible spectrum. In an indirect way, the data of Curry (1949) and of Meyer zum Gottesberge and Plath (1967) bear out this contention. Curry reports a high positive correlation (.802) between voiced numerals hearing ability and .5, 1, and 2 kHz tonal threshold average, whereas the correlation is merely .163 between whispered numerals and the same tonal average. By contrast, Meyer zum Gottesberge and Plath find a *lower* correlation between voiced numerals and 4 kHz tonal threshold (.433) than between whispered numerals and 4 kHz threshold (.641). The numerals test then will tend to correlate best with threshold at whatever frequencies are represented in the speech energy. The test fairly well mimics the tonal threshold test.

Various Other Speech Materials

Fowler

It is difficult to pin down the earliest report under this heading. Fowler's (1941) work is mentioned in Chapter 3 in connection with the invention of his system of percentage rating of "disability" (loss of capacity for hearing speech). In that paper, he provides results from 20 listeners comparing their percentage loss of capacity for hearing speech (calculated from tonal thresholds) and the distance at which "conversational speech was heard [p. 956]." The relationship between calculated and observed speech hearing ability is well-nigh perfect. Details of the speech material and test procedure are not given. The listeners were a variegated group ranging in age from 8 to 68 years, and their audiograms show various patterns of tonal threshold decrement. Scrutiny of the AC–BC traces suggests that 9 of the 20 had sensorineural disorder, 3 conductive disorder, and 3 mixed disorder. In the remaining 5 listeners, absence of BC data makes diagnosis uncertain, though the AC patterns of all 5 are consistent with a conductive picture. The selection of this particular group of 20 is not explained. However, it is odd that Fowler should even present such data. In his view, the reason for preferring the test of tonal threshold to establish percentage disability is that all other tests, including voice,

> are undependable, in fact useless for estimating percentage of disability . . . because . . . all are basically unsound and misleading. . . . Although . . . one might think it would be easier to obtain a percentage by testing with speech directly, careful experiments show speech tests are very unreliable; they may vary as much as 200 percent in distance even with trained examiners. . . . The ability to interpret speech varies to such an extent that all methods using actual speech are not really tests for loss of capacity to hear speech but rather tests for the ability to understand what is said [pp. 938–939, 941, 945].

Fowler's aim is to produce a system that allows the loss of capacity to hear speech to be calculated from the audiogram. Why he shows speech test data that accord with his calculations is beyond comprehension. Surely the last thing Fowler could expect would be a correspondence between his calculations and the results of an "undependable," "unreliable" speech test, and one he believes does not even measure "loss of capacity to hear speech."

In 1942, Fowler published his simplified scheme (using only four frequencies, .5, 1, 2, and 4 kHz) and included data from 7 listeners, 6 with AC–BC patterns consistent with sensorineural disorder, one with a conductive pattern. No other information is given about these cases, but the correspondence between calculated percentage loss of capacity and maximum distance for reception of *soft* conversational voice is virtually flawless. It is interesting to note that 5 of the 7 cases are ones whose data were previously used to validate the 1941 scheme using ordinary (not soft) conversational voice—hence the maximum distance figures are less than those given in 1941. The new calculation, however, fits these new speech test data.

For all that Fowler (1941, 1942) provides meager evidence in support of his schemes, it is interesting to note that he retains 4 kHz in the 1942 computation. Later study has, in fact, validated Fowler's 1942 formula in a heterogeneous clinical sample, and we will see that Fowler's is the first unwitting note in a battle over the value of including frequencies higher than 2 kHz in prediction of speech hearing ability.

Steinberg and Gardner

In 1940, Steinberg and Gardner of the Bell Telephone Laboratories presented results from 3 people with unilateral "mixed" hearing disorder. Articulation curves for Fletcher and Steinberg (1929) monosyllables were determined in the "poorer" ears of the 3 listeners and compared with the articulation curve of a group of listeners with normal hearing. The difference in average decibel level at threshold for tones of .5, 1, 2, and 4 kHz between each unilateral case and the normally hearing group was calculated. Similarly the increase in decibel level over the normal group required in each unilateral case to achieve 40% correct articulation was read off from the articulation curves. This latter measure, incidentally, can be taken as the earliest account of "speech reception threshold" as it is understood in present times. The agreement between SRT (40%) and average tonal threshold was very close in each case.

This is a painstaking study, and it is unfortunate that so few cases were examined. The diagnostic feature (mixed, i.e., partly conductive disorder) also makes generalization difficult. One feature of interest arising from the Steinberg and Gardner data (Figure 3, p. 272) is that the threshold levels at 4 kHz most reliably distinguish the three cases in terms of speech discrimination differences between them, and it is the inclusion of 4 kHz in the averaging calculation that allows agreement between SRT and tonal threshold to be so close in these cases. Fowler (1941, 1942) is well aware of the Bell Laboratories research, and it is not unlikely that his retention of 4 kHz tonal threshold is a result in part of these sorts of data.

Steinberg and Gardner (1940) give no details about how the speech material was administered in their study. It can be assumed, however, that the procedure recommended by Fletcher (1929) of monitored live voice with stepwise electrical attenuation of the spoken signal was adopted by them. This is certainly an advance on unmonitored attenuation gained via change of distance between listener and talker. And Hughson and Thompson (1942), whose study is considered next, made considerable efforts to ensure that consistent speech signals were presented by live voice to the listener.

Hughson and Thompson

These authors used Fletcher and Steinberg (1929) sentences given to a sample of persons who manifested various degrees of partial deafness. No diagnostic information about the group is reported. Their ages ranged from 14 to 83 years and the number of tested "ears" was 86. It is not known whether these come from 43 "whole" people or some larger number. One clue is that a normally hearing group of 56 people, acting as a control, provided 104 "ears." It can be assumed then that the 86 partially deaf "ears" came from at least 43 but perhaps not more than 50 people.

Hughson and Thompson divided their sample into 2 groups depending on shape of the tonal threshold trace over .125 to 8 kHz. One group (N_{ears} = 59) had essentially flat traces, the other (N_{ears} = 27) had traces showing unsymmetrical ("high tone loss") audiograms. These subgroups were further subdivided according to level at threshold. Only the arithmetic means for each (sub)subgroup are given, so there is no way of telling how the threshold levels of each are distributed, no way of knowing how distinct each is statistically. The result that Hughson and Thompson are most concerned with is the relation between mean SRT for the sentences (defined as level for correct repetition of at least two-thirds of the sentence lists) and mean percentage hearing loss (Fletcher .8 system) across the various (sub)subgroups. That relation is linear and regular, and the pattern of relationship is identical across the two major subgroups. Because of the manner in which this relationship is derived, it is unfortunately impossible to discern the actual correlation between the tonal and speech tests.

Goldman

An extensive survey of relations in military personnel between average tonal threshold (.25 to 2 kHz) and maximum distance for correct repetition of whispered speech was reported by Goldman in 1944. Although the speech material used is not described, it conformed with a general specification that it comprise, "numerals, names of places or other words or sentences" [p. 560]. Among the diagnostic groups was a sample of 53 cases of "nerve deafness." Goldman presents individual results but confines his data analysis to qualitative assessment, pointing out the more extreme cases of disagreement between the two test outcomes. In work already mentioned, Curry (1949) calculated a product–moment correlation of .553 for these particular data of Goldman's, but apparently he used each ear as a separate observation. Given that results from each ear are not necessarily independent (Elliott, 1963; Graham, 1960), such a procedure would tend to overestimate whatever relation exists between the two measures.

A Note on Sample Differentiation

The tactic of dividing the subjects in a study into various groups presumably has to conform with some underlying rationale. Where people are examined with respect to diagnosis and test results are reported, as by Goldman, for each diagnostic group separately, an argument can be made in favor of the rationale. It is readily understandable that *disorders* affecting different parts of the auditory system, or differently affecting the same parts, may well produce recognizably different *disturbances* of hearing.[1] Of course, it could require quite sensitive methods to unearth these differences in any satisfactorily objective way. One might hope only to come up with different patterns of audiometric response (*audiometric* meaning any measure of auditory function) even though these patterns themselves do not necessarily reveal the underlying qualitative differences in disturbance.

It is harder to make an argument supporting Hughson and Thompson's strategy, namely the division of people on the basis of tonal threshold profile. To do so is to assume a correspondence between audiogram shape and disturbance of hearing. While certain disorders of hearing fairly reliably manifest one type of audiogram profile rather than another, that profile cannot be taken by itself as a sure guide in diagnosis of disorder. There are types of disorder, such as otosclerosis, that manifest elevation of the level at threshold for high tones; types like Ménière's syndrome manifest uniform threshold elevation. While it might very well be that audiogram shape is critical in predicting the nature of hearing disturbance (and we will review evidence from more recent times pointing in that direction), there needs to be some theory of mechanism to explain the dependence. Unless this theory is forthcom-

---

[1] My distinction here and elsewhere between *disturbance* and *disorder* should be explained. By *disorder* I refer to a diagnosed pathology, by *disturbance* I mean a qualitative effect on auditory experience, reflected perhaps (perhaps not) in tests of auditory performance.

ing, on what basis are audiograms to be differentiated? What is a critical variation?

Carhart

These questions fairly beg to be answered in light of Carhart's study (1946b). Carhart notes Hughson and Thompson's (1942) finding that audiogram shape is immaterial in predicting SRT. He finds such an outcome "thought provoking" but does not say what thoughts it provoked. It is simply deemed desirable to explore the situation in more detail and to examine tonal–SR threshold relations in no less than *five* categories of audiogram shape. "Medical diagnosis . . . was ignored and may be considered random within the limits which are possible when groups are segregated according to contour of loss [Carhart, 1946b, p. 98]."

Thus any conclusions drawn about the interrelation between tone and speech thresholds on the basis of Carhart's evidence can have no bearing on the relationship between these measures in a specific population. And considering that Carhart's groups were military men and that one purpose of the study was to find out whether the then current AMA (1942) system was valid, it does seem counterproductive to lose sight of diagnostic categories in the exercise. After all, the people most likely to be presenting for assessment for compensation are those whose hearing is damaged from military combat and training. As a diagnostic category, this (noise or blast induced) injury ought surely to be singled out for special analysis.[2]

To be sure, in reiteration of the earlier point, certain types of disorder (and noise-induced injury is one of them) manifest characteristic audiographic profiles, but not exclusively. The fact is that not all noise deafness cases will show unsymmetrical, that is, high tone threshold elevation, or a "4 kHz notch" and, just as critical, neither will disorders *apart* from those induced by noise *refrain* from manifesting such patterns. Hence, if audiograms are classified and diagnosis ignored, any relations which emerge cannot reliably bear upon a diagnostic category.

All of which having been said, Carhart's (1946b) findings are worth

---

[2] The Veterans Administration in the United States does a great deal more, of course, than assess people's hearing for compensation purposes. Veterans with hearing disorders of whatever type, that is, "service-connected" or otherwise, enjoy the rehabilitative services of that agency. It is a legitimate exercise, therefore, for the Veterans Administration to try to find economic ways of estimating the likely difficulty these people will have. But the assessment-for-compensation feature of the Veterans Administration enterprise is its most crucial, for in these cases the outcome of the assessment fixes the pension that a veteran will receive. Thus it is vitally necessary that "service-connected" disorder be examined independently of other disorder so as to ensure that just decisions from all points of view are made in these cases. To have lumped all types of audiogram and disorder together to arrive at an overall picture is to have clouded the very special issue of "service-connected" disorder.

citing since they seem to bear out the point. There were five categories of audiogram identified in this study: "flat" profiles; "gradual" elevation of threshold with rising audio frequency; "marked" elevation of threshold with rising audio frequency; "notches" in audiograms beyond 2 kHz; and "untypical" or, in terms of the previous descriptions, uncategorizable audiograms. Correlation coefficients (statistic unstated) were computed inter alia between "better"[3] thresholds at .5, 1, and 2 kHz and binaural SRT for PAL disyllables. The choice of PAL disyllables and "better" tonal threshold at .5, 1, and 2 kHz was determined by another analysis of results (Carhart, 1946a). This study used case material provided by people in attendance at the army hospital, Deshon (where all these studies took place) for routine testing for assessment–rehabilitation purposes. The object of the 1946a analysis was to determine which tonal threshold–speech test material combination yielded the closest correspondence in a heterogeneous sample of partially deaf people. The mean tonal thresholds of 129 people also tested with Fletcher and Steinberg sentences (under conditions akin to those developed and used by Hughson and Thompson) were at .5 kHz, 45.5 dB ($SD = 19$); at 1 kHz, 50.9 ($SD = 17.4$); and at 2 kHz, 52.3 ($SD = 19.6$); clearly a heterogeneous group. Correlation (.69) was highest between sentence SRT and "better" threshold average at .5 to 2 kHz. In a very much larger group of randomly selected people from the same population, correlation was on average .75 between PAL disyllables and "better" .5 to 2 kHz tonal thresholds.[4]

Results of the 1946b study show high levels of relationship (.75 to .87) between "better" ear .5 to 2 kHz thresholds and disyllable SRT in all groups except that with "marked high tone loss" (.29; $N = 32$). Carhart does not report in this paper the point of origin (in terms of Hz) of "gradual" or "marked" high frequency rise in threshold. However, in an earlier paper (Carhart, 1945) describing the audiogram classification scheme, "gradual" and "marked" categories originate at very low frequencies (.125 or .25 kHz) and show linear increases in level at threshold with rising audio frequency.

A point that lacks clarity in the 1946b study is the sampling technique. Records were, "culled for good examples of each category [p. 97]." Fifty cases of each type were extracted, except for the "marked" category where N is 32. Questions of importance here are (a) the representativeness of the categories; and (b) the numbers in each category in relation to the population of cases as a whole. This latter remains unknown. Regard-

---

[3] Whichever was the lower level at the listener's threshold between the two ears at each frequency.

[4] The "on average" phrase refers to the fact that this large sample ($N = 682$) was made up from groups, each tested under slightly varying conditions and yielding correlations ranging from .71 to .82.

ing the former, Carhart (1946b), in addition to those specified, also selected 100 cases at random from the population, of whom 86 were said to be classifiable according to the 4 distinct categories, the remaining 14 falling into the "untypical" fifth group. The categories therefore seem to cover most instances in the population, but the distribution of the 86 cases within the four classifications is unknown.

What, then, can be made of Carhart's findings? He himself concludes that audiogram shape is an immaterial factor in prediction of SRT except where "marked" elevation of threshold with rising frequency is featured. In particular, .5, 1, and 2 kHz is as good a predictor of SRT as the then current AMA (1942) weighted averaging system which takes account of 4 kHz threshold. The "notched" category in particular bears out this point. While diagnosis is carefully avoided in this study, readers might not be blamed for concluding that the data show that "typical" noise injury audiogram profiles (the 4 kHz "notch") are no exception to the general .5, 1, and 2 kHz predictive scheme. Because diagnosis was ignored, however, no such conclusion is possible. The composition, in terms of pathology, of the "notched" group is unknown. The same is true for the "marked high tone loss" group.

One thing is certain: Noise injury cases of a beginning nature are more likely to be found in the "notched" group,[5] and cases which have become severe and overlaid with deterioration due to advancing age are more likely to be found in the "marked" group. Which group better represents noise injury is almost a matter of taste. I would submit, however, that the gross discrepancy between the two audiogram groups as regards relations with SRT underscores the point that diagnostic contamination, coupled with some critical effect of audiogram shape, is the reason for the difference. And I would make this final point: that in industrial cases at any rate claims for compensation would not emanate from people with early signs of noise injury (the law in many countries virtually prohibits this anyway; see Chapter 3) but rather from older people in whom the injury is severe and long term.

I have dwelt on Carhart's study at length because his data have been cited by many subsequent authors involved in drawing up schemes for assessment-for-compensation purposes as supportive of the use of tonal average at .5, 1, and 2 kHz for that purpose. I hope that the more complete exposition of Carhart's data presented here makes room now for some doubt about such a conclusion.

I have withheld discussion of another report by Carhart (1946c) until this point in order to show that the questions raised are fair ones arising directly out of his more publicized work. The 1946c report also raises

---

[5] "Specific effects [of selection] were probably operative to load group 4 ["notched"] with light loss cases [Carhart, 1946b, p. 100]."

other issues not directly connected with those dwelt on so far. It is opportune now, having made the foregoing points, to turn to Carhart (1946c), a work almost never mentioned by later authors, to provide some supporting evidence for the arguments about diagnosis made in the preceding discussion. In this paper, Carhart examined mean arithmetic differences in level at tonal and at SR thresholds as a function of diagnostic type. He found the greatest discrepancy in cases of noise-induced hearing disorder. Because he recorded only the mean arithmetic difference between the two measures, no clue is available about the actual degree of association between them as a function of diagnosis, though from statements made in the 1946c work one can infer that the "marked high tone loss" and "notched" groups of the 1946b paper indeed contain the bulk of noise injury cases.

In the noise-induced disorder sample ($N = 23$), the mean level at SRT was 5.6 dB lower than the mean level at .5 to 2 kHz tonal threshold. In other diagnostic groups, the means were within -1.7 to $+2.5$ dB. Thus Carhart's own data show that noise-induced disorder is out of step with other disorders.

Here a new feature is introduced to the discussion. Carhart points out that noise-induced disorder, being "service-connected," is likely to manifest a "functional" component. In other words, because of the assessment-for-compensation element, listeners with noise injury will exaggerate on tests. He argues that there can be no other rational explanation for lower levels at threshold for speech than for tones. We examine the general issue of "functional hearing loss" in Chapter 8, but certain technical arguments need to be settled here because this feature recurs in studies of speech–tone relations and the ghost needs to be laid from the start. There are two objections to Carhart's argument: First, it is illogical; second, other sets of his own data support alternative explanations.

To take the first objection: While exaggeration may occur in some cases, there is no evidence available in his data to allow that it is the underlying cause of the aberrant result in noise injury. It is as *logical* to conclude that the diagnostic category (noise-induced disorder) is explanatory of the difference and hence that the difference is as much a sign of that type of disorder as it is a sign of exaggeration. What is more critical, only *disagreement* between tonal and SR threshold levels is regarded as aberrant (especially in the direction SRT lower than tonal threshold); nondisagreement is accepted as a genuine response, but no reason is given as to why it should be so.

To take the second objection: Even supposing the inadmissable argument nonetheless pointed to a real effect, other data weaken the case for explanation in "functional" terms. For example, in Carhart (1946c) *all* groups of cases in which more than a minor sensorineural element was diagnosed showed mean SRT lower than tonal threshold, whereas the groups with a diagnosis of pure or predominantly conductive disorder show mean SRT higher than tonal threshold. Noise-induced injury is the only category that attracts compensation, so a "functional" explanation cannot apply to the other sensorineural groups. What is much more plausible, organic lesion in the form of sensorineural involvement can explain the effect since it is so reliably associated with it. Yet another set of data reported in 1946c show that the SRT-lower-than-tonal-threshold effect is much more marked when sentences rather than disyllables are used in listeners with noise injury. No explanation is offered for this different outcome.

All these data suggest an alternative explanation for the observed effect. Let us suppose that sensorineural disorder, as a general category, is characterized by disruption of the usual temporal integration properties of the cochlea and auditory nervous system (Corso, Wright, & Valerio, 1976). Let us assume further that in cochlear disorder caused by overstimulation by noise there is an increase in spontaneous discharging leading to increased "physiological noise" (Pugh, Horwitz, & Anderson, 1974). Because of the first condition, a relatively brief tone may not be detected at a level where a spoken disyllable can be detected. Adding the second condition, taking account of the fact of less effective masking for speech at SRT than tones at tonal threshold, would enhance the detectability of the speech signal. Presentation of a connected sentence in which redundancy is markedly increased would enhance it even more. Such an hypothesis may in fact be unsupported in a specific experimental test, but a priori it has as much going for it as any other, and it adequately accounts for *all* the results reported by Carhart (1946c).

From all these data we are still no nearer the facts of the matter regarding relations between tonal and SR threshold in people with noise-induced disorder. But we can conclude that audiogram shape is the sort of parameter which confounds with the diagnostic variable so that conclusions based on the former are unreliable in application to the latter.

Harris

In that fructuous year, 1946, Harris reported briefly on relations between SRT for prerecorded PAL disyllables and .5 to 2 kHz tonal threshold. In listeners with "feat" audiograms, the standard error of estimate (se_{est}) between the two measures was 3.9 dB. In listeners with unsymmetrical audiograms, the se_{est} increased to 5.8 dB.

Fletcher

Fletcher, who initiated the interest in .5, 1, and 2 kHz average in the first place (1929), returned to the scene in 1950 with a more searching analysis of the problem from a mathematical point of view and an impressive data base to back a conclusion that the .5 to 2 kHz (the "three-average") system was still valid in persons with relatively uniform elevations in level at threshold. In people with unsymmetrical audiograms, however, the average of the two lower threshold levels from .5, 1, and 2 kHz better predicted SRT. This has become known as the "two-average" system. The bulk of Fletcher's data came from persons tested with a phonograph recording of (PAL?) disyllables (precise origin unstated). The other data were Fletcher's (1929) original cases and data from Davis and colleagues (1947). In Fletcher's study, listeners were tested with numerals and in the Davis *et al.* study they were tested with monosyllables, disyllables, and sentences. Fletcher's data, like Carhart's, are of unknown value because diagnostic classification is ignored. Where cases of noise injury lie within the presented data is quite unknown, and so the precise relationship for these kinds of people remains masked.

Palva

The scene shifts at this point to Europe, where Palva (1952) in Finland reported an extensive investigation, inter alia, of relations between tonal threshold and SRT for recorded disyllables "representative of all Finnish speech sounds [p. 120]." Comparison was made between SRT levels (expressed relative to a normally hearing control group) and various tonal averages and calculi in several groups classified by diagnosis. Of special interest in the present context is the group having diagnoses of cochlear pathology other than that associated with Ménière's disease or presbycusis. This group ($N = 32$) had, "no history or signs of middle ear inflammation. . . . Some had been in noisy work for years [Palva, 1952, p. 66]." Others had been exposed to ototoxins, suffered cerebral injury, or suffered congenital degenerative cochlear disorder. In other words, within limits of diagnostic confidence, this group represents the first pure "perceptive" sample with cochlear disorder, including noise injury cases, to be tested with tones and speech. No details of the age structure or other characteristics of the sample are given, but it can be assumed they represent a heterogeneous group of people attending a clinic. Palva did not calculate a correlation between SRT and tonal threshold in his analysis but confined his interest to the closeness of correspondence between these data in this and other diagnostic groups. Audiometric data for each individual are given, showing SRT, tonal threshold at .25, .5, 1, 1.5, 2, 3, and 4 kHz; percentage loss of hearing capacity calculated from the Fowler and Sabine (AMA, 1947) formula; average threshold across .5, 1, and 2 kHz; and Fletcher's (1950) "theoretical prediction" of SRT. Palva found considerable underestimation of SRT by Fletcher's (1950) system and gross discrepancies, especially at the extremes, between measured SRT and the Fowler–Sabine percentage scale. This latter is hardly surprising, since the Fowler–Sabine scale was designed as a sigmoid so that observed lower-level SRT values will be apparently underestimated and observed higher level SRT values will be apparently overestimated. Correspondence between measured SRT and percentage incapacity will only tend to occur in the middle range. This is what Palva observes, and this is what Fowler and Sabine intended (see Chapter 3 for the rationale of the Fowler–Sabine scheme). Leaving aside this minor confusion, the most important result is that between straightforward .5, 1, and 2 kHz average and measured SRT. The relationship is almost perfect. Using only one ear of each listener (to avoid the inflationary effects mentioned earlier) and using completed records only (one listener could not provide a level at SRT), I calculated a Spearman rank correlation of .97 on data from 31 listeners.

This result is the first published evidence that tonal and speech thresholds are related almost to the point of identity in people with cochlear disorder, as opposed to people with specific audiogram profiles. Palva's data also provide a feature that bears upon the latter issue. It is evident that a sizable proportion of the audiograms in this sample show a relatively flat profile; others show increasing levels at threshold with rising frequency. These two types are plotted as composites in Figure 6.1 to demonstrate the distinctly different characteristics of each. It is clear from these data that cochlear disorder can present variously shaped audiographic traces, though it is obviously likely that noise injury cases are primarily represented by the second type of profile and ototoxic and congenital cases distributed through both types. Opportunity is here, though, to test the feature of audiographic shape and SRT prediction, with site (if not precise nature of disorder) constant. In fact, there is no difference observable between these two subgroups as regards closeness of agreement between tonal and SR threshold. Correlation, r_s, between the measures in the "flat" sample = .94 and in the "sloping" sample = .96. This is not too surprising of course. The virtual unity of correlation in the group as a whole allows little room for variability in subsamples thereof. Even so, there is not even the suggestion of a difference between them.

These data strongly support the finding of Hughson and Thompson (1942) and entirely contradict the findings of both Carhart (1946b) and Fletcher (1950). In a later study (Palva, 1955), no such close association emerged; and there is only one other study, to my knowledge, that shows a result akin to this one of Palva (1952). That is a relatively minor report by Simonton and Hedgecock (1953) in which data from 11 listeners with sensorineural disorder are given. Correlations between average "better ear" threshold at .5, 1, and 2 and .5, 1, 2, and 4 kHz and SRT gave r_s = .98 and .96, respectively. SRT was for recorded PAL disyllables delivered

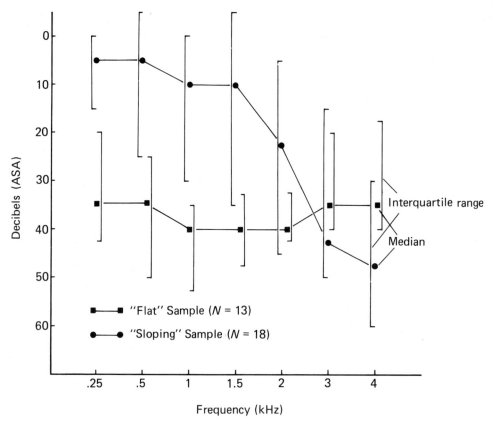

Figure 6.1. Data from Palva (1952) of levels at threshold in two groups of listeners with cochlear sensorineural disorders. Relations between tonal threshold and SRT in each group are separately analyzed in the text to investigate the possible effect of audiogram shape, with pathology held relatively constant.

binaurally in free field. Simonton and Hedgecock give no details of subject selection so one cannot say how representative their data are. Also, the listeners had various sensorineural disorders, so diagnosis is not as clear-cut as in Palva's study. Nonetheless, these data firmly support Palva's.

Harris, Haines, and Myers

Harris et al. (1956) reported results obtained from a large group of partially deaf listeners as well as analyses of how various predictive systems compared with observation. In other words, here are data in as much detail as in Palva's study from somewhat comparable populations, and it is therefore of interest to compare, where possible, the two sets of findings. Harris et al. (1956) do not cite the Palva work, and it is possible they were unaware of it at the time.

There are a couple of features of the Harris, Haines, and Myers study that make complete comparison with the Palva study impossible. First, Harris et al. give data for unidentified "ears," hence selection of only one ear per listener cannot be done. Second, the Harris et al. data are not tabulated as a function of diagnosis, hence a specifically "cochlear" group cannot be extracted. These are not major problems. As regards the second, enough information is given (namely AC and BC thresholds) to allow "pure" sensorineural cases to be extracted. Also, the sample is described in part by Harris et al. as follows:

> It should be pointed out that our population was not composed solely of relatively young servicemen.[6] About half our patients were not servicemen. There was, however, somewhat more noise trauma and somewhat less presbyacusis and severe childhood hypacusis than might be found in the usual hearing clinic [p. 165].

From this description the inference can be made that about half the listeners *were* relatively young servicemen, and presumably these are the ones who provide the disproportionate number of noise traumas. Pure sensorineural data will thus contain a high proportion of cochlear disorders, hence making comparison with Palva's data approximately valid. As regards the point about "ears," since the aim of the present exercise is to correlate tonal thresholds from "sloping" and "flat" audiograms with SRT in listeners with sensorineural disorder, then it is the differential outcome (if any) of this analysis that is of key interest, even if the actual correlation values cannot be wholly relied upon.

"Pure" sensorineural cases were defined for present purposes as "ears" showing identical AC–BC levels at threshold or no more than 5 dB lower level at BC than at AC threshold and at no more than two frequencies. Not many cases of "flat" sensorineural audiograms are observable in the Harris et al. group—and the criterion of "flatness" has to be relaxed somewhat to achieve reasonable numbers. The composite audiogram of 14 cases is shown in Figure 6.2. While the composite is obviously uneven compared with the composite from 13 of Palva's cases, a common feature is the lack of any high frequency elevation beyond .5 to 2 kHz. Even so, this "flat" sample contains a certain "sloping" component and hence is less purely "flat" than Palva's. The observed SRT in the Harris et al. study was the 50% articulation score for the Rush-Hughes recording of W-22 PB monosyllables. Correlation (Spearman) between .5, 1, and 2 kHz tonal threshold average and this measure in the 14 cases was .66. In contrast, in a group of 36 pure sensorineural cases manifesting threshold elevation with rising audio frequency, correlation between SRT and tonal threshold was .77. The composite audiogram for

---

[6] Harris et al. were operating at that time out of a United States Navy medical research laboratory.

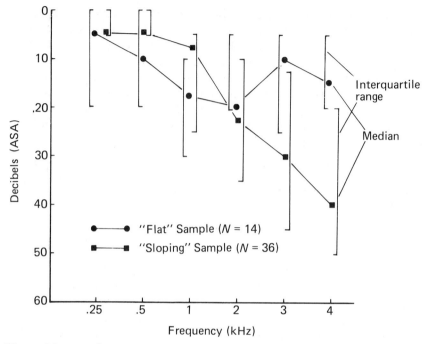

Figure 6.2. Data from Harris et al. (1956) of levels at threshold in two groups of listeners with sensorineural disorders. Tonal threshold–SRT relations separately analyzed to observe effect of audiogram shape, as in analysis of Palva (1952).

this group is also shown in Figure 6.2. The immediate features of interest emerging from this result are (a) a less than perfect relationship between the two measures in either sample; and (b) a different correlational outcome for the "sloping" as against the "flat" groups. No firm conclusion can be drawn from the latter finding as the somewhat higher correlation found in the "sloping" as against the "flat" sample goes quite against expectation (see, for example, Carhart, 1946b). However, the difference between the two coefficients (.66, .77) should not be emphasized unduly since the small N in the "flat" group, plus the slight "impurity" of that group from an audiogram-profile point of view, makes the correlational outcome in that case liable to sampling error. The outcome of more moment, one which can be relied upon, is the "sloppier" fit between the tonal and SRT data in either group. A relationship obviously obtains, but it is nowhere near the virtual identity observed by Palva. Results overall, in fact, conform more with those of Carhart. The obvious exception is the much higher correlation between .5, 1, and 2 kHz and SRT in the "sloping" sample than in Carhart's "marked high tone loss" sample. Once again, these two groups are not quite comparable since the sample extracted from the Harris et al. data contains "notched," "gradual," and "marked" cases and its composition is restricted to cases of pure sensorineural disorder.

What one is to make of the overall outcome remains uncertain. No consistent picture of tonal and SR threshold relations has emerged from research scrutinized thus far about cochlear disorder, particularly resulting from noise-induced hearing loss, and particularly affecting high frequencies. Obviously a relationship is there, but the precise conditions governing its manifestation are masked by confounding variables.

Harris *et al.* (1956) were not concerned with this sort of diagnostic question, even though they recognize that a purpose of the predictive exercise is to furnish evidence relating to the medicolegal issue (hence, by implication, evidence pertinent to those with noise-caused disorder, though Harris *et al.* do not make this point). These authors rather were concerned to test the predictive validity for SRT of various existing formulas derived from tonal threshold levels. Data from the 197 partially deafened "ears" were presented in three groups: those with a difference of at least 20 dB in AC threshold between .5 and 2 kHz ($N = 64$); those with a 15 dB difference ($N = 40$); and those with no more than a 10 dB difference ($N = 93$). This classification, which follows Fletcher's (1950), was made so that the predictive capability of each system on more and less unsymmetrical audiographic profiles could be observed. Statistic used was mean deviation of the differences between observed and predicted SRT. Note that this computation is different from mean absolute difference as it takes account of direction of difference. That is to say, the mean *arithmetic* difference between observed and predicted values is first calculated (i.e., accounting for sign) and the mean *arithmetic* difference from this mean is the mean deviation of the differences. Harris *et al.* examined the following predictive systems: Fowler's (1941, 1942); Fletcher's (1950, 1953); the Fletcher two-average and three-average systems; and an invention of the authors, "two-worst" (the average of the two higher levels at threshold of the three at .5, 1, and 2 kHz). A multiple regression analysis was also run on the .5, 1, 2, 4, and 6 kHz threshold data to find best overall fit between this average and observed SRT. From partial regression analyses, the weights applying to threshold at each frequency were then used as a predictive system.

One striking finding was that Fletcher's 1950 system, while as accurate as other systems in prediction of SRT in the third group of ears (no more than a 10 dB difference in AC threshold between .5 and 2 kHz), with a mean deviation of 6.6 dB, was grossly wide of the mark in the first group (the most unsymmetrical audiograms) with mean deviation of 16.8 dB. SRT was consistently underestimated in this latter group. The same was true of Fletcher's "two-average" system (mean deviation = 7 dB in Group 3; 13.9 dB in Group 1). Harris *et al.* note that Fletcher's 1950 system approximates the two-average system in that the more complex calculus is designed to highlight the two lowest levels at threshold in the .5 to 4 kHz range (which, in essence, means in the .5 to 2 kHz range). This result confirms Palva's (1952) observation.

Fletcher's (1953) system, which simply assigns weights to thresholds at octaves from .25 to 8 kHz, gave better predictions, with mean deviations of 6.9 dB in Group 1 and 6.5 dB in Group 3. The most consistently accurate system was that of Fowler (1942), with mean deviations of 6.4, 6.6, and 5.5 dB for Groups 1, 2, and 3, respectively. The "three-average" system gave mean deviations of 6.6, 7.3, and 6.3 dB, and the "two-worst" system gave 6.3, 7.1, and 6.2 dB. Fowler's 1941 system was applied only to Group 1 and was inaccurate (mean deviation = 9.5 dB). Fowler's 1942 system, whose rationale and validation had not heretofore been publicly demonstrated, is here given considerable support. The "three-average" system, previously validated in most situations by several authors, is once again shown to have good predictive validity. However, it is interesting that a system like Fowler's, in which 4 kHz plays a part, more accurately predicts SRT than the "three-average" from which 4 kHz of course is absent. This is most strikingly shown in Groups 2 and 3 where audiograms are relatively "flat" between .5 and 2 kHz then show considerable threshold elevations. In these two groups, Fowler (1942) predictions give mean deviations of 6.6 and 5.5 dB whereas the "three-average" gives values of 7.3 and 6.3 dB. Since it is the case that noise-induced disorder often shows relative lack of effect at .5 to 2 kHz and equally often a dramatic elevation above that range, a system like Fowler's seems more apt for these sorts of cases in predicting this sort of speech hearing performance.

Of course, the most accurate predictor of all was the one derived from multiple regression analysis. I comment at a later time on the multiple regression approach to this problem of predictive validity. It is sufficient at the moment to note that 25% of the weight applicable to different frequencies was assigned to 4 and 6 kHz. The data providing these weightings, remember, are from a mixed diagnostic group, but one with perhaps a larger than normal representation of noise trauma cases. It is of interest to note that in prediction of SRT for PB monosyllables the analysis reveals that so much weight should be given to frequencies higher than 2 kHz.

The study by Harris, Haines, and Myers is, from the present point of view, one of the most penetrating researches undertaken into relations between tonal and SR threshold. It shows without doubt that in a general population the two measures are closely connected. The detailed data presentation has also allowed different sorts of analyses to be made from the ones that interested the authors themselves and hence enabled us to show that subsamples within the population do not display the same level of agreement.

Further Study by Palva

In 1955, Palva reported an investigation of speech hearing ability of various groups. SRT was assessed in the manner described in the 1952 work. The main purpose of the study was to compare discrimination test results in ordinary, quiet test conditions and in background noise listening. We turn to this aspect of the study under the appropriate heading. The result of present interest is that individual tonal threshold data averaged over .5, 1, and 2 kHz and SRT assessed under ordinary test conditions are tabulated, allowing correlation analysis to be done on them. My analysis, using one ear only of each of 21 listeners diagnosed as having "perceptive" disorders, gives $r_s = .74$. Equally interesting is that 8 of the 21 listeners were diagnosed as having "acoustic trauma" or described as "noise workers." The latter (3 cases) show audiograms consistent with traumatic disorder, however. Correlation using one ear of these listeners between tonal average and SRT gives $r_s = .6$. The number of listeners is too small to allow any firm conclusions, but it is noteworthy that these results are quite different from the earlier ones reported by Palva (1952) and that they are also the first available data on persons specifically described as suffering noise-induced partial deafness.

Palva's two reports (1952, 1955) investigated relations besides that between tonal and SR thresholds. From about this period, in fact, we naturally see an increase in the use of "discrimination score" rather than "speech reception threshold" as the principal measure of speech hearing ability. The rationales of both these measures are discussed in Chapter 2. Many reports from the 1950s to the present continue to include SRT–tonal threshold comparisons, and some still examine that relationship exclusively; but the bulk of studies to be considered from this period will be reconsidered when discussion turns to DS–tonal threshold relations.

Further, this shift of research attention from SRT to DS means in some instances that analysis of SR and tonal threshold relations is sufficiently cursory to warrant no detailed description in this section. The study by Mullins and Bangs (1957), for instance, includes a minor analysis of SR–tone relations showing meager association between SRT and tonal threshold at 2 and 3 kHz (separately). That study figures more prominently in discussion of DS–tonal threshold comparison.

Quiggle, Glorig, Delk, and Summerfield

In the same year (1957), however, a study of major present interest was reported by Quiggle, Glorig, Delk, and Summerfield. Their aim was to find the best fit between SRT for disyllables (CID test W-1, CID recording) and tonal threshold using multiple regression analysis to obtain appropriate weights applicable to various audio frequencies. Recall that

Harris, Haines, and Myers the year before presented just such data (though using SRT for PB monosyllables). The populations of these two studies are different also. Quiggle *et al.* derived their equation from data obtained in right ears only of volunteer listeners, namely the 20–29-year-old group of males presenting for hearing tests at the 1954 Wisconsin State Fair ($N = 319$). Best fit by regression analysis was obtained between SRT and tonal threshold at .5, 1, and 1.5 kHz. Statistic was the standard error of estimate (se_{est}). The obtained se_{est} of 5 dB means that about two-thirds of observed SRT values lie within ±5 dB of predicted SRT and within ±10 dB (2 standard deviations) will lie about 95% of observed SRT values. The result of telling importance was the application of the equation to randomly selected samples of 30–39-year-old ($N = 40$) and 60–69-year-old ($N = 40$) listeners, also drawn from the 1954 Wisconsin State Fair sample. The se_{est} increased to 6.3 dB in the 30–39-year-old group and to 10.3 in the 60–69-year-old group. The authors rightly concluded that the predictive equation does not generalize to other samples, especially those greatly separated in age. Along with prediction of SRT using the multiple regression weightings, prediction was made in the two smaller samples using straightforward .5, 1, and 2 kHz average. The se_{est} by the latter means in the 30–39-year-old group was 7.7 dB and in the 60–69-year-old group was 10.5 dB. Hence, in these samples SRT for disyllables and .5, 1, and 2 kHz tonal average (one ear only) were not close.

This study exemplifies an important point. Multiple regression exercises naturally optimize, by intercorrelation analysis, whatever relationship obtains between measure X and measure Y *in the sample under consideration.* The regressions to obtain appropriate weights by audio frequency are, of necessity, dictated by whatever patterns of relationship within and between the measures happen to exist in the group being studied. By definition, these weightings cannot apply to other samples, because somewhat different patterns—caused simply by sampling variation—will obtain.

Notwithstanding the rather uncertain outcomes of this study, Quiggle *et al.* conclude from their own findings and from those of Harris *et al.* (1956) that "these observations are in complete agreement with the recommendation that 500, 1000 and 2000 cps adequately represent the 'speech' frequencies in calculations of speech disability due to hearing loss [p. 10]." This bold conclusion follows other revealing assertions. "The ear is most susceptible to noise-induced hearing loss at 3000, 4000 and 6000 cycles per second but these frequencies have no significant relation to the hearing *and understanding* of speech [p. 9; italics added]." The term *understanding* is an interesting one, appearing only once again in the authors' discussion. Throughout the paper, the authors emphasize the highly limited nature of disyllables (the material they used to test SRT) when it comes to representation of the speech of daily life. Further, they note that "most of the acoustic energy contained in spondee words is concentrated in the region of lower frequencies [p. 6]," and they go on to point out that, as regards multiple regression, "Different weights would be expected if one were predicting thresholds for samples of speech containing more energy in the high frequencies [p. 6]." Later there is the statement that "vowels are related to the sound power of speech, and consonants are related to the discrimination or *understanding* of speech [p. 10; italics added]." As every phonetician knows, the "sound power" of speech is largely to be found in the lower frequencies, the region mainly represented by disyllables, and consonants have energy throughout the spectrum, certainly well above 2 kHz.

Despite these fairly obvious contradictions, one could take it that Quiggle *et al.* felt justified in their conclusion by reference to the Harris *et al.* work using PB monosyllables. The time is not yet ripe for a major discussion of the nature of monosyllables and disyllables, but the former might be taken as more acoustically–phonetically representative of everyday speech than the latter.

Be that as it may, Harris *et al.* found that 25% of weight was required *beyond* 2 kHz for best fit multiple regression in their sample, and I calculated correlations of only .66 and .77 between .5 to 2 kHz tonal average and SRT in subsamples of pure perceptive hearing disorder drawn from their sample.

Were that not enough to make us pause before going along with the conclusion of Quiggle *et al.* (1957), their own data show only an awkward fit between observed SRT and that value predicted by .5, 1, and 2 kHz average. A proper conclusion then might be that SRT is most adequately predicted by .5 to 2 kHz but still *inadequately* represented by that prediction; and SRT in any case, certainly for disyllables, inadequately represents both everyday speech and everyday speech hearing ability.

A while back I mentioned a battle between advocates of different formulas for the prediction of "hearing loss for speech" (i.e., SRT). The battle has always been muted, and until very recent times, I would say, it has remained unobserved. The paper by Quiggle *et al.* represents a strong claim for use of .5 to 2 kHz. But it is not a solitary one: Harris *et al.* (1956) also support its use, though much less strongly. I think that in the Quiggle, Glorig, Delk, and Summerfield paper we witness the underlying reason for its advocacy. To repeat a passage from Quiggle *et al.* quoted earlier, "The ear is most susceptible to noise-induced hearing loss at 3000, 4000 and 6000 cycles per second [p. 9]." Years later, Glorig (1971) relates a story about an incident that occurred when he was a member of a labor–management committee in California deciding on what audiogram formula to use for compensation: "Management went along with the medical profession and said they wanted 500, 1000 and

2000 Hz used; but Labour, seeing the large losses at 4000, wanted 4000 Hz included [Glorig, 1971, p. 83]."

This is what the battle is really all about. Management (aided by the medical profession) wants to minimize its losses in noise deafness claims. Labor wants to maximize its gains. In this instance, we see "science" in the service of only one party to this dispute.

Miscellaneous Recent Studies

Two very interesting comments on all the foregoing are represented by the reports of Graham (1960) and of Quist-Hanssen and Steen (1960). Graham (1960) showed that Fletcher's "two-average" and "three-average" systems very closely correlated (.986; .981) with observed SRT in 100 listeners (one ear only) whose records he selected from those at the San Francisco Veterans Administration Hospital. Material for the speech test was presumably disyllables though no details are given. Graham comments that Quiggle *et al.* (1957) obtained similar though not so closely corresponding results. He goes on to comment that the Quiggle *et al.* formula, doing no better a job than the Fletcher two-average or three-average methods and being more arithmetically cumbersome, is somewhat redundant. In conclusion, he points out that high correlations notwithstanding predictions at the individual level will be considerably (i.e., at least ±10 dB) off target in 5% of cases (standard errors being ±4 to 5 dB in the major predictive systems he examined). This point is worth stressing. The purpose of prediction in the medicolegal, as opposed to the research, context is to allow an accurate assessment of handicap *in the individual case*. Unless the predictive system fairly accurately represents whatever is taken to be handicap *in every case*, then it cannot be valid for medicolegal purposes.

In relation to this point, Coles' (1970) argument with the present author is illustrative. Coles objected to my assertion that evidence was slight which showed a close association between tonal and speech tests, then stated: "While the relationship *was not as good as found among those with conductive lesions* there were *some overall rules*, and it was possible to use pure-tone thresholds as an indication of the *general level* of the speech communication handicap [Coles, in discussion of Noble, 1970, p. 75; italics added]." Precisely because there are only "overall rules" allowing estimates of "general level," because the relationship is untidy by comparison with what it might be, the prediction is too vague to allow justifiable use of pure tones in the legal context.

It is interesting to note the considerable discordance between Graham's analysis using the "two-average" and "three-average" systems and the results of Harris *et al.* (1956) using these same systems. Data are not directly comparable, as Graham uses se_{est} whereas Harris *et al.* use mean deviation—but it is clear that Harris *et al.* found much more discrepancy between observed and predicted SRT than Graham did. Graham considers that "functional hearing loss" has a contaminating influence on tonal–SR threshold relations. He calculates se_{est} with and without inclusion of such cases and shows an se_{est} of 12.2 between SRT and "three-average" prediction when "functional" cases are *included,* as against an se_{est} of 4.1 when they are *excluded.* It could be that Harris *et al.* had such "functional" cases in their sample, and this could explain the discrepancies they found. That cannot be the whole (hypothetical) explanation of the widely discrepant result, however, since differential outcomes for different systems were noted by Harris *et al.,* whereas presumably a "functional hearing loss" representation would foul up predictions across all systems, and this did not occur. We are left with an uncertain picture, therefore, regarding the merits of different predictive systems. The one point that should be mentioned is that the proportion of noise-induced disorder cases in the sample used by Harris *et al.* is probably higher than the proportion in Graham's sample.

As though to muddy up the picture thoroughly, Quist-Hanssen and Steen (1960) report results that agree with nobody else's. They compared predicted and observed SRT for various types of Norwegian speech material (Quist-Hanssen's lists—no reference given). Listeners were 27 boilermakers and aircraft pilots (age 27–61 years), and se_{est} between observed SRT for various speech materials and SRT predicted by various formulas produced the outcomes shown in Table 6.1.

TABLE 6.1

Results Obtained by Quist-Hanssen and Steen (1960) Showing Standard Error of Estimate, in Decibels, of SRT Predicted by Various Systems and for Various Speech Materials

	se_{est} (dB) of SRT for various speech materials			
Predictive system	Discourse	Monosyllables	Disyllables	Numerals
AMA (1947)	10.1	7.4	9.3	10.5
Harris *et al.* (1956)	9.6	6.5	8.8	9.9
Quiggle *et al.* (1957)	8.9	—	—	—

In all cases, prediction overestimated the SRT. We can conclude little from this result since the manner and material of speech testing is unknown. These data show, however, that generalization of results is nearly impossible; Quist-Hanssen and Steen's result is at odds with both Harris *et al.* and Graham. As to why disagreement in Quist-Hanssen and Steen's study should be so gross, no overall answer can be given. A partial answer is available and serves to illuminate a new feature of the whole tonal–speech interaction. Quite dramatic elevations in threshold are accompanied by only slight difficulty in speech hearing ability. The two cases cited to show this come from the sample of aircraft pilots. Comparison of the boilermakers and pilots as a whole shows far more overestimation by the AMA (1947) formula for the latter group. The authors consider that the pilots, more experienced in listening (no doubt through low-fidelity receivers or at least in poor acoustic conditions), are better able to detect speech signal information. Nor would one argue with this conclusion, though a motivational factor must surely be considered too, if these pilots were still active. What the result overall certainly shows is that nonauditory variables, such as job type, can interact in unexpected ways to confound relationships between tests of function.

Ward, Fleer, and Glorig (1961) conducted a most thorough study of the characteristics of noise-induced disorder. Their main concern was to investigate any qualitative differences between noise trauma induced by continuous noise and trauma induced by impulsive noise (they observed none to speak of); and part of the study involved assessment of tonal threshold and disyllable SRT. One ear only of each of 32 listeners was tested, and individual data were tabulated in the report. Listeners were police, including weapons trainers, and industrial workers, both groups exposed to high levels of both types of noise. Median age of the group was 37 years. A correlation (Spearman) by the present author between disyllable SRT (material unstated) and tonal threshold average at .5, 1, and 2 kHz gives $r_s = .695$.

These are the first substantial data on specifically noise-deafened listeners (Palva's 1955 data, it will be remembered, came from a very small number of people). But the correlation calculated on his data ($r_s = .6$) is similar to that on the Ward et al. (1961) data. Ward et al. might object to a correlation analysis of their data, as the listeners were selected from people showing a definite high-frequency threshold elevation and were also chosen from a younger age-group. Hence the data arguably are from a nonrepresentative sample of the noise-deafened population. The spread of data points is sufficiently dispersed so that restricted range effects are not creating a falsely loose correlational picture. Even acknowledging this point about the sample selection, one should note that these data, plus Palva's (1955), more closely represent the major population of interest than any other set published heretofore.

Whatever the strength of claims from studies in more heterogeneous samples about relations between tonal and speech thresholds, those rare reports on the people for whom this relationship is all-important do not, so far, lend substance to them.

The study by Ward et al. (1961) is a painstaking and more generally informative one about the characteristics of partial deafness due to noise. We will return to an extensive analysis of other aspects of their results at a later point in the chapter.

The study by Young and Gibbons (1962) mainly focuses on the tonal–

speech discrimination relationship: The Veterans Administration includes the latter test in its assessment-for-compensation program, and Young and Gibbons were interested to observe the extent of association between them. Part of the analysis included correlation between .5, 1, and 2 kHz tonal and SR thresholds (CID disyllables) in 100 men attending the Los Angeles Veterans Administration clinic. The sample, selected from a larger group, was screened to exclude people with suspected "functional hearing loss." A criterion for such suspicion was a difference in average .5 to 2 kHz tonal and SR thresholds of more than ±6 dB. The usual performance measures (delayed tone, Doerfler-Stewart, Stenger) were then run on these suspected cases. Young and Gibbons do not say what the exclusion rate was following this procedure, but obviously the initial selection is designed to reduce variability and hence increase the correlation between SR and tonal threshold at .5 to 2 kHz.

This should not be taken as critical of the Young and Gibbons design—their concern, as stated, was to study tonal–DS relations. Their procedure is mentioned because it helps explain the high (Pearson) correlations (.9 and .92) between tonal threshold at .5 and 1 kHz, respectively and SR threshold. It is mentioned too because it demonstrates one aspect of the faulty logic that the "functional hearing loss" concept brings in its train. The specific point to make here, as was made in reference to Carhart (1946c), is that discrepant patterns of audiometric response are taken as a sign of "functional hearing loss"—and some certainly will be; but nondiscrepant patterns are assumed, by what reasoning is unknown, to represent a genuine audiometric response. Despite the weeding-out process, correlation between 2 kHz tonal threshold and SRT was only .66.

In 1964, Siegenthaler and Strand analyzed data from 535 persons who had attended the Pennsylvania State University audiology clinic and received both tonal and one of a number of SRT tests. Data were separately analysed from 284 listeners tested with CID disyllables (W-2) and from 77 listeners tested with PAL disyllables. The study incorporated features of those by Harris *et al.* (1956) and by Carhart (1946b), in that the predictive validity of various formulas derived from the audiogram was examined as a function of audiogram shape—using Carhart's (1945) classification system. Correlation (Pearson) between calculated and observed SRT ranged from .8 to .9 in both of these larger groups of listeners. The relationship, although less consistent (.5 to .8) in the subgroups of listeners with "marked high tone loss," was closer than Carhart (1946b) observed. Of all systems, Fletcher's (1950) two-average was a consistently good predictor for most audiogram types and speech tests. Siegenthaler and Strand's (1964) work adds little to the body of information except to rescue Fletcher's two-average system, which had fared badly in the Harris *et al.* study. It is interesting too that Fowler's 1942 system fares poorly, whereas it had emerged strongly in the work of Harris *et al.* The major difference between the study by Harris *et al.* and that by Siegenthaler and Strand is that the latter authors used disyllables and the former used monosyllables. We have already, in discussion of Quiggle *et al.* (1957), referred to the lower frequency predominance in disyllables as compared with monosyllables. These results bear out the point.

Engelberg (1965) followed up Siegenthaler and Strand's work with a report on disyllable SRT prediction from records of 700 veterans attending the Cleveland Veterans Administration audiology clinic. By a complex process of inclusion and exclusion that could not be unraveled by this reader, Engelberg reports that his 700 cases produced a sample of 1434 records ("ears"). The vast bulk (93.7%) of SR thresholds lay within ±5 dB of *either* the "two-average" or "three-average" predictions. Engelberg notes that this mopping-up is considerably greater than that reported by anyone else using only one predictor. In those instances, ±5 dB is typically the standard error of estimate, hence catching only about 68% of differences. He does not seem to realize that by taking two bites of his data he is bound to improve the odds of getting agreement. The question is, *which* frequency average (2 or 3) will better predict SRT? In an individual case, "two-average" will produce a level of X dB, "three-average" will produce a level of $X \pm n$ dB. Which of these better predicts SRT? Engelberg can only reply, "Both"!

In Norway, Gjaevenes (1969) calculated a multiple regression equation from tonal thresholds at .5, 1, 2, and 3 kHz which best fit SRT for Quist-Hanssen's Norwegian PB monosyllables. The number of listeners is unknown, but there were 300 "ears"; 100 of each in the following diagnostic categories: conductive, cochlear, and presbycusis. Details of diagnostic procedure are not given. The se_{est} across all groups was 6.36 dB. The interquartile range of differences was 7.5 dB, compared with an interquartile range of 9.3 dB when the three-average was used to predict the SRT. Regression analysis has already been dealt with in this section. A feature of interest in Gjaevenes' study is that inclusion of 3 kHz improves the fit between monosyllable SRT and tonal threshold, compared with the "three-average" (.5 to 2 kHz) fit.

The most recent study of which I am aware of SR–tonal threshold relations is again a multiple regression analysis, reported by Carhart and Porter (1971). Audiogram shape is still a feature of this report. From records at the Northwestern University hearing clinic, the audiograms of almost 2000 clients were classified (somewhat roughly) into Carhart's (1945) groups, and multiple regression equations were run on these to achieve best fit with measured SRT (for locally recorded disyllables). It was found that two frequencies out of .5, 1, and 2 kHz in the "better ear" were optimal in first-order regression to achieve correlations of between .89 and .98 with SRT in the various audiogram groups. "Marked high tone loss" cases showed the lowest correlation.

These results are on a par with others obtained by regression analysis, but in audiographically as well as diagnostically heterogeneous groups. It is unfortunate that Carhart and Porter did not run their regressions controlling for both of these factors in turn.

Summary and Discussion

The reader will appreciate that we are only part way into the forest of tonal–speech predictive validity. Be that so, a summary statement is needed at this stage as a landmark before we proceed to a brief theoretical excursion into the nature of SRT for words, followed by our expedition into tonal–DS relations.

It seems that in a heterogeneous population, SRT for disyllables is predictable from average or weighted average tonal threshold in the .5 to 1 or 2 kHz region. That prediction will typically be erroneous by up to ±5 dB in 60–70% of cases. It will be erroneous by more than ±10 dB in 5% of cases. When monosyllables are used, frequencies higher than 2 kHz play an influential role. When a population is divided according to audiogram shape, SRT for disyllables is still predictable from frequencies in the .5 to 2 kHz region, but certain configurations, such as asymmetrical (rising or falling) audiograms, are less consistently associated in the .5 to 2 kHz range with SRT. Monosyllabic material has not been used in studies in which audiograms are classified by shape. If a population is divided according to diagnosis, the picture is much less certain. Cochlear disorder sometimes shows very close SR–tonal threshold association, sometimes not. Sensorineural disorder, as a broader category, has a similar showing. But no report *specifically* involving listeners with noise-induced hearing disorder has produced the high correlations between .5 to 2 kHz tonal and SR thresholds that are found in more heterogeneous groups. Typically, correlations in those sorts of samples are in the .6 to .7 region.

Assuming that this is a reliable finding (and results from "configuration" studies do not contradict the idea that it is), we nevertheless cannot firmly state why it should be so. The research considered in Chapter 8 and the discussion at the end of this chapter can illuminate the problem to an extent. Of more immediate theoretical concern is the place of SRT and that of monosyllables and disyllables in the assessment of speech hearing ability. The disyllable test was designed to provide a modulated low frequency energy contour. Familiarization of the listener with a small set of words helps reduce the "information content" in the signal; use of two equally stressed syllables gives the listener, in a sense, two chances to pick up the whole word message. Finally, the feature of uniform delivery in terms of loudness enhances the lower frequency vowel energy in the word. It could thus be said that the test is a contrivance which does no more than present lower frequency amplitude and frequency-modulated energy which the listener has simply to be able to detect in order to "comprehend." It could be argued further that the special qualities of speech, relying on discrimination of phonemes whose features and modulations cover a wider audio-frequency spectrum, are not being represented in the disyllable test. In addition, the uncertainties of speech, its unpredictability, are not fully represented by such a test.

In contrast, it might be argued that monosyllables delivered in "free" voice capture more of the essence of speech. Their greater consonantal content and lessened redundancy make them better substitutes for "everyday speech."

Finally, as regards the SRT itself for whatever material, the argument could be made that a 50% detection rate is nonrepresentative of daily life. We surely do not strive to listen in circumstances where only half the spoken message can be understood. Preference must be for a transmission system that broadcasts information at a comfortable level of listening—in which the bulk of the energy is well above SRT.

There is, notwithstanding, a case to be put that gives more credibility to the disyllable SRT than is apparent from the foregoing arguments. I admit that this case is based on hindsight, but it is a case all the same. We come to it in Chapter 10. In the final event, I think the SRT *is* insufficient as an everyday speech hearing measure, precisely because of all these arguments. But insufficiency is not to be equated with nonvalidity. The SRT for disyllables tells part of the everyday speech hearing story in its own limited code. The discrimination score tells another part. The whole story can only be told by the people themselves, but the exposition of that notion must wait until existing ideas and evidence are more radically reviewed.

TONAL THRESHOLD AND DISCRIMINATION SCORE

The nature of discrimination testing is detailed in Chapter 2. The only reminders needed here are that discrimination score (DS) is a measure of percentage of correct or incorrect identifications of a list of words (or their parts), either disconnected monosyllables or words of various syllable length embedded in sentences or words from a closed set of possible alternatives known to the listener. Discrimination score is obtained by presenting some sort of list at an acoustic level determined by the listener's SRT. Typically, DS is measured 25–40 dB above SRT, but variants of this procedure have been used, as we will see. Some authors measure the complete articulation (intelligibility) function, not simply DS at a single level above the SRT. In these cases, PB-max (the maximum DS obtained) or some integrated score may be presented.

Early Studies

Among earlier measures of discrimination (Fletcher & Steinberg, 1929) were sentences to be repeated or questions the listener had to answer, the answer's correctness being dependent on the listener's having successfully discriminated key words in the question. I am aware of no reported study relating tonal threshold with this earlier type of sentence discrimination. Fletcher and Steinberg (1929) also devised lists of monosyllables, and Fletcher (1929, p. 302) noted that monosyllable articulation functions of people with sensorineural disorder not only were shifted in terms of intensity like those of people with conductive disorder but also were distorted in shape. No investigation of tonal threshold–articulation function was carried out at that time. In fact, as far as I am aware, it was not until Steinberg and Gardner's small study (1940) that these two measures were looked at in juxtaposition.

Steinberg and Gardner used the Fletcher and Steinberg monosyllables to obtain articulation functions in three listeners with unilateral mixed disorder of hearing. These functions were relatively uniformly shaped compared with the normal function. It will be recalled from our earlier discussion of this paper that at the 40% correct identification point (SRT) the articulation functions were separated by amounts of intensity that fairly well matched the listeners' average tonal thresholds at .5 to 4 kHz. Other features of the articulation curves are tabulated along with tonal threshold and SRT data in Table 6.2.

TABLE 6.2

Calculated Values, from Figure 3 in Steinberg and Gardner (1940), for Tonal Threshold and Various Features of the Articulation Functions of Three Listeners

	Listener		
Tonal threshold	A	B	C
$\bar{x}$ .5– 4 kHz	46	64	77 dB (re: normal sample)
.5 kHz	48	48	58
1 kHz	50	60	60
2 kHz	45	85	85
4 kHz	37	60	100
SRT (40% correct identification)	49	55	76
PB-max (errors)	98 (2)	87 (13)	73 (27)%
DS at 30 dB re: SRT (errors)	95 (5)	87 (13)	72 (28)%

It can be seen that discrimination measures parallel the average tonal and speech threshold measures. It is interesting to note once again that 4 kHz tonal thresholds most clearly differentiate the three listeners and hence most closely match both expressions of the discrimination scores.

French and Steinberg (1947) published an important study of speech intelligibility and factors affecting it. In this paper they described the articulation index, a system for estimating the probable intelligibility of speech under various conditions of transmission. While they allude to the effect of individual differences in sensitivity as an obviously important variable in the calculation, they themselves did not examine discrimination as a function of tonal threshold; and it was not until many years later that MacRae and Brigden (1973) brought French and Steinberg's (1947) work to bear on the speech discrimination–tonal threshold issue.

The Steinberg and Gardner (1940) study is fairly limited, and it is discussed here simply because it probably represents the earliest such work. Siegenthaler (1949) made the first systematic investigation of discrimination as a function of audiogram type. Earlier, Walsh and Silverman (1946) had confirmed Fletcher's (1929) informal observation that listeners with a sensorineural component in mixed disorder and a higher frequency threshold elevation showed distorted articulation functions (asymptotic rather than sigmoid). Siegenthaler does not refer to that work, but his study nonetheless focuses on the feature of flat as opposed to unsymmetrical threshold profiles. Three groups of five listeners were tested: Group A with "flat" audiograms; Group B with marked elevation of threshold at 2 to 8 kHz; and Group C with thresholds in the "normal" range. The main speech material was pairs of monosyllables matched on all except one characteristic, such as *voicing*, (talk [tok]; dog [dog]) *attack* (see [si]; tea [ti]), and *consonant–vowel order* (bad [baed]; dab [daeb]). The third type produced differences in place of articulation of the vowel. Listeners were presented with one of the words from each pair (by monitored live voice) at +5 dB re: SRT; −5 dB re: SRT, and at SRT level. SRT was determined using monitored live-voice disyllables. Listeners had to indicate from written lists of each word pair, which of the pair had been presented over a loudspeaker. In addition, discrimination score for a scrambled list of all words in these pair groups was measured at ±5 dB re: SRT and at SRT level. Listeners in Groups A ("flat") and C ("normal") provided approximately similar results (though Group C had generally higher scores), but listeners in Group B showed considerably lower discrimination ability on all word lists except the voiced–unvoiced consonant pairs. This latter finding is explicable in the fact that voicing of consonants involves low frequency energy, so listeners with high levels at threshold in the higher frequencies would be able to distinguish the voiced–unvoiced difference by detecting or failing to detect the consonant component in the word.

Siegenthaler's (1949) study demonstrates that discrimination can be considerably affected in people who show high frequency threshold elevation but have little elevation of threshold in the .5 to 2 kHz range. Because types of audiogram rather than types of disorder formed the basis of subject selection, no firm conclusion can be drawn from these data about the latter.

Emergence of Systematic Studies

In Palva's (1952) study, already described in the previous section, is found the first readily available statistical study of tonal–DS relations. Correlation, using one ear only of listeners with cochlear disorder, between DS and .5 to 2 kHz tonal average yields an $r_s = .89$. This is a close relationship, though it contrasts with the near unity relation in Palva's tonal–SR data, suggesting therefore that DS is not so predictable as SRT from the audiogram.

In 1953, two nonstatistical reports appeared, one by Simonton and Hedgecock, the other by Cawthorne and Harvey. These two reports are relatively minor as regards the present purpose. In the Cawthorne and Harvey work, there is careful differentiation of listeners into diagnostic groups and measurements of the complete articulation function. But to our eternal frustration, only a few raw results are presented, nor is any statistical analysis performed by the authors. They conclude, however, that in cochlear disorder due to noise exposure and Ménière's disease there is no discernible relation between the tonal audiogram and the articulation function, measured using United Kingdom Medical Research Council PB words. By contrast, that function is fairly regularly related to tonal threshold in conductive disorder. Without the data, there is no way of scrutinizing results to see whether any nonobvious pattern of interrelationship between tonal and speech test results might be recoverable from them.

Simonton and Hedgecock (1953) at least present their data, even though they themselves make no numerical analysis of it. Simonton and Hedgecock, it will be recalled, reported tonal–SRT data, calculation on which provided a near unity outcome and thus supported, though from a somewhat differently composed sample, the result of Palva (1952). Features of present interest regarding tonal threshold–speech test results, which can also be extracted from their reported results, are given in Table 6.3.

Data are from a small sample representing various sensorineural disorders, but the fit between tonal threshold and DS (for PAL PB lists at the most comfortable listening level) is remarkably close. How representative the data are remains unknown as no details of how these cases were selected for presentation are given. However, one feature of inter-

TABLE 6.3

Correlation (r_s) Coefficients, Derived from Results of Simonton and Hedgecock (1953), between Tonal Threshold Averages and Various Speech Measures ($N = 11$)

	Speech test		
Tonal average	SRT	DS in quiet	DS in noise
.5, 1, 2 kHz	.98	.91	.81
.5, 1, 2, 4 kHz	.96	.97	.86

est is that .5 to 2 kHz average is very slightly closer than .5 to 4 kHz in prediction of PAL disyllables but drops to consistently lower levels than .5 to 4 kHz in prediction of DS for monosyllables. These data support the view that 4 kHz tonal threshold has an important role to play in people with sensorineural disorder when it comes to prediction of discrimination ability. The majority of Simonton and Hedgecock's cases show marked and sudden elevation of higher frequency threshold, hence these data bear out Siegenthaler's finding of poor discrimination associated with that sort of audiogram profile. But from both Cawthorne and Harvey's (1953) and Simonton and Hedgecock's results it is clear that people who do not display this configuration (as in Ménière's disease) also have poor discrimination. So audiogram shape is not the only guide to poor discrimination, though I argue later that it may be one route to such a problem—along with other, possibly independent routes. Another interesting feature of these data is that DS was assessed in high-level noise as well as in quiet conditions. This procedure is used by quite a few subsequent authors, and its various rationales need to be examined.

Simonton and Hedgecock, for example, wanted to find out whether airline pilots with minor degrees of sensorineural disorder would fare badly on discrimination in the noisy conditions typical of an aircraft cockpit. They found that high-level noise of this kind adversely affected listeners with bilateral cochlear disorder to a greater extent than listeners with either unilateral disorder, conductive disorder, or no disorder. Their data were insufficiently numerous, however, to allow firm conclusions.

Palva (1955), who also examined speech discrimination in a background of noise, was interested to find some means of differentiating within sensorineural disorders. Hood (1950) found abnormal loudness adaptation to noise in the affected ears of 20 of 25 listeners with unilateral Ménière's disease, whereas no such effect was evident in people with unilateral conductive disorder. Hallpike and Hood (1951) reasoned that this result was intimately connected with recruitment of loudness. Palva's (1955) view therefore was that ongoing noise, having an abnormal adaptation effect on recruiting ears, should affect discrimination to a greater extent than in nonrecruiting ears—because of increased masking of the lower-energy consonant sounds vital to the discrimination process. Palva was unaware of the work of Lansberg (1954) who reported that in people with noise-induced disorder, and hence rerecruitment, he could nevertheless find no sign of abnormal adaptation. He also reports that Langenbeck, in personal communication, got the same null result. This result is hard to reconcile with Hallpike and Hood's tie-up of recruitment of loudness with the abnormal adaptation effect. It certainly confounds Palva's attempt to distinguish recruiting from nonrecruiting ears in listeners, some of whom had Ménière's and some noise-induced disorder.

Two features of present interest in Palva's (1955) data are first, DS and tonal threshold measurements in a group of listeners with sensorineural disorder and in a group with conductive disorder. These data allow a quantitative substantiation of the asserted difference in discrimination between the two major types of lesion. Another feature of major present interest is of course the data concerning relations between tonal threshold and DS in the listeners with sensorineural disorder, especially in those with disorder induced by noise. It will be recalled that there were not many people in Palva's (1955) study with a diagnosis of noise deafness or a history of noise exposure. It is still worthwhile, however, to compare tonal threshold–DS relations with tonal–SR threshold relations in the same sample.

Both these features are given in Table 6.4. One ear only of each listener gives 20 observations for conductive, 21 for sensorineural disorder. It is evident that though conductive SRT is on average at a 15 dB higher level than sensorineural SRT, discrimination is only 7% as against

TABLE 6.4

Calculations on Palva's (1955) Data Showing (a) the Distinction between Conductive and Sensorineural Discrimination Ability; and (b) the Correlations between Tonal Threshold and DS in Sensorineural and Noise-Induced Cases (N = number of listeners)

	(a)			(b) Correlations	
	Conductive	Sensori-neural		Sensori-neural	Noise induced
N	20	21	N	21	8
Mean SRT (dB)	56	41			
Mean DS (%)	93	84	Tonal average		
			.5–2 kHz	.425	.264
			.5–4 kHz	.627	.425
			1–4 kHz	.617	.35
			1–8 kHz	.665	.4

16% impaired. The picture of conductive versus sensorineural disorder as regards the effect on discrimination ability is here verified.

The correlations also shown in Table 6.4 reveal an instructive pattern. Between .5, 1, and 2 kHz tonal average and DS under quiet listening conditions in the group of 21 listeners with sensorineural disorder, r_s = .425. When 4 kHz threshold is included in the average, this correlation increases; it remains similar when .5 kHz threshold is then removed from the average; and it increases further when 8 kHz threshold is then included. In no case is the correlation particularly close. The important outcome is that high frequency tonal threshold has an instrumental influence upon it. This pattern is maintained to some extent when correlations are run using one ear of each of the 8 noise exposure cases within the group. The relations are much weaker, but that is partly attributable to the restricted range of DSs in this subgroup. We cannot, in other words, take this result as indicative of relations between tonal threshold and DS in noise-induced disorder, but we can see that high frequency threshold is influential in this subgroup as in the larger group. We can conclude from both sets of results that tonal threshold and DS are not so well related in sensorineural disorder as are tonal and SR thresholds, since correlations between the latter were in the .65 to .75 range in these same samples.

The Effect of Recruitment versus Higher Frequency Threshold

I have not analyzed the data obtained by Palva in noisy listening conditions, as these were intended to provide a hoped-for differential fatigue effect. The noise level, therefore, was very high and unrepresentative of the sort of background noise encountered in most everyday speech hearing conditions. Subsequent authors have attempted to simulate everyday conditions, and it is more relevant to the present purpose to scrutinize their "noise" data than Palva's. It is worthwhile, however, to take a look at the recruitment effect. Recruitment allegedly has a malevolent influence on discrimination of speech. Palva found no differentiation of recruiting from nonrecruiting ears as far as discrimination shift in noise was concerned, and we have already discussed a possible reason why. In Chapter 8, we consider the recruitment phenomenon more critically; but it is appropriate to see what emerges here as regards the influence of recruitment. In other work discussed in this section, an alternative hypothesis regarding the discrimination difficulty of people with sensorineural disorder is examined, so it is fair to look at data that may illuminate the recruitment case.

Unfortunately, Palva does not publish his recruitment data as such but simply identifies listeners in whom it was complete and in whom it was totally absent. Of the 21 listeners, 13 showed complete recruitment and 8 showed none. Certain associated effects ought reasonably to be manifest in the first group but not in the second if recruitment really is a critical governor of discrimination difficulty. Most straightforward of these is a lower DS in the recruitment group than in the nonrecruitment. Of course one must be satisfied that the two groups are fairly matched otherwise.

A less obvious but still reasonable expectation would be a closer correlation in recruiting ears between discrimination difficulty and level at tonal threshold in those regions where recruitment is most likely to be manifest in Palva's sample, namely 1 to 4 kHz. This would be expected because where recruitment is manifest its degree is fairly regularly related to the level at tonal threshold (Hood, 1960). Hence the higher the level at threshold, the greater the degree of recruitment, and so by inference the greater the effect on discrimination. Obviously one cannot expect any correlation to be a true index of the relationship because it is unknown where recruitment was most manifest in each listener. Using 1, 2, and 4 kHz average fairly safely covers the major recruitment area, but is not refined enough to get a reliable gauge of the relationship. The critical outcome, however, is the comparison of that relationship in recruiting and nonrecruiting ears. The data relating to both these hypotheses are given in Table 6.5.

TABLE 6.5

Calculations on Palva's (1955) Data to Examine the Difference in DS and the Difference in DS–Tonal Threshold Correlation between Listeners with Sensorineural Disorder Showing and Not Showing Recruitment

	N	1–4 kHz average	DS average	r_s (1–4, DS)
Recruitment	13	30 dB	86.2%	.483*
No recruitment	8	37 dB	82.5%	.405

* $p < .05$.

We can see that trends are only partly in the direction favoring a recruitment hypothesis. The recruitment group show a slightly lower 1 to 4 kHz average threshold level and a slightly higher average discrimination score. Neither difference between recruiting and nonrecruiting groups is significant. The correlation data do support the recruitment hypothesis but not in any marked way. The first finding would be expected if recruitment had no special influence, the second suggests such an influence.

Mullins and Bangs (1957) reported results from 199 "ears" abstracted from 167 veterans attending the Houston Speech and Hearing Center in Texas. The original number of listeners was reduced in a screen for suspected "functional hearing loss" and absence of observable disorder, but Mullins and Bangs do not say how many people finally supplied the 199 "ears" in their correlational study. For this reason, the correlations reported cannot be taken as representing the actual level of association between the various measures used. The pattern of relationship is still informative, however.

Mullins and Bangs report correlations between percentage loss in DS for monitored live-voice PAL monosyllables at the listener's most comfortable listening level and a variety of other performance tests and indexes. Level at threshold at individual audio-frequencies (.25, .5, 1, 2, 3, and 4 kHz) as well as the .25 to 4 kHz average was correlated (Pearson) with DS. A recruitment measure was made, namely the range between level at threshold and level at the threshold of discomfort at .5, 1, 2, 3, and 4 kHz. An index of intra-aural masking was calculated on the assumption that higher frequency threshold elevation signifies masking of the less audible higher frequency speech components by louder lower frequency components. The AC–BC gap at each frequency from .25 to 4 kHz was also correlated with DS, and the DS–SRT relation was calculated. Finally, the five highest coefficients were pooled for a multiple correlation with DS.

The overall outcome was that relations between each measure and DS were negligible to medium. Average tonal threshold correlated at .279, with individual frequencies ranging from −.144 (.25 kHz) to .467 (3 kHz). The masking index (over .5 to 2 kHz) gave the highest result, $r = .506$. The index involved subtraction of level at threshold for the frequencies below each frequency in turn—hence an increasing elevation of threshold through .25 to 2 kHz correlated most "closely" with DS in this study.

The AC–BC gap correlations ranged from −.138 to −.315. Negative correlations are the expectable outcome here since deterioration of DS was the discrimination measure, so it would be expected that such loss would increase with decreasing AC–BC gap. The recruitment measure ranged from −.113 to .084. SRT correlated at $r = .362$. Multiple correlation with DS using SRT, 2 and 3 kHz tonal threshold, masking index at .5 to 2 kHz, and AC–BC gap at .5 kHz yielded a value of .873. When AC–BC gap was omitted, the multiple correlation was .716. The authors regard this latter as the more reliable value, since the AC–BC gap result was negative and apparently inclusion of negative correlation values in an otherwise positive correlation matrix spuriously improves the multiple correlation picture.

The information to be extracted from this study is that higher frequency tonal threshold and a sloping audiographic profile seem more influential than lower frequency tonal threshold or the occurrence of recruitment in affecting speech discrimination. But it is also evident from this study that speech discrimination fits very loosely with other test results. Not enough is known about the diagnostic composition of the group (age levels and so on), but presumably it is the usual "veteran mix." The results are discordant with those of Palva (1952) and more in accord with those of Palva (1955).

The study by Ward et al. (1961) has already been mentioned in the section on tonal–SR threshold relations. Listeners were 32 men with a history of substantial exposure to high-level noise. Two measures of discrimination were used in this study: DS for PB monosyllables (origin unstated) and a highly complex consonant-confusion test. The latter test represents a rather unhappy marriage of Fairbanks' (1958) rhyme test principle with more easily confusable consonants, as derived from data by Miller and Nicely (1955).

Two groups of listeners were involved—16 policemen (including weapons trainers) and 16 industrial workers. The two groups were closely matched for the purpose of the study, which was to find out whether any differences could be observed between people habitually exposed either to impulsive or to continuous noise. The two groups showed no difference in response to a large battery of audiological tests except for the two tests of discrimination. In both of these, the police sample showed significantly less impairment than the industrial sample. The authors point to the observed difference in educational level between the two groups as perhaps the reason for this difference. The evidence they adduce from the consonant-confusion test data of the two groups to rule out any other explanation is not altogether clear. In addition, an argument in terms of educational level, which implies different familiarity with the more obscure words of the consonant-confusion test, may be supportable, but it cannot be extended to the words in PB lists. These were designed originally (see Chapter 2) to comprise highly familiar words.

One hesitates to put forward any alternative explanation for the difference. It would be wisest to have results comparing listeners exposed to impulsive (as against continuous) noise in whom educational as well as other variables were matched. Meantime, it might be considered as a possibility, and one I advocate in detail presently, that since policemen are engaged in jobs with a high listening demand they may have an enhanced ability to perceive isolated words in unfamiliar settings. This sort of effect was observed by Quist-Hanssen and Steen (1960) in comparing aircraft pilots and boilermakers.

Whatever the explanation, this outcome is both instructive and somewhat unfortunate. It is instructive in showing that extraneous nonaudiological factors may operate differentially to affect speech discrimination ability in otherwise matched groups. It means, unfortunately, that speech discrimination results from the industrial and police samples must be analyzed separately. The latter requirement has its positive aspect, though, in permitting the consistency of correlation between speech discrimination and other test data to be observed between one group and the other.

A test of recruitment (Alternate Monaural Loudness Balancing) was included in the Ward et al. study, and again we have opportunity to compare the recruitment case with a case based on tonal threshold level.

The PB monosyllables used to measure DS were given at 40 dB above the listener's SRT and the consonant-confusion test was administered at four levels above SRT (10, 20, 30, and 40 dB). Tonal threshold was determined at 8 audio frequencies (.5, 1, 1.5, 2, 3, 4, 6, and 8 kHz). A first approach to the analysis involves computation of correlations between each tonal and speech variable (error rate). As this provides 40 coefficients for each of the two groups of listeners, it is probably simpler to present results schematically as a set of line diagrams. Data are also tabulated (Table 6.6) as a reference. In Figures 6.3–6.5, coefficients for tonal threshold–DS (errors) and tonal threshold–consonant-confusion (errors) correlations are presented.

TABLE 6.6

Correlation Coefficients (r_s), Calculated from Ward, Fleer, and Glorig's (1961) Data, between Tonal Threshold and Various Speech Discrimination (Error) Measures in Two Groups of Listeners with Noise-Induced Disorder

Test	Frequency (kHz)							
	.5	1	1.5	2	3	4	6	8
Police and weapons trainers								
DS monosyllables								
40 dB re: SRT	−.008	.183	.512**	.717*	.736*	.017	−.259	−.267
Consonant-confusion								
40 dB re: SRT	.471**	.297	.352	.636*	.393	.5**	.244	.186
30 dB re: SRT	.079	.161	.530**	.752*	.571**	.473**	.073	.125
20 dB re: SRT	.191	.21	.469**	.707*	.558**	.509**	.148	.150
10 dB re: SRT	−.339	−.2	.221	.487**	.35	−.001	−.343	−.306
Industrial workers								
DS monosyllables								
40 dB re: SRT	.094	−.024	.529**	.749*	.683*	.419	−.035	−.041
Consonant-confusion								
40 dB re: SRT	−.076	−.246	.523**	.406	.535**	.604*	.583**	.430**
30 dB re: SRT	−.323	−.324	.358	.254	.532**	.265	.434**	.225
20 dB re: SRT	−.313	−.311	.072	.046	.211	−.034	.204	−.029
10 dB re: SRT	−.237	−.357	.384	.56**	.724*	.454**	.449**	355

* $p < .01$.
** $p < .05$.

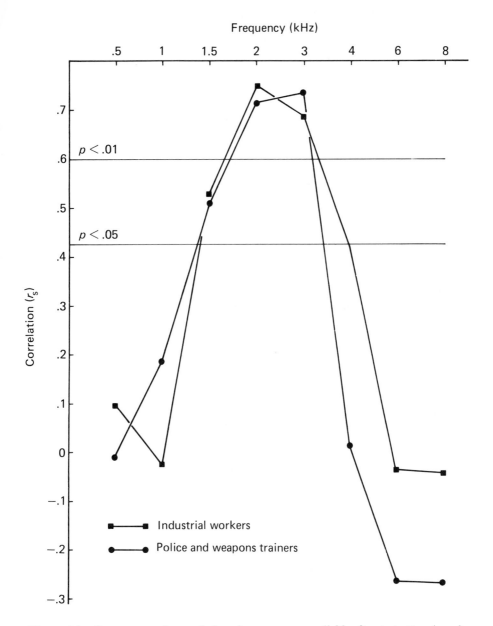

Figure 6.3. Spearman rank correlations between monosyllable discrimination (error) scores at 40 dB re: SRT and tonal threshold levels at individual frequencies in two groups of listeners (N = 16 in each group). Data from Ward *et al.* (1961).

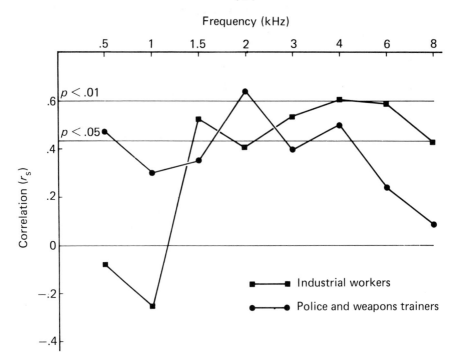

(a)

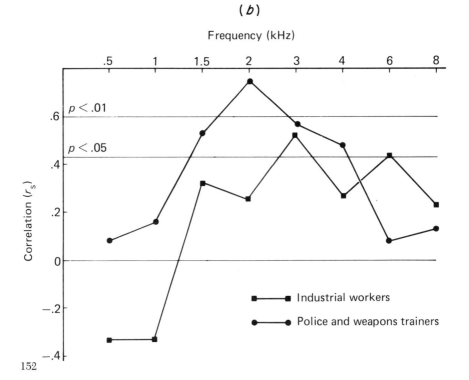

(b)

The feature of most importance is that the significant relations between speech and tone measures are in the 2 to 3 kHz region, with involvement of 1.5 and 4 kHz in some instances. Frequencies above and below these levels figure hardly at all. This result bears out the finding of Mullins and Bangs (1957). As with their study, data should not be regarded as providing a definitive estimate of the association between the two types of test. In the present instance, this is because small numbers and a somewhat restricted range will produce unevenness in the data. The *pattern* of association is the critical element and can be relied on.

Other features of interest in the results are (*a*) the trend toward involvement of thresholds at higher audio frequencies in the consonant-confusion–tonal threshold than in the DS–tonal threshold picture; and

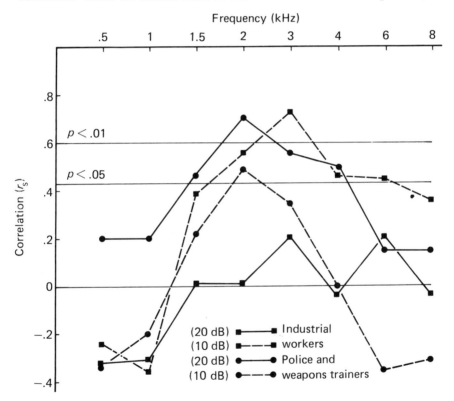

Figure 6.5. Spearman rank correlations between consonant-confusion (errors) at 20 dB (SRT) and 10 dB (SRT) and tonal threshold in Ward *et al.* (1961), two groups of listeners.

Figure 6.4. (*a*) Spearman rank correlations between consonant-confusion (error) scores at 40 dB re: SRT and tonal threshold in Ward *et al.* (1961), two groups of listeners. (*b*) Correlations between consonant-confusion (errors) at 30 dB (SRT) and data from Ward *et al.* (1961), two groups of listeners.

(b) the difference in relational pattern between the two groups of listeners. The tendency is for consonant-confusion data from the industrial sample to show the higher frequency effect to a greater extent than data from the police sample, with a contrary trend, namely more lower frequency involvement, in the data pattern from the latter group.

These trends are reflected to some extent in correlational analysis (Table 6.7) of various tonal averages against both DS and consonant-

TABLE 6.7

Correlation Coefficients (r_s), Calculated from Ward et al. (1961), between Various Tonal Averages and Discrimination and Consonant-Confusion Error Scores

Tonal average	Police and weapons trainers		Industrial workers	
	DS	Consonant-confusion (40 dB)	DS	Consonant-confusion (40 dB)
.5, 1, 2 kHz	.449**	.422	.627*	.142
1, 2, 3 kHz	.716*	.520**	.757*	.465**
1.5, 2, 3 kHz	.758*	.550**	.765*	.461**
1.5, 2, 3, 4 kHz	.653*	.574**	.728*	.563**
2, 3, 4 kHz	.702*	.581**	.754*	.527**

* $p < .01$.
** $p < .05$.

confusion at 40 dB re: SRT. We see in Table 6.7 that all averages are significantly associated with DS, but those involving 1.5 and 3 kHz show closest associations. By contrast, those involving 3 and 4 kHz show closest associations with consonant-confusion (40 dB). In the latter comparison, closer association is achieved in the industrial group by inclusion of 4 kHz, whereas in the police group association is roughly the same whether 4 kHz is included or not. And while there is no relation between consonant-confusion and .5, 1, and 2 kHz average in the industrial sample, there is a slight association in the police sample.

The first and most obvious point is that higher frequency tonal threshold is critically influential in speech discrimination in these samples of people with noise disorder. It is worth mentioning, too, that the finding by Ward et al. of no apparent differences between their two groups of listeners may have been premature. It is clear from Figures 6.3 through 6.5 and Tables 6.6 and 6.7 that a fairly consistent relational difference emerges from the present analysis.

The relational difference between the two groups may well underscore the hypothesized reason given earlier for their different levels of speech test performance. French and Steinberg's (1947) work and much subsequent study have shown that quite drastic frequency distortion is required to affect speech intelligibility. Licklider and Pollack (1948) showed that complete removal of frequency–intensity transitions nonetheless did not render speech totally unintelligible. However, these authors noted quite a marked practice effect. This latter point is critical in considering speech processing. Harris (1960) discusses the multiplicity of information sources in speech such that removal of a single source does not make the signal irretrievable. But he overlooks the social–occupational variables that must differentially constrain opportunity to maximize use of the information in these alternative sources. Since practice has a demonstrable effect, variable opportunity for such practice will produce different levels of success at listening in the everyday world. If we can apply all this to the Ward et al. (1961) samples, the account we come up with is that the police group, with occupational opportunity (even necessity) to practice at listening, will learn to use lower frequency information to retrieve the speech message. The industrial group, performing a different role, will not learn to use these clues to the same extent. Variable constraints of this kind are reflected in the different speech–tonal threshold interrelationships observed across the two groups. Since there are no pathological differences between them, this explanation for the relational difference has some force; and it gains further weight when we note that the relational difference is much more marked for the unfamiliar words of the consonant-confusion test compared with the difference in relations on the highly familiar words of the PB lists.

The fundamental implication of this sort of finding, whether or not the foregoing interpretation is accurate, is that assessment based solely on threshold sensitivity cannot reveal the sorts of effects shown in the correlation analysis. I show in Chapter 11 how another information source, lip-reading, is subject to the same sort of extrinsic influence as seems to be operating here. It could also be that the kind of influence I suggest here is at work to help produce the quite inconsistent results between tonal threshold and discrimination score not only within but between samples.

Finally, there is the recruitment measure to consider. As is evident from the results in Table 6.8, this measure bears no relation to any of the speech discrimination measures.

The "Filter" Hypothesis and Cue Reduction

As I mention earlier, recruitment is discussed in detail in Chapter 8. It is worthwhile including it here because other explanations for speech discrimination difficulty have been supported by authors concerned only with the tonal threshold–discrimination relationship. One such explanation is tied in with higher frequency threshold elevation, a common

TABLE 6.8

Correlation Coefficients (r_s), Calculated from Ward et al. (1961), between Recruitment Assessed by AMLB and Speech Discrimination

	Police	Industrial workers
DS	.079	.015
Consonant-confusion		
40 dB	.031	.301
30 dB	−.321	.28
20 dB	−.212	.324
10 dB	.26	.274

audiographic accompaniment to noise-induced disorder. The precise terms of this explanation are varyingly presented. French and Steinberg (1947) advanced the notion that high frequency threshold rise has the same effect as a low-pass filter. However, as mentioned in the last section, low-pass filtering has to be quite severe before any effect on discrimination for sentence or other connected material is apparent to normally hearing listeners. And yet, as Harris, Haines, and Myers (1960) point out, people with high frequency threshold elevation nowhere as restricted as the filtering required in the latter experimental conditions report considerable difficulty in understanding everyday communication. And presumably everyday communication is approximated by sentences or other connected discourse.

Harris et al. (1960) therefore approach the issue from a different standpoint. They reason that everyday speech signals, being highly redundant, can yet be interpreted by a person with good hearing in some part of the speech spectrum. If, however, the speech is itself distorted in some way, muffled, interrupted, or presented rapidly or in competitive conditions, then a person with higher frequency threshold elevation is more susceptible to this reduction in the cues physically presented to the auditory system. Harris (1960) confirmed Licklider and Pollack's (1948) finding that a variety of sources of distortion of speech signals when presented singly result in little reduction in intelligibility for normally hearing listeners but that combinations of two or more types of distortion have a marked effect. It therefore follows that if elevation of higher frequency threshold can be considered a source of frequency distortion then introduction of another type of distortion to the speech signal itself should have a marked effect. From pilot experiments it was found that the combination of fast word rates plus low-pass filtering produced a deleterious effect, thus supporting the above point.

Armed with this paradigm, Harris et al. (1960) assessed the speech discrimination ability of listeners with high frequency rises in threshold at different frequency "cutoff" points. The material used was interrogative sentences of an everyday colloquial nature recorded several times by the same speaker, who varied his word rate on each recording. The sentences were designed along the lines of Fletcher and Steinberg's (1929) but requiring less searching knowledge of the listener in order to get the correct answer (alternative answers were supplied on a checklist for the listener's reference). The lists were tried on a group of normally hearing people, and it was observed that increasing word rate was associated with a slight falloff in performance. When the sentences were given to people with even marked threshold elevations starting at 4 kHz and higher, the same outcome occurred. But in listeners with elevations of threshold starting at 3 kHz, a considerable performance decrement was observed at the faster word rates. This effect was more obvious still in listeners with elevations starting at 2 kHz. Scattergrams of threshold level at 3 kHz and 2 kHz against discrimination impairment at the fastest word rate in the respective groups showed a fairly regular positive relationship.

Harris *et al.* (1960) do not wish to invoke a filtering explanation as such for their result; they prefer to talk of cue reduction and loss of redundancy. While I have no wish to quarrel with that conclusion, it is nonetheless fair to say that their result does not deny a filtering hypothesis. I do not want to sidetrack the narrative at this stage to consider reasons for discrimination impairment. We will discuss possibilities once all relevant data are presented; but data that bear directly on the finding of Harris *et al.* come once again from Ward *et al.* (1961), and they are data, furthermore, that could certainly be used to advance a "filtering" argument. Ward *et al.* noted the cutoff frequency on the audiograms of their noise-exposed listeners. The range of such frequencies was from 1.7 to 3.9 kHz. This range is insufficiently broad to allow complete comparison with the Harris *et al.* study, but two analyses are permitted: (*a*) correlation of both DS and consonant-confusion with cutoff frequency; and (*b*) comparison of DS and consonant-confusion between listeners with cutoff frequencies above or below 3 kHz. The former analysis needs to be done separately for the two groups in the Ward *et al.* study, for the same reason as before, and the latter analysis depends on the outcome of the former. Obviously, a nonrelation or low-level correlation between cutoff frequency and discrimination will also likely mean no major difference in discrimination performance between higher and lower cutoff subgroups.

The correlations between cutoff frequency and DS are .649 in the industrial sample and .719 in the police sample. Correlations between cutoff frequency and consonant-confusion at 40 dB (SRT) are lower, at .566 and .317, respectively. Pooled data from all 32 listeners show that the average number of errors in DS in the subgroup with cutoff at and above 3 kHz ($N = 15$) is 3.8 whereas in the subgroup with cutoff below 3 kHz ($N = 17$) the average is 10. This difference is highly significant (Mann–Whitney, $p < .005$). A significant difference, but less marked is apparent in errors on the consonant-confusion test between the two cutoff groups (at or above 3 kHz, 6.7 errors; below 3 kHz, 9.5 errors. Mann–Whitney, $p < .025$).

In the Harris et al. (1960) study, listeners had reportedly no material threshold elevation at frequencies below the critical cutoff points. In the Ward et al. (1961) sample, there were of course different elevations in threshold level up to 2 kHz, hence the cutoff effect might be mediated by this variable. This is feasible since a certain degree of relation exists between .5 to 2 kHz average and DS in both groups (see Table 6.7). The mediating effect is not probable regarding cutoff–consonant-confusion relations since the association between .5 to 2 kHz threshold and consonant confusion is minor (see Table 6.7). Partial correlations run on the two samples to find the relation between cutoff frequency and DS, with .5 to 2 kHz threshold level controlled for, gave negligible variations in the original coefficients (changes of $-.008$ and $.029$ in the industrial and police groups, respectively). Hence it can be fairly safely concluded that cutoff frequency is directly associated with DS in these samples.

The important observation from this analysis is that DS was measured under nondistorted conditions, and the outcome is indeed remarkably similar to the filtering effects for the same speech material (monosyllables) noted by French and Steinberg (1947). Since no other source of distortion was introduced, an explanation in terms of filtering is quite feasible. This is not at odds with the conclusion of Harris et al. (1960). It is presented to show that a single distortion source originating in the auditory system can affect discrimination for undistorted speech. Furthermore, the type of effect suggests a mechanism akin to acoustic filtering. Sher and Owens (1974) have presented results which confirm this point. These authors found discrimination difficulty among listeners with threshold elevation at 2 kHz and above comparable to that found among listeners receiving speech through a 2 kHz low-pass filter. It should be noted, however, that the former group showed more variable performance than the latter, suggesting mediatory influences of the kind already discussed.

One flaw in this thesis is prompted by analysis of yet another set of data from the limitless warehouse of the Ward et al. report. They calculated the threshold trace slope at the frequency cutoff point in terms of decibels per octave. It might be expected (and the data on intra-aural masking of Mullins and Bangs (1957) suggest) that in a pure filtering situation a sharply sloping filter "skirt" would show a more pronounced effect than a shallow one. Hence there should be an interaction between slope and DS which confounds the relation between cutoff frequency and

DS. Partial correlation of DS–cutoff frequency, controlling for slope, had little effect, however, reducing the coefficient in the industrial sample from .649 to .634 and increasing the coefficient in the police sample from .719 to .730. Thus a variable that might be expected to influence cutoff–DS relations if a "filter" hypothesis were to be strongly supported does not in fact seem to do so. There may be additional postulates that can get around this anomaly to save the filtering hypothesis. In the final event, however, the hypothesis probably has only an operational strength rather than an explanatory one.

I suggested earlier that audiogram shape may be only one of several routes to lowered discrimination ability. Data from people with sensorineural disorder but displaying uniform threshold elevation as a function of frequency also show poor discrimination. A brief report bearing out this very point was made by Thompson and Hoel (1962). Listeners with "flat" audiograms (varying by no more than 10 dB between any test frequency) and sensorineural diagnosis (no more than 10 dB AC–BC gap) showed a regular reduction in DS (CID monosyllables) with increasing tonal threshold level. No individual data are given, unfortunately, only averaged results from different subgroups arranged by increasing threshold level. But the point to be made is that the shape of the audiogram is no criterion of discrimination difficulty or the lack of it.

"The Battle of the Frequencies"

Young and Gibbons (1962) carried out an extensive comparative study of tonal threshold and DS for recorded CID monosyllables. This study was conducted among veterans who had been assessed for compensation, and its purpose was to discover the predictability of DS from tonal threshold data and vice versa. Three independent analyses were made, and the results are of course centrally relevant to our purpose in that listeners were virtually all people exposed to noise.

The first analysis was a correlation study of tonal threshold at .5, 1, 2, and 4 kHz; SRT; and DS. Records of 100 people (aged 21–60 years) were abstracted, and in half of these the "better" ear was used, in the other half the "worse" ear ("better" and "worse" being determined by DS). The range of performance responses was very wide, and no one in the sample showed evidence of exaggerated test performance.

The correlations (Pearson) between DS and .5, 1, 2, and 4 kHz were .36, .48, .65, and .45, respectively, a result that partly agrees with earlier findings, particularly as regards the influence of 2 and 4 kHz threshold on DS. Multiple correlations between DS and various combinations of 2 other test results did not produce any closer fit of the data than the best relation shown above.

In the second analysis, records were searched to find cases closely matched in terms of DS within three distinct ranges: 92–96%; 80–84% and 68–72%. There were 125 records used altogether, 50 in each of the first two DS groups, 25 in the third. The purpose of the analysis was to observe the dispersion of other test data, given the restriction of DS range. The overlap was considerable, and indeed between the groups with DS = 80–84% and DS = 68–72%, the only statistically significant differences from my calculation were in tonal threshold at 2 kHz ($t = 5.1; df = 73, p < .01$) and at 1 kHz ($t = 2.29; df = 73, p < .05$). Young and Gibbons, however, report a t value of 2.59 derived from the smallest of the observed differences in performance between these two groups, namely, at .5 kHz. Present calculation from means and standard deviations in their published table (p. 28) does not confirm this result. Be that as it may, the data themselves show that distinctness of DS is not accompanied by distinctness of other test data.

Their third analysis was the corollary of the second. The DS records of 50 people showing levels all within 0 to 5 dB at .5 kHz and within 50 to 55 dB at 2 kHz tonal threshold were abstracted. Their DSs ranged from 70 to 96% with standard deviation, based on present visual inspection of the middle two-thirds of scores, of ±7%. Clearly a considerable spread of data from listeners with identical audiograms.

Young and Gibbons not surprisingly conclude that DS is only vaguely related to threshold measures and can by no means be predicted from them. Their analysis in the second and third parts of the study certainly bears out the point most clearly and shows the value of other ways of studying data apart from correlation or predictive calculation. For it is rare in a research report to find a given variable held constant so that the variance of the independent factor can be clearly seen.

Kryter, Williams, and Green (1962) reported on a mammoth study involving linear and multiple correlation between tonal threshold at .5, 1, 2, 3, 4, and 6 kHz and speech discrimination measured using recorded PAL monosyllables and sentences. Speech material was presented under the usual conditions, as well as through a 2 kHz low-pass filter and at various signal-to-noise ratios. Listeners were 114 male servicemen. Composite audiograms show that the bulk of listeners had high frequency threshold elevation at 2 kHz and above, and from clinical examination the authors concluded that nearly all with "significant hearing loss were suffering a permanent, predominantly nerve-type of deafness, presumably due to exposure to intense gun and vehicular noise [p. 1218]." For the purpose of linear and multiple regression analysis, listeners with no deviation in threshold below the "normal" range were excluded, leaving 162 "ears." This feature of the study is unfortunate since both ears of each listener were used independently in correlation analysis and thus the actual values obtained cannot be taken as a reliable guide to relations between tests. However, the pattern of relationship can be relied upon as that pattern would have emerged whether data from one or both ears of each listener had been used for correlation.

An important aspect of the speech test administration is that all material was at fixed output levels. Palva (1955) initiated this procedure when testing DS in a constant high-level noise. This departure from the usual practice (which is to estimate DS at a level fixed according to the listener's SRT) is worth commenting upon. Indeed, it is odd that neither Palva nor Kryter *et al.* take time out to discuss it. The original purpose in assessing DS somewhere between 25 and 40 dB re: SRT was to check whether speech at a level that ordinarily should be almost fully comprehensible is indeed so. Departures from almost 100% DS at 40 dB (SRT) indicate that discrimination is impaired. However, it can be argued that in listeners in whom it is presumed a discrimination problem exists a fixed output level makes sense. If it is also known that almost no conductive element is involved in the disorder, then the procedure is sensible, for under these conditions a similar input to the cochlea will occur for all listeners (within the variability of antecochlear structures).

The further point might be made that listeners with impaired hearing suffer handicap in everyday life because they cannot arrange to hear at levels appropriate to their SRT. Hence it is arguably more realistic to find out how people fare with a fixed signal rather than with one that is amplified to meet their requirements. It can be seen immediately, of course, that both of these conditions prevail in daily life. Sometimes one is stuck with a less than adequate signal level, and sometimes one can manipulate the level or the prevailing conditions to make the message more intelligible.

As it turns out from the Kryter *et al.* study, their procedure did not produce a pattern of results much at variance with those of either Mullins and Bangs (1957), who presented speech at the listeners "most comfortable listening level," or Ward *et al.* (1961), who presented it at 40 dB re: SRT.

No marked difference in relational pattern was observed by Kryter *et al.* between tonal threshold and different speech tests–test conditions. The average correlations between DS over all tests and tonal threshold in $N_{ears} = 162$ were

Frequency (kHz)	.5	1	2	3	4	6
Correlation	.31	.48	.76	.75	.62	.39

In listeners with high frequency threshold rises at and beyond 3 kHz ($N_{ears} = 71$), the correlations were lower than these, and 3 and 4 kHz thresholds showed the only significant associations (.443 and .434). There was no separate analysis for listeners with threshold rises at 2 kHz and above, so direct comparison with my analysis of the Ward *et al.* results is not feasible. But the two sets of correlations nicely bracket the set given for DS–tonal threshold from Ward *et al.* in Table 6.7.

Kryter *et al.* (1962) from this and multiple regression analysis concluded that the average threshold at 2, 3, and 4 kHz (or 1, 2, and 3 kHz as a compromise) was the most reliable guide to speech hearing ability in people with noise disorder. These authors recognize that SRT is best predicted by .5, 1, and 2 kHz average but challenge the validity of SRT as a measure of everyday speech hearing. They argue that sentence intelligibility particularly is surely a more valid guide to everyday speech conditions.

It is instructive to note what happened following the publication of Kryter *et al.* (1962). Webster (1964) took considerable care to undermine their recommendation to modify the then (and now) current averaging procedure of .5, 1, and 2 kHz recommended by AAOO. One particularly noteworthy observation made by Webster is that the Kryter *et al.* (1962) data are unrepresentative, being only from people with noise-induced disorder. Consequently the data show a restricted range effect at .5 and 1 kHz which naturally depresses the correlation in that region. By contrast, Webster asserts, Harris *et al.* (1956), studying a heterogeneous population, were able to show the significance of .5 to 2 kHz. The fact is, of course, that Harris *et al.* gave not inconsiderable weight (25%) to the 4 and 6 kHz threshold combination in their best-fit equation. Leaving that aside, the gist of Webster's criticism of the Kryter *et al.* recommendation is that it would be invalid for any but noise-induced cases, whereas the aim of the AAOO formula is to "encompass all types and shapes of hearing loss due to any cause [p. 497]." This expansive purpose is all very well, but it smacks a little of the "tyranny of the majority." One should not get too carried away with the AAOO ideal. For the purpose of the AAOO may be to gather everyone under the same umbrella, but the only people who actually use the AAOO formula are legislators regulating compensation for deafness, typically caused by noise. People who otherwise attend hearing clinics have no need to learn that they are X% handicapped according to some grand but nonspecific design. It is faulty in principle and wrong in fact to advance such an argument.

The kind of statement Webster makes helps to conceal the true purpose of the AAOO-type exercise as I explain it in Chapter 3 and in the previous section. What Kryter did was sound a fresh note in the "battle of the frequencies," and the forces of the .5 to 2 kHz brigade, the region in which little noise damage occurs, were quick to return the call. Webster (1964) goes on to show that the interfering effect of noise-masked speech for normally hearing listeners is best predicted by its levels in the .5 to 2 kHz region. Webster equates noise masking with hearing disorder, but it is doubtful whether this is legitimate. In any case, whatever may be true of performance with noise-masked speech by normally hearing persons, if it does not square with performance among people with disorder of hearing, then it is unfortunate by thereby rendered irrelevant.

Webster cites, as apparent support for his conclusions, the work of Elliott (1964) who showed that the correlation between monosyllable DS and 1, 2, and 3 kHz tonal average was not significantly better than DS–.5 to 2 kHz threshold correlation in listeners with sensorineural disorder. No details are available regarding these listeners, but the criteria used for diagnosis as sensorineural rather than mixed or even conductive were rather liberal (Elliott, 1963). Chances are that a fair overlap occurred between one diagnostic group and another, so Elliott's (1964) data probably refer to heterogeneous rather than homogeneous groups.

Ross, Huntington, Newby, and Dixon (1965) reported results from an extensive study of normally hearing listeners and listeners with sensorineural hearing disorder. No diagnostic or personal details about the latter group were given. Among the wealth of interrelations between tests in their study are correlations between DS (recorded CID monosyllables at 40 dB re: SRT) and tonal threshold at .5, 2, and 4 kHz, separately calculated on left and right ears in the sensorineural group. The correlation values (transposed from negative to positive) are

Frequency (kHz)	.5	2	4
DS left ear	.19	.44	.58
DS right ear	.16	.59	.38

In the absence of details about these listeners, we cannot say much about the results found by Ross et al. other than that they bear out previous findings. Among the tests applied in the Ross et al. study was one of differential intensity threshold. Reduction in this threshold is a sign of loudness recruitment, and results showed a significant reduction at 2 kHz in the sensorineural as against normally hearing group. Correlations between DL for intensity at 2 kHz and DS in the former group were −.01 in the right ear and .1 in the left ear.

A paper by Harris (1965) follows up both that author's own work (Harris et al., 1960) and the report by Kryter et al. (1962). Harris used speech test material of two kinds: the interrogative sentences used previously by Harris et al. (1960), delivered both normally and at the highest talker rate; and the everday speech sentences described by Silverman and Hirsh (1955) and given in Davis and Silverman (1970). As far as I know, this is the first time the latter materials have been used in a comparative study, and I believe too that they have had only one subsequent use of a similar kind. The key words of the Silverman and Hirsh sentences were recast by Harris in different but still meaningful permutations to provide 300 sentences from the original 100. They were then recorded in variously distorted ways. Harris's argument in this paper and in other publications regarding distortion is that it is quite common for speech to be heard in nonoptimal conditions, or badly enunciated, or in competitive noise. This is a plausible argument, but it is unfortunate that like the Kryter *et al.* (1962) procedure it is not substantiated with empirical evidence. It is simply asserted that speech is probably heard about half the time in distorted ways. Thus comparison was made between tonal threshold and DS for distorted speech, undistorted speech, and the mean DS for both types to give 100%, 0%, and 50% distortion conditions, respectively.

Listeners were 52 men with sensorineural disorder. No details are given about the origin, age structure, or other characteristics of these men, and it is not entirely clear whether both ears of each man were tested or only one (or if so, which one). Harris states only that each person's "appropriate ear was tested," but it is not clear what that means. The tonal threshold data presented in the paper show marked threshold elevations at 3 kHz and beyond but with a fair though positively skewed distribution of threshold levels at 1, 1.5, and 2 kHz. The sample is therefore akin to that of Kryter *et al.* (1962), and the bulk of it probably comprises men with noise-induced disorder. Table 6.9 is adapted from Harris (1965) and shows the correlations obtained between DS and tonal threshold at various frequencies in the 0%, 50%, and 100% distortion conditions.

It is clear that with increasing distortion higher frequency threshold becomes more influential. In conclusion, Harris observes that if one takes the 50% distortion condition as representative of everyday speech transmission conditions, correlation between the mean threshold at .5, 1,

TABLE 6.9

Correlation Coefficients (*r*) between Tonal Threshold and Discrimination Score (Errors) under Different Degrees of Distortion[a]

Type of distortion (%)	Frequency[b]					
	.5	1	1.5	2	3	4
0	.19	.32	*.52*	*.34*	.09	.1
50	.19	.31	*.50*	*.48*	*.38*	.36
100	.16	.24	.39	*.50*	*.53*	*.49*

[a] Adapted from J. D. Harris, Pure-tone acuity and the intelligibility of everyday speech. © American Institute of Physics, *Journal of the Acoustical Society of America*, 37 (1965), and reprinted with permission

[b] Figures in italics are the three highest correlation values in each case.

and 2 kHz and DS gives $r = .55$, whereas $r = .74$ between DS and the average of 1, 2, and 3 kHz threshold. Harris's finding, then, concurs with that of Kryter *et al.* and he joins Kryter in advocating the adoption of 1, 2, and 3 kHz average for assessment of speech hearing ability in everday conditions.

Recent Studies

Niemeyer (1967) confirmed the findings of Ward *et al.* (1961); Harris *et al.* (1960); and indirectly Harris (1965). He showed that sentence intelligibility in people with noise-induced disorder is reduced as the cutoff frequency point revealed by the tonal audiogram gets lower. In listeners with a 4 kHz "notch," no effect is seen on articulation function for sentences in either quiet or slightly noisy conditions. As the cutoff frequency approaches 2 to 3 kHz, an effect is noticeable in quiet conditions and a marked effect is noticeable in noisy conditions. With lower and lower cutoff points, intelligibility approaches closer and closer to zero. It is unfortunate that Niemeyer gives no details of test material or of the number and origin of his listeners. Nor is the actual relationship between tonal threshold and sentence intelligibility presented in other than aggregate graphed data. The author remarks that the tonal threshold–DS relationship is not distinct and that in people with higher frequency rises in threshold at less than 4 kHz a discrimination test is essential since the audiogram is not a certain guide in the individual case. Niemeyer asserts the filter hypothesis to explain the differential cutoff effect and explains the deleterious effect of background noise by a masking principle. In this case, such an explanation is plausible as the major component of the noise used in his study was in the .1 to 1 kHz region.

Lindeman (1969) reported results using an abbreviated speech discrimination test. Recorded Dutch monosyllables were presented in groups of 10 at a fixed signal level (70 dB SPL) against noise presented at signal-to-noise ratios varying in 5-dB steps from $+10$ to -5 dB. In all, 679 listeners with various degrees of noise-induced disorder were tested in this way, and they also provided self-recording tonal audiograms. Multiple correlation between DS at 10 dB signal-to-noise ratio and tonal threshold revealed the closest relation to involve average threshold at 2 and 6.3 kHz ($r = .787$). Correlation between DS and 2 kHz alone was .769. The .5, 1, and 2 kHz average correlated with DS at .726.

Hood and Poole (1971) presented results from a group of 43 people with Ménière's disease. Data were presented for subgroups of listeners categorized according to average .5, 1, and 2 kHz tonal threshold. There were 5 subgroups with average thresholds in 10-dB ranges from 26 to 75 dB. The average maximum DS for PB monosyllables for each subgroup lay in linear relation to the average tonal threshold level of each subgroup. This report is akin to Hughson and Thompson's (1942) though it is a bit more informative in that the considerable range of articulation functions within each threshold subgroup can be seen in the graphed data. No correlation analysis was made, however, nor were raw data presented. The authors remark that "the obvious explanation for the poor speech discrimination in the Ménière's Group is the presence of loudness recruitment [p. 33]." The obviousness of this relationship is not manifest to the reader, nor do Hood and Poole present any evidence to support the assertion. If anything, their data show that it is reduced level at .5, 1, and 2 kHz threshold that "explains" the poor speech discrimination.

The final study to be considered here is the first of the kind, that I know of, to be carried out in Australia. It is quite fitting that this should be a local work and that it should be one of the most interesting studies carried out on relations between tonal threshold and DS. MacRae and Brigden (1973) recorded the Silverman and Hirsh (1955) sentences then presented them at fixed levels (60 and 80 dB SPL) in quiet and against a background of shaped random noise or a background of noise recorded in a large cafeteria during a typical busy period. The SPL of both these noises was 70 dB. The shaped noise had a level of 57 dB(A); the cafeteria noise 67 dB(A). Four lists of sentences were used—each listener having to repeat one list played at 80 dB in quiet conditions; then another list at 60 dB; a third list at 80 dB in noise; a fourth at 60 dB in noise. Conditions were thus similar to those in Lindeman's (1969) study except that sentences were used instead of monosyllables.

Listeners were 309 male veterans screened to exclude suspected "malingering." There was predominance of sensorineural disorder (80%) in this sample, the great proportion of which would be caused by noise exposure. Ages ranged from 23 to 86 years (average 54). Average tonal thresholds at .5, 1, and 2 kHz in the ear of each listener showing lower average threshold level were spread over the entire intensity range but showed an expectable negative skew.

Data were reduced from raw results to incidence frequencies within blocks of DS and tonal averages. This is an exercise similar to that carried out by Hood and Poole (1971), except that data on both variables were handled in that way. The incidence of results lying within 10% DS ranges from 0% to 100%, as a function of .5, 1, and 2 kHz average (blocked in 10-dB ranges from 0 to 120) was tabulated. Curves were fitted to the nonextreme ranges of these frequency tables. It was found that in most cases the relationship between tonal average and DS for sentences was nonlinear and indeed that a double-exponential (Gompertz) function best described the variability of results on one test in relation to the other. The Gompertz function produces somewhat sigmoid curves. No correlation was calculated between the two sets of results, but from one frequency table published it is evident that in the region described by the Gompertz curve the actual relationship between .5, 1, and 2 kHz threshold and DS is not close. The interesting feature of the result is the curvilinear outcome, and we return to this later.

MacRae and Brigden went on to a second analysis of their data, and it is this feature of their report which is of considerable interest. They approached the intelligibility–tonal threshold relationship by means of the articulation index (French & Steinberg, 1947). Kryter (1970) demonstrated, using ideal–typical tonal threshold data, the theoretical interrelation between articulation index and speech intelligibility and hence pointed the way for use of this system in assessment of speech hearing difficulty. MacRae and Brigden (1973) applied the index for the first time to actual threshold data. The articulation index in quiet was calculated by the 20-band method for the 2 speech signal levels using the idealized speech spectrum given in Kryter (1962). The estimated average spectrum levels in one-third octaves of the 2 types of noise were calculated and overlaid on the speech spectrum plot to allow calculation of the AI of the speech in noise. The "normal threshold of audibility" curve given in Kryter's (1962) revision of the articulation index was replaced by an individual listener's "better ear" threshold trace whenever that trace level exceeded either the estimated spectrum level of a given background noise or the idealized speech spectrum. In this way the articulation index of the speech signal for each particular listener was derived. It was then plotted against actual discrimination score. Once again the shape of the function describing these two variables was of double exponential form. The other major feature was that the articulation index emerged as a considerably better predictor of speech discrimination than .5, 1, and 2 kHz average. Standard error of estimate of DS from AI was between 4% and 7% (varying between listening conditions) whereas se_{est} of DS from .5, 1, and 2 kHz threshold average was 12%.

Now the important feature about the articulation index is that frequencies from 2 to 6 kHz contribute almost as much as frequencies between .5 and 2 kHz to the calculation (8 bands and 10 bands, respectively). Thus prediction of DS from tonal threshold that takes account of the whole threshold trace rather than its lower half emerges as twice as accurate. Furthermore, the system suffers none of the disadvantages of multiple regression because the weightings of each frequency band are independent of the data from the population. The actual predictability of DS from the articulation index needs to be viewed cautiously. A major reason for the high correlations reported by MacRae and Brigden and the small standard errors of estimate lies in the bulky representation within the data of an extremity effect. In their correlation table, reproduced below as Table 6.10, DS is shown as a function of AI, and we can see that

TABLE 6.10

Correlation Table of Word Score on List H of the CID Everyday Sentence Lists at 60 dB in Quiet Listening as a Function of Articulation Index Calculation[a]

Score on List H	Articulation index										
	0	.01–.1	.11–.2	.21–.3	.31–.4	.41–.5	.51–.6	.61–.7	.71–.8	.81–.9	.91–1
91–100				3	8	27	23	18	29	17	48
81–90			2	9	7	3	1				
71–80			2	5	1						
61–70			4	1							
51–60			2	2							
41–50		1	1	1							
31–40		1	3								
21–30		2	2	1							
11–20		5	1								
1–10		2	1								
0	66	9	1								

[a] From MacRae and Bridgen (1973); © S. Karger, A.G., and reproduced with permission.

a very large number of data points lie at the extreme ends of the distribution. Within the body of the distribution, there is considerable spread of results. A person presenting an AI of between .11 and .3 could have a DS anywhere between 0% and 100%. Precisely these cases would be the ones at the tail of the se_{est} distribution. People at the extremes are the ones whose results go to making the smallish standard error of estimate. The predictability of the DS of a person presenting a nonextreme tonal threshold trace is probably not so certain.

A finding of considerable interest in the MacRae and Brigden report is the curvilinear relation between sentence DS and tonal threshold by whichever average is used. If sentence DS can be taken as a more valid index of everyday hearing handicap than other types of material, then this result suggests that the Fowler and Sabine (AMA, 1947) system had some validity also. Their scheme had a sigmoid relation between observed threshold average and percentage handicap. While a Gompertz function is not the same as a sigmoid, it approximates that form. A curvilinear rather than a linear threshold–handicap relation would seem to be more accurate.

DISCUSSION AND CONCLUSIONS

Results bearing upon the tonal threshold–DS interrelationship are, for obvious reasons, primarily obtained among people suffering sensorineural disorder, especially noise-induced disorder. This means that the date base available for review is centrally located in the region of present interest. Instead of having to tease out data specifically on noise-induced disorder, as was the case with reports on tonal–SR threshold relations, we find the evidence here patently on hand and in need of no extensive reworking.

Two conclusions about tonal threshold–DS relations can be firmly drawn. First, as regards noise induced disorder the involvement of frequencies higher than 2 kHz is established beyond question. Indeed, in a major proportion of reported cases, thresholds at these higher frequencies are the only ones showing more than chance association with discrimination ability. Secondly, with only occasional exceptions, the evidence shows a relatively low level of association between tonal threshold and discrimination ability. Almost all the exceptional results come from reports whose evidential status is uncertain. The exception to this exception is the result reported by MacRae and Brigden (1973). However, while their report shows that a new and viable approach to the tonal threshold–discrimination score issue can be made through application of the articulation index, their results with regard to actual predictability of the one from the other must be treated cautiously.

Two further conclusions inevitably follow from those just drawn. If hearing handicap is validly represented by discrimination score, in particular discrimination score for sentences in both quiet and noisy listening conditions, then (a) the practice of using the three-average (.5, 1, and 2 kHz) system is invalid; and (b) the use of tonal threshold systems in general is inaccurate.

The question that becomes of vital concern, given these conclusions, is whether DS is valid as a measure of everyday hearing handicap. Furthermore, is DS more valid than SRT? For if a case can be made that SRT is the more valid, then of course conclusions (a) and (b) above cease to have such compelling force. They still have some force because as regards listeners with noise deafness frequencies somewhat higher than 2 kHz are influential in tonal–SR threshold interrelations. And as regards these same listeners, the level of association between tonal and SR thresholds is by no means close enough to allow prediction of the one from the other.

As to the question whether DS is more valid than SRT, I think no answer is available at this stage. On the face of it, a test that looks to success at understanding ordinary words embedded in sentences heard at a fixed acoustic level against a babble of other noise should represent the most valid approach of its kind to everyday hearing handicap. We look at some evidence that bears on this point in Chapter 10.

Whatever might be the case—and empirical testing is needed before any firm conclusion can be drawn—it is impossible to deny the face validity of sentence material heard in situations that simulate everyday conditions; and it is impossible to defend the face validity of the disyllable material typically used in SRT determination. But face validity and operational validity are not the same, so the argument cannot really go further than that at this stage.

Other questions that can be tackled are concerned with why DS, for monosyllables at least, and tonal threshold are poorly related and what mechanism can account for the reduced discrimination observed in sensorineural disorder. In relation to the first question, the answer seems to be that as soon as the meaningfulness and information content of the material increases, then the task for the listener involves more than detection of a signal. More central mechanisms are necessarily brought into play to aid in the retrieval of the message. Not least of these would be the structure and content of an individual's lexicon (or "dictionary in the head"). How words are arranged in memory and which words are there in easily retrievable form will have critical bearing on the ease of recognition of a degraded signal of unpredictable content. Also, as was argued in relation to data presented on pages 149–155, extrinsic variables affecting practice at listening critically influence DS while they obviously have no impact on threshold.

To the extent that auditory disturbance such as discrimination breakdown may be a part-threshold phenomenon, then there is a link between threshold and intelligibility. This begs the second question, however. How is discrimination breakdown to be explained? I do not intend to come at this question all at once. Evidence relating to cochlear mechanisms, which is discussed in Chapter 8, has a critical part to play. We can here examine certain hypotheses on the strength of evidence presented in this chapter.

Suprathreshold effects such as loudness distortion seem to bear no relation to discrimination breakdown in people with noise-induced disorder. This picture consistently emerges from studies reviewed here. Other evidence, which relates to Ménière's disease, might encourage a somewhat different conclusion (see Chapter 8). We therefore postpone a conclusion regarding the general role of recruitment until then, but we can safely take it that recruitment and speech discrimination difficulty are quite unrelated in cases of noise disorder.

This leaves us with the "filter" hypothesis and the "reduction of cues" hypothesis. As I indicate earlier, these hypotheses are not antagonistic. The filter theory has it simply that differential attenuation, especially attenuation of the all-important consonant sounds, leads to reduced discrimination because information has been lost. It is, then, a purely acoustical mechanism, and its effect can be witnessed in optimal transmission conditions where the performance of listeners with sharp high frequency threshold rise is similar to that of people listening through low-pass filters. The filter effect is noticeable only when the signal has high information content (unconnected and hence unpredictable words).

It ceases to be so clear-cut as soon as words have predictability by being embedded in sentences.

The cue-reduction hypothesis contains the filter hypothesis and takes it to be a precondition for discrimination breakdown once distortion is introduced into the transmission system. In these circumstances, the redundancy in a connected message is reduced by degrading the cues available in that message. This is an acoustical–informational mechanism. One problem for these hypotheses is that the discrimination response of listeners with unsymmetrical hearing loss is not as predictable as the response of listeners receiving through filters. The breakdown is not precisely the same. Another problem is that discrimination is severely affected in people who have cochlear disorder but show no threshold asymmetry or even a particularly gross threshold elevation.

More is going wrong in the cochleas of people with noise disorder than the mere knocking out of cells normally stimulated by high frequency energy (Stephens, 1976). Martin (1974) showed that there is a widening of "critical bands" in the ears of such people. Corso et al. (1976) report impairment of the normal temporal integration characteristic for tones. Martin's finding suggests a degradation of the tuning properties of the cochlea, and animal experiments clearly bear out this effect. We return to this work in Chapter 8.

The interaction between higher frequency threshold level and discrimination may thus reflect something more than, or other than, a direct relation between these two qualities. It may be that elevation of high frequency threshold is a somewhat reliable sign of damage within the cochlea, which damage is of more than one kind. Thus high frequency threshold may have an operational rather than, or as much as, a causal function. In noise disorder at least, it may reflect its own effect—cue reduction, filtering—and/or it may signal other effects—detuning, temporal breakdown. At this stage, we really cannot be sure what is going on.

The main aim of this chapter was not so much consideration of these issues, vital as they are, as of the more straightforwardly technical matter of predictive validity. In conclusion, it seems clear that in the people for whom this predictiveness is of most concern very little reliance can be placed upon the tonal test. Certainly, no reliance can be placed upon the .5, 1, and 2 kHz average so strongly advocated by certain parties; but even beyond that, the tonal test, whatever its other virtues, has limited usefulness in assessment of hearing for compensation or other purposes.

7

Ancillary Problems: I. Normal Hearing

THE MEANING OF NORMAL

In this text the term *normal* has been used as a shorthand way of describing levels at threshold for tones or speech that are not elevated beyond certain recognized limits. Where possible I have avoided use of the term altogether for two major reasons. First, the term has connotations of "proper," "correct," etc., and its use in place of *hearing* (as opposed to *deaf* or *partially deaf*) perpetuates the evaluative labeling that adheres to the latter states. It is only hearing people who are "normal"; deaf people are thus "abnormal." It is time such evaluative descriptions were done away with, so that "hearing" can be recognized as having a different but no lesser or greater status than "deaf."

The other reason for trying to avoid the use of *normal* is because the term refers to a person's response on tests. One's hearing is "normal" if the level at threshold is at or around 0 dB on an audiogram. The bulk of this chapter is taken up with a rather convoluted exploration of this state of affairs. Let me point out from the start that application of the term *normal* to the audiogram trace begs the question about that trace's validity in differentiating hearing from partially hearing listeners. We have seen in the previous chapter that the audiogram trace may at times bear only a tenuous connection with speech hearing ability, and if we suppose this also represents a hearing impairment measure, then the validity of the former is called in question. But traditionally, *normal* refers to zero level at tonal threshold, hence it applies as a label not broadly to people who hear but quite narrowly to people who hear tones at very low output levels. If we bracket, for the moment, the issue of validity and take it that this capability (hearing acuteness) is a sufficient measure of hearing capacity in general, then it follows that *normal* applies only to people with highly acute hearing. This application of the term is fitting, in that *normal* means *not deviating from a standard*. But the term *normal* also means *ordinary* or *as a rule*. The question then is, can audiometric zero function as a "normal standard"? Does it represent *ordinary* hearing? I will show, after a necessarily circuitous critique, that a certain zero level no longer in use can be taken to represent an "ordinary standard" for hearing, but that the currently used zero represents highly acute and hence nonnormal hearing.

Despite my misgivings about use of the term, there is a context in which a related concept is quite justifiable: that is, the hearing which a listener would "normally be expected" to present in the absence of exposure to some noxious or injurious agent. In assessment of hearing for compensation, that concept is all-important, for it is needed to help judge whether and to what extent a person's hearing has been impaired.

The concept of normal expectation is familiar to epidemiologists. The classical technique of epidemiology involves comparison of populations or representative samples of populations in which all other features are as similar as possible so that the effect of the agent to which only one sample is exposed can be observed. If possible, several samples are compared in which the agent in question has been present in varying degrees. By this means, a more precise observation can be made of any relationship between extent of presence of the agent and prevalence or degree of suspected effect that the agent produces. In the case of noise, the latter kind of survey is all too readily feasible. People at work in some occupations are perpetually exposed to finely graded injurious levels of noise, depending on the type of work involved, and have been for quite some time. Indeed, as mentioned in Chapter 2, the first reported epidemiological study of noise-induced deafness was conducted by Barr in 1886 in Glasgow. Barr was not the first to report on deafness among people working in noisy trades or surviving the tumult of war; but his study is the first reasonably systematic investigation of the injury, and its prime virtue lay in the comparison of the hearing of three samples of men drawn, respectively, from quiet, relatively noisy, and extremely noisy trades. It is unfortunate that it is not known whether the men were comparable in terms of age distribution, although the average age (about 35 years) of each group is similar.

Barr assessed the auditory thresholds of 100 letter carriers (mailmen), 100 ironmolders, and 100 boilermakers using the maximum distance, in inches, from each ear at which the tick of his pocket watch could just be heard. The hearing ability of each group was then expressed as the total number of inches for that group. The letter carriers scored 5694 inches; the moulders, 3291 inches, and the boilermakers 704 inches. It is instructive to note that these values were also expressed as percentages of a "normal hearing" distance of 7200 inches. The derivation of "normal" here is unstated, but 7200 inches is given by Barr as the combined value at which 100 men having normal hearing *should* hear the tick of a watch. Given usual clinical practice of the times, it is not unlikely that

Barr simply multiplied the distance at which he himself could hear the watch and declared the value obtained to be "normal" hearing. The argument could well be made that the letter carriers and not the author represented a more appropriate norm against which to judge the hearing of the other groups. But the dilemma arising from this early report about what value should represent normal (in the sense of expectable) is precisely the one which has dogged the practice of audiology ever since.

It is precisely the same because research has been directed both toward determining "the best hearing available" and toward "the best hearing expectable." And it is my contention that our taken-for-granted concept of highly acute hearing as "normal" has led at times to the adoption of unsuitable norms of expected hearing against which to judge the injurious effect of noise or some other harmful agent. The example of "sociocusis," which is considered in detail pages 193 to 195. D typifies the dilemma in the present time. It appears, depending on how you look at it, as though accelerated deterioration of hearing can result from mere habitation in an urban, mechanized environment, and on the face of it such an outcome seems quite feasible. But this could never be regarded as *normal* because *normal* has always been taken to mean *highly acute*. Hence, in some cases, results from studies which observe hearing uncontaminated by any known agent have been chosen to provide standards with which to judge other people. In other cases, the opposite step has been taken, and average levels for unselected populations have been used as the expectable level. In yet another instance, almost all reported data have been lumped together to form a conglomerate norm—presumably in the hope of minimizing error.

Clearly, each of these strategies is unacceptable, for each is likely to involve comparison between incomparable samples. There seems to be no way out of the dilemma, however, as long as a single norm is demanded against which to judge someone. Perhaps it would be considered too cumbersome (or somehow unjust) to establish different norms for different populations, but unless this is done or until all populations have environmental and genetic identity, fallacious (and equally unjust) assessments may be made.

In the next section, there is a review of work that has been carried out to establish the so-called "normal threshold of hearing" and a discussion of why there is a difference in average normal thresholds, despite the tight constraints on the investigations, between the old United States standard and virtually all other normal standards. In the third section, there is a review of the threshold of hearing as an age-related variable, a property which has produced even greater disparity than the "normal threshold." In the final section there is a discussion of nonnormal—the point, if there be such, beyond which hearing is poorer than normally expectable.

AUDIOMETRIC ZERO

Origin of the "Normal" Zero

According to Davis (1970c), when the first commercially produced audiometer was designed in the 1920s, the standardization of output was to have been based on acoustic zero (0 dB = 20 μP). But E. P. Fowler, the otological consultant involved, was adamant that the instrument should fulfill a diagnostic–assessment function and that zero output should represent "normal" hearing. Fowler figured quite prominently in the early days of audiology, and this surely must be the worst conceptual legacy he has bequeathed to the field. The zero level on the early audiometer was accordingly fixed at the average threshold level of listeners at the Bell Telephone Laboratory. Other manufacturers may or may not have used this reference in constructing audiometers over the next 15 years or so, but they all fixed the zero output along the same conceptual lines. It then required the results of a vast survey of the population to provide a standard to which all manufacturers could reliably adhere.

The Former United States "Normal" Zero (ASA, 1951)

In 1938, results were reported which had been obtained as part of the monolithic 1935–1936 National Health Survey organized by the United States Public Health Service (USPHS). The Hearing Study Series was directed by W. C. Beasley. A representative sample of about 9000 people from the United States populace had their levels at various tonal thresholds determined. The threshold levels of those who reported "no noticeable difficulty with hearing" ($N = 4662$) were taken as the data pool for "normal" threshold of hearing in that country. Actually, according to Beasley (1957), the distributions of the "normal" threshold results were controlled for skewness by use of modal values after the results had been trimmed so as to exclude audiograms "exceeding a 20 dB variation for all frequencies, with reference to the average characteristic of the distributions with skewness eliminated from the distributions for high frequency tones [Beasley, 1957, p. 669]." Quite what this means is unclear. In the same paper (p. 665), it is taken by Davis and Usher (1957) to mean results from people in whom threshold level at any frequency was more than 20 dB above the mean. Harris (1954), however, states that data were from people "whose air conduction audiograms for both ears did not exceed a variation of 20 dB [p. 930]."

Whatever was done, the effect was to eliminate extreme values from the data pool. By this procedure, the original "normal" sample of 4662 people was reduced to 1242. A further constraint was placed on data from this smaller group, namely use of threshold values only from the "better" (lower threshold level) ear, or from both ears if they showed the same values. The surprisingly high attrition rate (from 4662 to 1242) is perhaps explicable by the fact that the values under consideration were drawn from people of all ages (8 to 76 years), hence in the older groups levels at threshold at higher frequencies varying by more than 20 dB from threshold level at other frequencies (or from the group mean) would be fairly common. The feature of age structure is one we will return to presently. Its being left uncontrolled in the "screened" sample of 1242 people has created no small confusion regarding the final composition of the USPHS survey "normal" sample. An age-stratified analysis was reported, but using the data from the original 4662 listeners. These data, as Harris (1954) points out, do not coincide with the data base of the later standard adopted in the United States. That standard is based on the data from the 1242 persons remaining after the screen. Nonetheless, the age-stratified data from the 4662 listeners have been taken by other authors as "normal" values (Spoor, 1967; Sunderman & Boerner, 1950).

In 1939, according to Watson and Tolan (1949), Beasley's screened "normal" values were adopted by the National Bureau of Standards. But while subsequent investigations produce results in confirmation of that standard (Watson and Tolan's own data, for example), according to these same authors, data from the New York World's Fair of 1939 (Steinberg, Montgomery, & Gardner, 1940) and from Bunch (1943) seemed to provide average values up to 10 dB lower than the USPHS survey "normal" values. Despite these apparent discrepancies, the American Standards Association (1951) adopted the USPHS survey data as the specification for audiometers.

It is at this point that the water becomes a little murky. ASA (1951) clearly states (p. 7, paragraph 1.2) that "normal threshold" is defined as the modal value of the level at threshold in normal ears of people *aged 18–30 years*, to be taken for these purposes as the level observed in the USPHS survey of 1935—1936. The appearance of an age range of 18–30 years in ASA (1951) is a puzzle. It is beyond dispute that ASA (1951) is based on the screened sample of 1242 listeners in the USPHS survey and that their ages ranged from 8 to 76 years. However, as I stated earlier, the older contingent in that sample would doubtless have formed the bulk of the people screened out of the original group of 4662, but no clues as to the age structure of the screened sample are publicly available. What remains is a strange discrepancy in age range between ASA (1951) and USPHS survey (1938).

In spite of this curious puzzle, it seems clear that the USPHS survey was carefully conducted and results (giving rise to an ASA specification) were painstakingly treated. As from 1939, with the adoption of the survey standard by the United States National Bureau of Standards (Watson &

Tolan, 1949), and certainly from 1951, American audiometers conformed with the "USPHS zero." These instruments were both exported and used in the United States, and it was supposedly the dissatisfaction voiced by otologists in the United Kingdom and Europe, to the effect that the "normal zero" was too high, which led to the search for a new standard.

The Former British "Normal" Zero (BSI, 1954)

Two independent but cooperating research teams in the United Kingdom set about determining threshold values in highly selected young people. Their reports (Dadson & King, 1952; Wheeler & Dickson, 1952) showed results that agreed almost perfectly with each other and disagreed quite markedly with the American standard. It was undoubtedly the similarity of two independent data sets that silenced any argument against setting up a new British standard. The data of the two teams confirmed the Anglo-European complaint that ASA (1951) "zero" was at too high a level. The mean difference across the usual audiometric frequencies between ASA (1951) and the British data was about 10 dB.

Naturally, as soon as the British standard was established (British Standards Institution, 1954), British audiometer manufacturers had to conform to it. In Germany, a separate standard midway between British and American was established, and indeed in many countries different zero levels have been used, apparently covering a considerable acoustic range. The International Organization for Standardization has finally produced a document (1964) which supposedly provides a single international zero (R 389). We have already (Chapter 5) touched on the probable uncertainty of the locus of that zero, but the point in present context is that ISO "zero" conforms more to British than to American zero. Furthermore, independent investigation by many subsequent authors has tended to confirm the British standard rather than the American. ASA (1951) is now defunct, and the new American National Standards Institute (1969) specification is ISO R 389 (1964).

Following publication of the British Standard (1954), a considerable amount of agonizing took place to try to account for the discrepancy between American and British results. This culminated in a meeting held under the auspices of the Armed Forces–National Research Council Committee on Hearing and Bioacoustics (CHABA). Davis and Usher (1957) edited synopses of the papers delivered by various authoritative persons at this meeting, as well as provided their own observations One of the contributors to the symposium was none other than Dr. W. C. Beasley, the man whose data formed the ASA (1951) zero. While it would perhaps put the wrong light on proceedings to say that Beasley was "grilled" at the meeting, it would be fair to say he was called upon to try to account for the discrepancy between American and British results.

Despite all this effort, no satisfactory explanation for the difference was forthcoming.

The Controversy about the Former Anglo-American Mismatch

Readers may ask why the whole business should not be let subside into history while attention is turned to the problem of establishing a reliable international audiometric zero that will do away with all discrepancies.

To such readers I can only bow and seek indulgence to unfold what to me has been an illuminating inquiry into the Anglo-American controversy. In addition, the reason I propose later in this section for the difference between the USPHS and other data bears critically upon the central theme of this book; namely the valid assessment of hearing ability. I think it is irrelevant what value zero takes on the audiometer; but it is not irrelevant to inquire why one value is thrown over in preference for another.

Finally, had there been no follow-up scrutiny of the Anglo-American difference, and of the USPHS survey in particular, I would have more contentedly dismissed the difference with a shrug of "who knows why?" But the fact is, after fairly intensive limelighting of survey and data—of a kind that would probably embarrass a great deal of audiological survey-type research—no fault could be found, no convincing explanation made for the difference.

The "Survey–Laboratory" Myth

To be sure, Davis (in Davis & Usher, 1957), when summing up, produced an explanation for the difference as lying within a difference in the attitudes of both audiologist and listener to the measurement task. Supposedly this attitude is more serious-minded in "laboratory–research" studies (the British approach to normal hearing determination) than in "survey–clinical" studies (the American approach). This "explanation" is simply drawn out of the air, no evidence for it having been adduced anywhere in the body of the report. A highly illuminating comment on it comes from Harris (1954). He reports that Davis *et al.* (1947) had produced the "laboratory–survey" distinction upon reporting seemingly higher levels at threshold in listeners tested by the "survey–clinical" approach than in those tested by the "laboratory–research" approach. But Harris notes that the reference zero for data by the two procedures was different and that there was in fact a negligible difference between the two sets of results produced by Davis *et al.* Harris states (1954) that data of his own show no difference between "survey" and "laboratory" contexts. It is instructive that Davis (in Davis and Usher, 1957, and 1970c) goes on relying on this nonexistent distinction.

A final and very important point needs to be emphasized. The ASA (1951) standard is apparently isolated from other survey results. But according to Harris (1954) once again, when earphone calibration differences are correctly accounted for, data from the New York World's Fair, for example, are in quite close agreement with the USPHS survey results. The ASA (1951) standard is not necessarily out on its own.

The only reasonable conclusion to be drawn at this stage, in light of the quite intense inquiry into the conduct and conditions of the USPHS survey, is that the Anglo-American difference is a real one, not explicable by some flaw in one program or another.

This conclusion stands despite the remarks of Glorig, Quiggle, Wheeler, and Grings (1956) and Glorig (1958). These authors showed that the USPHS survey results are in close agreement with results from the 1954 Wisconsin State Fair (Glorig, 1958) whereas results from the 1955 Wisconsin State Fair (Glorig, 1958) are more in accord with the British standard data. Glorig et al. (1956) and Glorig (1958) point out that the 1954 Wisconsin procedure was less strict, more hurried, etc. than the 1955 procedure. Without claiming anything one way or the other, the authors allow the implication that the USPHS survey procedure is somehow akin to that of the 1954 Wisconsin State Fair, whereas the British study has more in common procedurally with the 1955 fair. No evidence backs up the former claim, and the conclusion that the USPHS survey result is attributable to the same sloppy procedure as occurred in the 1954 Wisconsin State Fair cannot be made. Apart from the fact that this method of argument, relying on implication without proof, is quite inadmissable, Beasley (1940b) provides the following refutation:

> Careful attention was given to securing reliable measurements on each subject. For over one-half of the 9324 subjects studied, . . . two complete sets of audiograms were obtained for both ears by air conduction and by bone conduction for both the ascending and descending approach to threshold. For the remainder of the subjects, one complete set of audiograms was obtained for the ascending and descending approach to threshold. Although more time than was really necessary was devoted to the audiometric tests, it is considered that the higher degree of reliability resulting from this procedure fully compensated for the additional time spent in testing [p. 117].

The final point to be made is that ASA (1951) and BSI (1954) zeros do not reflect an actual difference in hearing threshold acuity between the two national groups. Subsequent American study has confirmed the British data. There must be some other explanation.

The Politics of "Normal" Hearing

I prefer to take a circuitous route to an alternative explanation because it is important to include in this discussion a consideration of the consequences of using a "louder" or "softer" audiometric zero. It was stated by Davis and Usher (1957) that growing dissatisfaction in Europe with American audiometric zero led to new investigations of normal hearing. Why should it trouble otologists in Europe to have a "loud" zero? Because, it would be argued, the audiometer is relied upon as an instrument to allow discrimination of normally hearing from hearing-impaired persons. If zero is taken to represent the normal standard, then the higher its acoustical level the greater the chances of nonnormally hearing listeners slipping through the screen. Consider the graph (Figure 7.1) from the USPHS survey (1938). It shows the relation between equal–better ear threshold and three degrees of self-reported ability to hear. The spread of threshold values at each level of ability means that threshold levels in the range 0 to 10 dB (.5 kHz) could occur, though not with equal likelihood, in persons reporting "normal," "slightly impaired," and even "moderately impaired" hearing. Threshold level in the range −10 to 0 dB on the other hand, though less representative of the self-reportedly "normal" group, would be unlikely to be found in any but those reporting normal or slightly impaired hearing.

If the aim of audiometry is to try to detect people with impairments of hearing, a strict standard of normal will facilitate the task, a liberal standard will not. It makes otological sense, then, to push for a strict standard. But does it? The only place a strict standard actually makes sense is in the armed forces and certain other occupations that demand good hearing. Only in these will there be concern to separate those with good hearing from those with possible impairments. In all other circumstances, there is no need for such vigilance. Clients in a clinical setting seek the services of otologists presumably because they recognize that something is wrong with their hearing, and diagnosis of the complaint is then the prime issue, the location of audiometric threshold is of secondary concern. It is only conceivably in situations where good hearing is an occupational requirement that precautions are needed to reduce the likelihood of the inclusion of partially deaf persons. And of course a strict standard cuts two ways: While it may block more of those with partial deafness, it also blocks more with good hearing. Many more people than need be will be excluded from occupations if a strict standard operates. Although it could be argued that this is unfortunate but necessary if one wants to exclude people who cannot hear well, of course this is true only if reliance is placed on audiometric measurement in the first place.

The whole problem emerges because despite the USPHS data the otological and audiological world has taken it that a given audiometric level actually corresponds to a given experienced hearing level when, as is obvious both from the data in Figure 7.1 and from the discussion in Chapter 6, no such state of affairs can be said to exist.

Nonetheless, given this presumption, however dubious, the argument

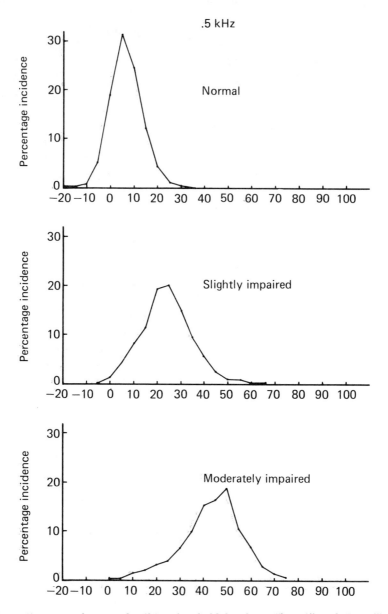

Figure 7.1. Distribution of .5 kHz threshold levels in "better" and "equal" ears of listeners reporting "no noticeable difficulty" ($N = 7310$), "slight impairment" ($N = 2454$), and "moderate impairment" ($N = 1697$) of hearing. Data from USPHS 1935–1936 survey. Reference zero level for dB scale is the Western Electric 2A value given by Fletcher (1953, p. 122) as 39 dB(SPL).

presumably runs that "normal" hearing is audiometrically defined as X dB. Observations of $X + n$ dB presumably are derived from those with nonnormal hearing. More than occasionally, X dB will also be observed in those with nonnormal hearing, but rarely will $X - n$ dB occur in such folk. A standard of "normal" at $X - n$ dB is desirable, then, to ensure reliable exclusion. The question then becomes how to gain such a standard.

There are ways of ensuring that only persons with low acoustic levels at threshold are included in a standardization sample, hence providing legitimately strict normizing levels. The basis of selection would be such as to exclude persons of certain socioeconomic background, age, occupation, and clinical otological state. The effects of noise exposure, childhood middle-ear infection, aging, and minor "attenuative" states of the outer ear (wax, scarring, etc.) all contribute to a raising of sound level at threshold. Standardization samples, with one exception, have always been carefully stripped of such cases. That exception of course, is the USPHS survey. A *report* of normal was sufficient for inclusion in that group.

From his summary report, Beasley (1957) could be taken to contradict this assertion. He reports how the larger sample of 4662 people who reported "no noticeable difficulty in hearing" was screened to provide the "reference normal" sample of 1242 people. He goes on to remark that current practice favors the use of young "ears" with a "clean" otological and environmental (noise) history for purposes of standardization (bearing out my point). In view of this, the records of 953 people aged 15–24 years were selected from the larger group (of 4662 people). Of these, 329 had unblemished otological and environmental records. Their threshold levels did not differ significantly from those of the "reference normal" group except at 4 and 8 kHz. This might be taken to mean that screening otologically and for noise history makes no difference to the threshold outcome. But of course the comparison is between people selected from the larger, *unselected* sample (4662), and people making up the "reference normal" sample (1242). In the latter, audiometric screening had already been done, so the comparison is inappropriate.

If one subscribes to the view that "normal" hearing is merely related to but not identical with "good" hearing, then it comes as no surprise that ASA (1951) zero is higher than any other. The assumption that elevation of threshold is a sign of reduction of hearing ability necessarily leads to the conclusion that elevation of threshold must imply a departure from *normality* when of course all that it may mean is a departure from *good*. One might still *report* normality of hearing because, of course, normality of hearing can mean anything from good hearing to adequacy of hearing for one's general life purposes.

We can see an immediate general implication of this argument, namely that what I assert about my hearing is ignored in favor of what I do in response to the tests of an audiologist. In the determination of normal hearing, we witness the conflict between functional tests and self-report. We see too, in the "good-to-adequate" concept, one reason why there is lack of correspondence between self-report and functional test.

Let me make it clear once again that I care little which acoustic level is used as audiometric zero. What I am concerned to show is the interest being served by determination of a strict standard and the means adopted to legitimate such a standard. I wish to show further that although strict standards may fulfill a discriminative function they should not be taken to represent the universe of "normal hearing." Wheeler and Dickson (1952) recognized this in presenting the data which largely dictated the British standard. Their description of the thresholds as representing "normal *good* hearing" (my italic) is an acknowledgment that the standard typifies not the norm of hearing but an extreme aspect of that norm.

Why has this seemingly simple explanation of the Anglo-American difference not been recognized before? For the reason, I think, that the concept of "self-reportedly normal" has not been realized as different from the concept of "otologically normal." Researchers have so closely identified the audiogram trace with the state of a person's hearing that a self-report of "normal" has come automatically to mean "audiometrically in and around 0 dB."

The advent of an international zero (R 389) has not settled the issue. Indeed, in confirming the British standard it has merely enhanced the legitimacy of regarding highly acute thresholds as the norm. Leaving aside the matter of R 389's inherent uncertainty (Delaney & Whittle, 1967), the crucial point is that R 389 will become unshakable by virtue of being internationally agreed upon. If the foregoing arguments have any persuasive force, the point will have been taken that ISO zero does not represent any truer characterization of normal hearing than British zero. The only virtue of R 389, once its precise transformations are defined, is that eventually audiometers will have a common nominated output and the arguments can then concentrate on the still unresolved issue—what constitutes normal hearing or partial deafness. Of course, had Fowler not had his way and audiometers been calibrated to "acoustic zero," or even more sensibly to dB (A) zero, and had the issue of normal hearing been tackled separately, none of these problems would have arisen. Such an idea, of course, is at odds with the very assumptions of audiometry. Even so, the point must be forcibly put that pure tone audiometric threshold does not provide a reliable guide to the normality or otherwise of a person's hearing.

NORMAL HEARING AS AN AGE-RELATED VARIABLE

The Purpose of "Presbycusis" Curves

It was asserted earlier that the only reason why one would wish to try to arrive at a standard of normal is for purposes of discrimination in selecting personnel for occupations demanding normal hearing. A major restriction placed on normal hearing determination is that of age. With increasing age, a higher and higher proportion of people manifest disorders of hearing (Corso, 1963). This, as Schmidt (1967) has pointed out, is an expectable result of tissue and nerve degeneration and injury, increased susceptibility to infection, secondary effects of drugs, and the like. It seems that sheer passage toward death brings inevitable side effects, and the concept of presbycusis embodies the idea of "aging hearing." Whether or not "aging" is an actual intrinsic process separable from historical effects on the person (and this is virtually an issue of nomenclature), the result is observable as a decline in sensory function among other things. And of course from an actuarial point of view, such things are predictable, unavoidable, and hence expectable. The observed change in hearing is not generally regarded as "normal," because of course it represents a departure from norms such as British and ISO zeros, established to the exclusion of the age effect. We will, however, consider a confusion about the normality–age issue in the last section.

The effect of age needs to be quantified when the time comes to gauge the hearing of a person claiming industrial or service injury benefit who is no longer in the 18–24-year-old bracket. The question then asked is what this person's hearing would be like had it not been affected by the trauma alleged to have produced partial deafness.

To put this question opens up a fairly large issue. People live in different environments and have different dietary habits, and these, according to Schmidt (1967) after reviewing the whole issue, are two factors which seem to influence hearing as an age-related variable. A person claiming compensation for occupational deafness should presumably be compared to a counterpart with the same general background but unexposed to any deafening trauma or agency. Whatever effects on their hearing the backgrounds of these two persons may have produced will presumably be common to them both, and the effect of the occupational agent on the first individual will reveal itself in the difference in hearing between them. This is no more than a restatement of the epidemiological principle outlined at the beginning of this chapter.

It is unfortunate that this kind of precise information is unavailable. There are abundant data from various samples, in some cases selected with great demographic care, which nonetheless represent the hearing of only specific populations, and not of various sectors of the population as a whole. In particular, the kinds of populations comparable with those from which the majority of claims for occupational deafness are likely to emerge have never been properly surveyed.

The Problem of Sampling

The philosophy of age-related hearing research has suffered from the same sort of definitional problem as that of research into normal hearing. Representativeness has been considered in terms of finding the optimum level of hearing in age-stratified populations, hence research has gone to those sectors of the population likely not to have suffered any ill effects of, for instance, an urban environment.

Rosen, Bergman, Plester, El-Mofty, and Satti (1962) reported data on tonal threshold levels in an entire group of Sudanese people, desert dwellers unexposed to sustained high noise levels and consuming a diet lower in cholesterol than is typical of European or North American diet. A striking finding of their study was the apparently negligible average change in level at lower threshold with advancing age. Moreover, this was the case for both males and females. The latter feature contrasts with many European and North American reports that show a greater deterioration of hearing with age among males than among females. It has generally become accepted that more extensive exposure to noise among men in technological cultures accounts for this sex difference. Rosen *et al.* (1962) thus described their finding of nondifference in hearing between the sexes, along with the overall finding of no real age effect, as evidence that technological culture adversely affects hearing. Two sets of age-stratified North American data were used by Rosen *et al.* for comparison with the Sudanese: One was data from the 1954 Wisconsin State Fair (Glorig & Nixon, 1960); the other was data from a sample of "non-noise exposed" males also described by Glorig and Nixon (1960). A gross difference was to be observed between the Sudanese and 1954 Wisconsin State Fair data, the latter showing marked age effects. A lesser but still noticeable difference was to be seen from comparison of the Sudanese and nonnoise exposed groups.

A later publication by one of Rosen's original coauthors (Bergman, 1966) criticized these comparisons as being epidemiologically unsound. In regard to the 1954 Wisconsin data, Bergman made the point that these were from a self-selected sample drawn, in any case, from the heavy-industry region of Milwaukee and hence likely to contain a high proportion of people with occupational noise disorder. As regards the "non-noise exposed" sample, Bergman asserts that Nixon, Glorig, and High (1962) described these as in fact quite contaminated by cases of occupational and other hearing impairment, so once again they are an epidemiologically unsuitable comparison sample.

It appears that Bergman (1966) may be confused over this latter issue, though he cannot be blamed, for the issue is hard to tease out. Scrutiny of the Nixon, Glorig, and High (1962) report makes it doubtful that these authors were referring to the nonnoise exposed group that Rosen *et al.* (1962) used for comparison. It seems rather that a subsample of "office-workers" was extracted from the 1954 Wisconsin sample, and this was the group later found to be contaminated in the manner described in the foregoing discussion. Rosen *et al.* compared the Sudanese with a sample described by Glorig and Nixon (1960) and by Glorig and Davis (1961) as being drawn from groups of office and professional workers in the vicinity of Los Angeles. This sample was very carefully screened to exclude anyone with a history of occupational or service noise exposure, etc. Ironically, Bergman (1966) goes on to compare the Sudanese with this very group, to prove that the Sudanese do not really show lower levels at threshold than a properly selected North American sample. Yet Rosen *et al.* were somehow able to use this same sample to show the opposite to be the case. How do we explain the contradiction?

A feature of the study by Rosen *et al.* which is unemphasized in the original report pertains to the high acoustic levels at the "zero output" level of the audiometer. The SPL conversion figures given in the report show that zero was some 10–15 dB higher than ASA (1951) zero. When the threshold values for the male Sudanese are converted to dB SPL and then compared with the Glorig and Nixon (1960) values for males similarly converted (which is what Bergman did), the two sets of data are quite similar. And between the younger men of each sample, the Sudanese show higher levels at threshold than the Glorig and Nixon (1960) listeners. This, of course, follows since "zero" was defined by Rosen *et al.* as the level at threshold for the younger Sudanese.

But this outcome raises several questions. If young Sudanese show, if anything, higher levels at threshold than young North Americans, why do the older groups merely show deterioration comparable with that of the older North Americans? In fact, Bergman's reanalysis shows that the older Sudanese present a narrower range of levels at threshold than the older people in the Glorig and Nixon sample.

There is no single answer to this question. We can only speculate about possible explanations. One such speculation might be that whereas the Sudanese people, for genetic or constitutional reasons, begin life with hearing levels only approaching those of non-noise-exposed North Americans, prevailing environmental conditions do indeed favor the continued integrity of that hearing ability, whereas the prevailing North American environment is more hostile to hearing, even without specific occupational or service noise exposure.

Another speculation centers on the issue of age determination. No reliable, independent record of age was available for the Sudanese people. Only indirect evidence could be obtained, no single reported source of which could be considered foolproof. If the average lifespan of the Sudanese were less than that of the North Americans and if individuals were wrongly categorized as to age by the researchers, these two factors alone could account for all the observed differences in data between the Sudanese and North American samples. Thus a higher acoustic level at threshold for the "younger" Sudanese could have resulted from contamination of that subsample by older people; vice versa for the "older" subsamples. The narrower range in the "older" subsample could simply reflect a shorter lifespan. In other words, an unreliable and falsely elongated age stratification could produce the observed outcome.

One observation by Rosen et al. (1962) supports this latter speculation, namely that the people "generally look younger than their chronological age [p. 732]." Since chronological age was based on indirect evidence, the younger appearance could mean that the evidence for actual age was faulty. The foregoing explanation has no more weight than the previous one, but it remains unassailable on present evidence. Hence, on the basis of data presented by Rosen et al. (1962), we are left no nearer a conclusion that a desert environment is necessarily associated with the better preservation of hearing ability. Only one piece of evidence suggests the likelihood of such beneficence—the lack of difference in hearing between males and females. This particular outcome supports the idea that the environment of the Sudanese has a nonharmful effect, in view of the harmful effect of a technological environment on the hearing of males.

Rosen and various associates subsequently studied hearing ability in a variety of samples of people: in the island of Crete, in Finland, and in the Bahamas. These studies are reviewed in summary by Rosen (1969). The issue pursued in these investigations largely involved characteristic differences in diet reflected in differences in age-related loss of hearing. Quite marked differences were observed between the various samples, and these seemed to be reliably associated with differences in level of blood cholesterol. Independent physiological experimentation supports an hypothesis that diminished blood supply to the cochlea is critical in the etiology of sensorineural hearing disorder (Hawkins, 1971). According to Rosen (1969), cholesterol is one agent which would bring about such malnutrition.

More recently, Rosen, Preobrajensky, Khechinashvili, Glazunov, Kipshidze, and Rosen (1970) compared the hearing levels of groups of clerical workers in Moscow with those of agricultural, clerical, and factory workers in Georgia, Soviet Union. The importance of the 1970 study is that apparently reliable age records were available so that the groups could be compared without possible confounding from this source. Levels at threshold were consistently lower among subjects in the rural area; and while Rosen *et al.* wish to argue for a dietetic explanation of the difference, acoustic–environmental differences between the two samples cannot be ruled out.

With the exception of findings in the Sudanese sample (whose uncertain nature has already been discussed), the data of Rosen and associates consistently show an increase in level at threshold, especially at higher frequencies, as a function of age. That is to say, irrespective of dietary–environmental factors, increasing age inevitably seems to bring reduction in hearing ability. That reduction, however, is arguably mitigated or exacerbated by characteristic ecological factors. Schmidt (1967) proposes that any sign of age-related hearing loss must be explicable by one or more disease forms found in the general population and simply happening to occur among or intensify and converge upon people of increasing age. Corso (1976), on the other hand, proposes that presbycusis is a pathology in its own right, distinguishable from other types of ear disease or injury. As stated earlier, this seems to me to reduce to a semantic issue, but Corso's claim needs to be examined in detail, for he produces certain administrative proposals as regards "presbycusis correction" in cases of compensation that he sees as emerging from this claim.

Corso (1976) points out one assumption behind "presbycusis corrections," namely that the pure tone audiogram expresses the effect of occupational noise injury *plus* the effect of age. Hence by determining the effect of age alone, one can make appropriate subtractions to arrive at the "presumed noise induced hearing loss" component in the audiogram. Corso raises the possibility of an interactive rather than purely additive picture, however. Such interaction could hypothetically take the following forms: Age (and hence amount of preexisting presbycusis) at the time of first exposure to injurious noise could affect the degree of hearing loss sustained; or exposure to noise could hasten (or retard) other degenerative change. Corso cites evidence to suggest that neither of these patterns actually occurs, however. A further point is that presbycusis, by reason of being a degeneration throughout the whole auditory system, brings about reduction in speech discrimination ability with no necessarily accompanying elevation in level at tonal threshold. Hence the audiogram of an older person may not reflect that person's speech hearing ability. On this point, of course, one can only agree. Corso's proposed solution, however, is to suggest that beyond a certain age presbycusis correction should remain constant. The reasoning behind this proposal is hard to grasp. A further proposal, that more than the pure tone audiogram should be used to assess hearing impairment, does make more sense in light of the foregoing point.

Another proposal is to modify existing "correction" practice, which in general is to subtract a linearly increasing percentage from the calculated percentage hearing loss with increasing age. Instead, the "correction" should actually mirror the nonlinear increment in level at threshold observed in non-noise-exposed groups.

As to which presbycusis data should be used to calculate corrections, Corso (1976) suggests either the conglomerate curves produced by Spoor (1967) based on eight studies carried out in Europe and North America or his own data (1963) which he considers, and cites Kryter (1973) as considering, to be the most reliable observations of pure tone thresholds from a non-noise-exposed sample in the United States.

Spoor's (1967) composite curves are a problem for administrator and student of presbycusis alike. Because of the variability between different sets of data, especially variability due to different reference "zeros," Spoor assumed uniformity of data from the youngest age group in each of the eight samples he included in the analysis. All age-stratified data were expressed with reference to levels at threshold for the 18–30-year-old group in each sample. Zero thereby is an arbitrary point of origin whose acoustic counterpart is unknown. If person X, aged 60 years, were to have a tonal threshold measurement, results would be expressed relative to some known "zero" point. To correct the result for presbycusis would require data also expressed according to that reference. Because this is impossible from Spoor's representation, one is left in the dark about what to do. According to Corso (1976), Lebo and Reddell (1972) converted Spoor's data into the 1969 United States reference.

Lebo and Reddell's (1972) figures show a conversion of Spoor's (1967) composite curves to the ANSI (1969) reference in TDH-39 earphones; but the only way in which that could be done is by returning to the original data, in effect bypassing Spoor's collapsing technique. Scrutiny of Lebo and Reddell (1972) gives no clues as to what they actually did. They state that their presbycusis curves were prepared by "application of the ANSI-1969 calibration to Spoor's ASA calibrated tables [p. 1404]." Spoor's (1967) tables are not calibrated to anything, as I have pointed out, so this statement makes no sense. Even assuming that Lebo and Reddell (1972) did take Spoor's zero to represent ASA (1951), application of the appropriate ASA–ANSI correction to any of Spoor's tabulated values does not provide the same result as Lebo and Reddell published (pp. 1402–1403). The exercise therefore remains a mystery, but the reader is cautioned not to take Lebo and Reddell's data as meaningful at this stage.

The Male–Female Difference

Spoor's (1967) technique is potentially of interest (though it has no practical worth) to the legal administrator. To the student of age-related hearing, it represents nothing exceptional simply because the outcome of the exercise is a composite shorthand in which any aberration or systematic difference between research outcomes is hidden in the curve fitting. The marked and systematic difference between the age-related thresholds of men and women is the only source of major variability retained.

The male–female issue is an interesting one in audiology, as it is indeed in so many other ways. The basic question raised by data is whether the lesser effect on hearing with increasing age generally observed in women is biological or environmental. Earlier I noted in passing that the effect is environmental. That assertion needs to be examined more critically because it may not necessarily be true, and whatever the reason for the male–female difference, it could have implications for medicolegal administration. A woman exposed to as much noise as a man and presenting identical loss of hearing by tonal test could gain more compensation were different expected levels of hearing to be applied In each case. I am not aware of such practice, but it has been recommended (Corso, 1963) and we need to examine its basis.

Hinchcliffe (1959) reported results from a stratified sample of people living in a rural area of the United Kingdom. Data from males and females showed the same sort of difference found by surveys among urban dwellers. Hinchcliffe nonetheless provided evidence to support a differential noise-exposure case even in this relatively noise-free sample. Corso (1959, 1963) reported results from a relatively noise-free suburban sample, randomly selected and very carefully screened to exclude persons with previous or current noise exposure, either occupational, from military service, or in daily life. The sex difference was still quite apparent in the results.

Flodgren and Kylin (1961) used a multiple regression technique to partial out the effect of age in groups of 66 women and 60 men employed in a textile mill. When years of employment were matched with threshold level, controlling for age, there remained a significant difference between results for men and women. Flodgren and Kylin concluded that men are more injured by noise than women and that the two groups needed to be considered independently. In a similar study, Atherley (1967) found a different picture. The fact that female weavers have time out in their late teens and twenties to bear children suggested to him that the longer-term effects may be caused by discontinuity in employment in the trade. When this feature was taken into account by comparing 13 matched pairs of male and female weavers, all with unbroken employment, the male–female difference was no longer evident. Kylin (1960) mentions the feature of broken exposure as more common in female employees but considers it an unimportant variable. Atherley's (1967) result suggests otherwise.

A side issue, but not an irrelevant one to this question, is raised by Flodgren and Kylin's results. They remark that previous military service might have contaminated the results for men in their sample to give the appearance of greater hearing injury. However, they briefly note that no differences were apparent between male and female listeners in a group occupied in quiet jobs, yet the males in the group had the typical remote histories of military experience. They infer from this observation that the same would presumably be the case in the textile-worker groups.

Many authors assume that samples must be screened to exclude remote histories of noise exposure, despite evidence that even after a lifetime of noise exposure some recovery can yet take place (Taylor et al., 1965). Corso's (1963) results also show that after carefully screening his suburban sample to exclude remote histories of noise exposure, very little change occurs in his data. Exceptionally, results from the older age groups show a mean reduction in threshold following screening, but this is explicable by the fact that among older age groups an increasing proportion of people were excluded on the grounds of signs indicating otological "impurity." Atherley and Noble (1969) could find no difference in the thresholds of various, otherwise matched groups of listeners in whom a remote history of military gunfire exposure was or was not presented.

These results therefore suggest that remote exposure to noise is not long lasting, unless presumably it is extremely severe. This result nevertheless sits oddly with Flodgren and Kylin's (1961) claim that men are more injured by noise than women. Were that the case, one might have expected a difference to be apparent between males and females in the quiet-occupation groups surveyed by these authors. Ward, Glorig, and Sklar (1959) found no significant difference between 15 male and 15 female listeners in susceptibility to short-term noise episodes, though the difference between the 2 samples was in the predicted direction.

Results are therefore contradictory. Corso's (1963) result, following careful screening, could be taken as the most substantial evidence favoring a differential (biological) effect; Flodgren and Kylin's result is the most substantial favoring differential susceptibility to noise in the long term. All other results showing male–female difference are explicable in terms of differential noise exposure. Rosen et al. (1962) found no male–female difference among desert dwellers; Atherley (1967) found no male–female difference in weavers after accounting for time out. It is possible that Flodgren and Kylin's (1961) employment–time data were affected in this way or by differential overtime working. Unfortunately, no details are given. Corso's (1963) data for men, even when screened to exclude those with noise exposure etc., show a distinct drop in the older groups, with notching around 4 kHz typical of noise disorder.

The impression one comes away with is that the picture will remain unclear while men and women engage in different life styles in our culture. Male–female aging effects are not differentially recorded in regard to other sensory systems (Sunderman & Boerner, 1950), a fact which suggests that differential biology cannot satisfactorily account for the male–female difference in age-related hearing.

It thus seems wisest at this stage to make no differential allowance for aging between the sexes. Wiser still, perhaps, and a policy advocated by not a few authorities, is to ignore the aging effect and concentrate on extent of injury. We return to this issue in the final section of the chapter.

Many fewer women are assessed for compensation purposes than men. This mainly reflects the fact that women in our culture do not occupy the jobs which are most harmful to hearing. This is probably changing as more women take on traditionally male occupational roles. With that change will perhaps come other changes in women's life styles so that the sexes become relatively similar in occupational and social performance. Once that happens, the time will have come to discover whether men and women really do show differences in aging independent of differences in environmental experience. It is to be hoped that by then the interest will be purely academic, living and working conditions having been so improved that the need for inquiry is no longer in regard to fair compensation for women deafened by industrial din.

Sociocusis

Because of the fact that men are most commonly the people to be assessed for compensation, expected hearing levels for that group have been reported more often than expected levels for women.

One major issue which has emerged in discussion of these sorts of data is that labeled "sociocusis" by Glorig and Nixon (1962). This is a general term describing the age-related hearing of people not exposed to any occupationally injurious agent but rather exposed to the noises of technological society as part of the daily round. It is this which Rosen *et al.* (1962) tried to highlight when showing the difference between desert dwellers and North American urban dwellers.

As a result of comparisons made by Glorig and Nixon (1962) between a screened sample of urban-dwelling professional men and the suburban sample of Corso (1959) as well as the rural sample of Hinchcliffe (1959), it seems that sociocusis is not apparent. It might be expected that suburban and rural dwellers should show lower age-related threshold levels than urban dwellers if sociocusis were a reality. Recall that Bergman's (1966) comparison of the Rosen *et al.* (1962) data from the desert dwellers with the samples from Glorig and Nixon (1962) showed no differences.

For this reason presumably, legislators have been advised to use data from rural dwellers as expected values for age-related hearing. Advisors have also pointed to the 1954 Wisconsin State Fair data (Symons, 1958) as showing that age-related thresholds deteriorate markedly in the population as a whole, so the case for occupational loss of hearing should not be overstated. No one, of course, has pursued that line too seriously, given what is known about the composition of the 1954 Wisconsin sample and the report by Glorig et al. (1956) of its inadequate procedures. Recall why the 1954 and 1955 Wisconsin surveys were undertaken in the first place: Following the 1953 decision in favor of Wojcik and against the Green Bay Drop Forge Co. by the Wisconsin Supreme Court (see Chapter 3), an enormous spate of claims was made in that state. Management of both industry and insurance companies needed to know what they were up against. The 1954 data very likely came from people all too conscious of the legal struggle going on, so the audiological test booths probably were disproportionately filled with industrial workers.

The surveys from Wisconsin have, nevertheless, been regarded as showing sociocusis alongside occupational hypacusis, and I think there is a case to support that view. The absence of difference between upper-middle-class urban dwellers and randomly selected rural dwellers says nothing as regards city noise and other agents potentially damaging to hearing. Upper-middle-class people live in secluded suburban residences, travel in well-insulated automobiles, enjoy high quality food and drink, smoke only a little tobacco, and generally are in better health than the lower-middle-class and working-class people who form the bulk of society. The latter, by contrast, live in crowded areas, often alongside noisy factories, highways, railroads, or airports. They travel in cheaper automobiles or on noisy buses and trains. They are exposed to the racket of the machine culture to a far greater extent than the upper middle class and enjoy poorer diets, poorer health, and so forth. It would be an amazing discovery if it were reliably shown that these two groups of people can hear equally well throughout their lives. From the 1935–1936 USPHS survey, Beasley (1940b) in fact reported that "prevalence rates for impaired hearing among families of lower income are from 25 percent to 112 percent higher than among those with higher income [p. 121]." But of course most people claiming compensation came from lower-income groups. Far be it from me to argue for an administrative reduction of these claims by any amount, and this is not my intention in making this point. My point is simply that if expectable values are to be brought seriously into the picture, let these values truly reflect expectation in each case and not be mere tokens, as they are presently, to pare down compensation claims.

As things stand at the moment, some agencies subtract an increasing percentage from an assessed handicap the older the claimant, others do not. The rationale behind such subtraction is usually administrative. No recognition is given to real actuarial values, perhaps for the very reason that these real values are not known. The best advice seems to have been that of Glorig and Davis (1961) that no subtraction for age be made, that a "low fence" is sufficient to deal with expectable effects. The ensuing section examines the "low fence" concept.

THE "LIMITS OF NORMAL"

Two concepts apply to the "limits of normal": the limits of variability around an audiometric norm and the point of "beginning impairment." These two concepts have been confused, especially when expectable age-related threshold change is brought into play. I deal with the confusion at the close of this section. The two concepts themselves are best illustrated by Beasley's analysis of the USPHS survey data; indeed it is these data that have largely informed agencies like AAOO about the level of "handicap" supposedly associated with a given level at threshold. Some of these results have already been given in Figure 7.1. The graphed results to which I refer the reader for present purposes are shown in Figures 10.2 through 10.4 (pp. 273–275). These and other results are given in that chapter because the major analysis of the USPHS 1935–1936 survey is made there whereas the present point is a more minor one. In Figures 10.2 through 10.4, the distributions of threshold levels at .5, 1, and 2 kHz associated with various stages of self-reported hearing impairment for speech are plotted.

It can be seen that up to a level about 15 dB above the modal value lie roughly 98% of the values obtained from ears reported as "normal," i.e., from respondents who declared they had "no noticeable difficulty in hearing speech." A level of 15 dB (ASA) has therefore been taken as the upper limit of the normal range for these three frequencies (Davis, 1960, p.257). The rules for estimation of handicap drawn up by the AAOO and later adopted by the AMA specified the beginning point of impairment, and thus of handicap, as an average over .5, 1, and 2 kHz of 16 dB (ASA). This was the "low fence": a construct that (as can be seen) had both biological and administrative meaning. A problem that can immediately be seen however, arises from the variability of threshold values at stages of self-reported hearing impairment. The percentages of "ears" in Stages 1 and 2 of impairment whose levels at threshold are 15 dB and less, are as follows:

Stage	Frequency (kHz)		
	.5	1	2
1	25.3%	39.2%	28.0%
2	4.3%	.3%	.2%

At least a quarter of the "ears" and by implication of the people with Stage 1 impairment, i.e., "preventing a person from understanding speech in a public auditorium . . . or in a conference between five or six people," have threshold levels below the "low fence." There is even a slight percentage of people with Stage 2 impairment, i.e., "preventing a person from understanding speech originating from a distance two or three feet directly in front of him [USPHS, 1938, p. 2]."

While the "low fence" successfully excludes from consideration most of those who report no noticeable difficulty in hearing, it *unsuccessfully* excludes a fair proportion of people with more than a slight disturbance of auditory ability. This situation illustrates the bind that reliance on tonal threshold can get us into. While there seem to be upper limits to "normal," there do not seem to be lower limits to "nonnormal," We return to consideration of these findings in Chapters 10 and 11.

The purely administrative nature of the "low fence" becomes apparent when we note that with the switch to ISO zero (on average about 10 dB lower than ASA) the "low fence" was fixed at 25 dB (ISO). In other words while the arguments were loud in proclaiming that "normal" hearing is best represented by ISO zero, a curious silence is observable over the fact that the limit of normal is now magically stretched to the same point as previously. What it means is that the same overlap problem remains. However, certain words were required to "fill in" the 10 dB gap because statistically it could not happily be filled with "normal" data. So we find that a 8 "fence" of 25 dB (ISO) is now accompanied by a description like, "no significant difficulty with faint speech [Davis, 1970b, p. 255]." The precise point of the normal limit is now uncertain, sometimes being portrayed as about 20 to 23 dB (ISO) (Davis & Kranz, 1964), sometimes nowhere in particular (Davis, 1971, p. 10).

The original concept of a "low fence" has thus been contaminated, and agencies in different parts of the world feel free to fix its limit according to administrative or actuarial convenience. It is quite openly recognized in the United Kingdom, for example, that the fence, 50 dB ISO average at 1, 2, and 3 kHz, is at that level to limit claims so that the public purse is not overstretched. I frankly prefer this purely economic approach, which pretends no biological validity, to one that does imply such validity.

The fence principle becomes confused when age-related threshold levels are taken into account. Both Glorig and Davis (1961) and Ward (1971) advocate abandonment of an age-correction principle in assessment for compensation. Their reason for so doing demonstates the confusion in regard to the "fence," namely whether its role is to account for "normal" variability or whether it is fixed for administrative convenience. For if the "fence" is seen as the "normal" limit, then of course that limit must change with increasing age. The conceptualization of the "fence" as a variable construct is shown in Figure 7.2a. Both Glorig and

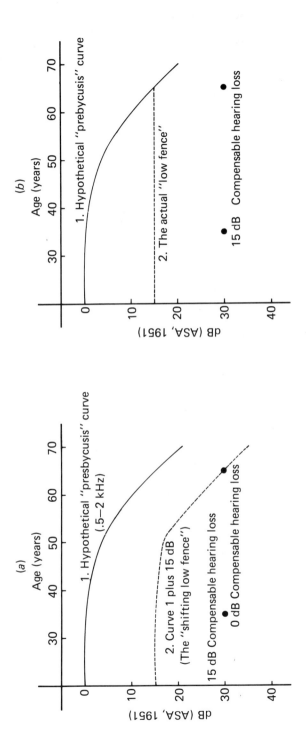

Figure 7.2. Two schematic models of the "low fence": (a) as a shifting locus that parallels the average change in .5–2 kHz threshold with age (a "biological" fence); (b) as a constant locus that accounts for some of the age effect (an "administrative" fence—the more equitable conceptualization).

Davis (1961) and Ward (1971) argue from this conceptualization that a person aged 35 having a 30 dB average threshold will have 15 dB of compensable hearing loss. But if a person aged 65 has a threshold average of 30 dB and 15 dB is subtracted as the expectable age effect (Curve 1 in Figure 7.2a), then that leaves 15 dB of hearing loss attributable to noise or whatever; and since that is merely at the fence, the loss is noncompensable.

To these writers, this seems unjust, and I am sure it is. But the reasoning that leads to this posited outcome depends upon a shifting fence tied to the variability about the "normal" threshold for 65-year-olds. If, however, the fence is correctly conceptualized as merely an administrative line, then its locus is as shown in Figure 7.2b. Our 35-year-old will get 15 dB of compensable hearing loss, and our 65-year-old will *also* get 15 dB of compensable hearing loss because the aging effect merely reaches the fence, and he has 15 dB on top of the expectable limit. At age 70, he would perhaps get only 12 dB compensable hearing loss with a 30 dB average threshold level, because 3 dB of that suprafence loss would be expectable. The fence, in other words, has already taken care of the bulk of expectable effects.

Why should such distinguished authors' have made the fairly obvious error schematized in Figure 7.2a? One reason is that they themselves originally conceived the fence, and they conceived it as the "limit of normal." They subsequently failed to adjust to its reconstruction. The other reason is that "normal" hearing, audiometrically defined, continues to be seen as "normal" with increasing age simply because it is *normative*. The audiogram once again restricts the perception of hearing to the line on a piece of paper. The term *normal* in fact is being asked to do double duty once age-related hearing is under consideration. Whereas *normally expectable* and *ordinary* are the concepts applicable to age-related hearing, the concept *normal*, actually meaning *pure* or *unblemished*, is the only one applicable to audiometric zero.

This confusion would never have arisen, let us realize in conclusion, has the USPHS data given in Figures 10.2 through 10.4 been used as normal (i.e., *ordinary*). These data come from the reports by people of all ages and can therefore be used to gauge expectable hearing level at any age.

When we discuss certain applications of the technique of self-reported scaling of hearing loss in Chapter 11, a different concept of the "low fence" will be advocated, one which gets away from the upper limit of "normal" and examines the lower limit of "nonnormal."

8

Ancillary Problems: II. Recruitment and "Functional Hearing Loss"

INTRODUCTION AND APOLOGY

The critical reader might infer that by putting *recruitment* and *"functional hearing loss"* together in a single chapter and further by prefixing their conjunction with the term *ancillary problems*, I have already shown a disagreeable bias in regard to these phenomena. In the first place, the two issues bear no practical relation to each other (with one fortuitous exceptional link). Hence it seems that lumping them in one chapter suggests a careless attitude not in keeping with the structural precision sought throughout the work. In the second place, the two issues are seen to be portrayed sketchily, lacking the need for a separate chapter for each; and finally, seeing them as ancillary (subservient, auxiliary) is to have assigned them a minor role in the assessment scene.

This opening gambit is obviously intended to disarm the critic, if not by offering a defense at least by acknowledging that one may be called for. Clearly I am not all that apologetic, else an alternative arrangement and titling would have been made. In explanation then of the existing plan I point out that the phenomena of recruitment and of "functional hearing loss," like that of "normal hearing," are ancillary in the sense of being attendant issues in the assessment of hearing loss, issues which must be discussed in that context but in the final event represent theoretical constructs not central to the problem of assessment *per se*. I do not anticipate that the foregoing assertion will fall in with the views of some researchers in the hearing assessment field. My view reflects a personal appraisal of the range of problems worth tackling within that field and, more important, the range of problems apparently settled that I see as needing to be unearthed and looked at again. Normal hearing, recruitment, "functional hearing loss," all need to be examined critically, but too great an emphasis on these matters would deflect effort and attention away from fundamental issues about the nature of hearing and the assessment of its impairment.

Recruitment might arguably stand as a fundamental issue. In spite of the picture of things painted in Chapter 6, there are apparently data which show its role in creating or at least aggravating the special problems associated with certain sensorineural disorders of hearing. We will seek out these data in due time.

NATURE AND HYPOTHESIZED MECHANISM OF RECRUITMENT

One cannot hope critically or comprehensively to report on physiological processes associated with recruitment. Current understanding of auditory physiology is going through quite rapid transformation, and it is unsafe to assert that a given mechanism somehow explains the phenomenon. The best one can offer is an account of prevailing views on the subject. In any event, mechanism is of secondary concern in present context. It is the evidence to support a supposed *effect* of recruitment on hearing that must be critically scrutinized. Only insofar as claims are made about the adverse effects of recruitment on auditory information input must one try to understand its mode of mischievous operation. As a separate exercise we examine the evidence submitted to underpin the alleged effect.

Manifestation

First, however, the nature of recruitment needs to be specified. In the classical version, "recruitment of loudness" is the description casually given by Fowler (1937) to a compressed loudness–intensity relationship in certain aural pathologies. This odd term has, in addition to the more usual meaning, a dictionary definition of, "recovery in health, restoration, reinvigoration." Common sense tells us that a person with partial deafness is less able to hear sounds, even at levels above lower threshold, than a person with more acute hearing, and in some cases this is true: We have to shout to make ourselves understood in face-to-face conversation with people who are partially deaf. Surely, the common sense view would declare, this is what we mean by partial deafness! True—yet consider a partial deafness that is more like a masking situation, whereby sounds below the masking noise level are inaudible whereas sounds above it are audible *at the same level of loudness* as they would be even without the masking. That circumstance is analogous to the recruitment phenomenon. In a person with recruitment, auditory signals above threshold in the impaired ear can sound as loud as they do in the unimpaired ear (supposing the person is partially deaf in one ear only).

The two illustrations in Figure 8.1 represent, respectively, the picture in nonrecruiting and recruiting unilateral hearing impairment in the right ear. In Figure 8.1a, the uppermost points represent lower threshold in the left and right ears. These points, at different levels of acoustic intensity (0 and 15 dB) can be taken to represent 0 dB sensation level in each case (the values in parenthesis). Equal loudness contours at levels above threshold are represented by the dashed lines, and there is a regular relation between sensation level and acoustic intensity. No recruitment is evident then. Loudness (sensation level) increases in parallel fashion between the impaired and unimpaired ears. In Figure 8.1b, by contrast, the growth of loudness in the right ear is accelerated relative to the left ear, and this is reflected in greater increases in sensation level as a function of intensity change in that ear, compared with increases in sensation level in the left ear.

Fowler (1936) claims to have discovered the method of alternate binaural loudness balancing which is the technique modeled in the illustrations. In the 1936 paper, he also describes the phenomenon which later gained the label *recruitment*, for he noted that people with sensorineural disorder often provided the compressed growth function described in the preceding paragraph. He did not at that time explore the possibility in such cases further. Fowler's (1936) purpose was in fact to use the balance technique as a way of aiding early diagnosis of otosclerosis. His hypothesis was that the very opposite of the "recruitment" effect may be manifest in that disorder. In its early stages, he reasoned, no threshold change is apparent nor any loudness distortion at levels slightly above threshold. But as loudness increases, the stapes footplate in the potentially otosclerotic ear should meet increasing resistance caused by beginning ankylosis, and loudness should thus increase more slowly in the disordered ear. While he demonstrated such an effect in some cases of people with a family history of otosclerosis, he never observed it in anyone with a confirmed case of the disorder. Typically, loudness in each ear increased as shown in Figure 8.1a.

The diagnostic significance of compressed loudness in regard to sensorineural disorder was recognized by Fowler (1937), and a major study of the differential presence of the effect was reported by de Bruïne-Altes (1946). The crucial feature of de Bruïne-Altes' research was to show that recruitment is virtually absent in people with presbycusis—the mechanism of which is presumed to affect the neural pathway of the auditory system as a whole—but present in people with sensorineural disorders affecting cochlear and labyrinthine structures, such as noise trauma and Ménière's disease. Hence recruitment was not simply a distinguishing feature of sensorineural disorder, but seemingly of only certain sen-

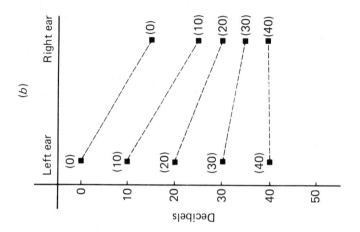
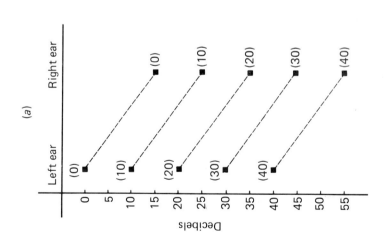

Figure 8.1. Schema (a) of nonrecruitment between an unimpaired (left) ear and an impaired (right) ear, and (b) of recruitment in the impaired (right) ear.

sorineural disorders. This notion was confirmed by Dix, Hallpike, and Hood (1948) and by Eby and Williams (1951) who compared people suffering Ménière's disease with people suffering various diseases of *retro*cochlear origin. These researchers found the phenomenon in the former group but not always in the latter. The diagnostic utility of recruitment became more marked, and it is now taken by some authors (Hallpike, 1967) that *absence* of recruitment signifies absence of cochlear disorder, especially Ménière's disease, and in conjunction with other signs of pure sensorineural disorder, its absence may signify (though less reliably) the presence of retrocochlear dysfunction.

Fowler's original postulate (1936) about recruitment of loudness and otosclerosis was not borne out, but his striking results from people with sensorineural disorder perhaps overshadowed any emergent data from otosclerosis sufferers. Anderson and Barr (1966), using the acoustic reflex threshold technique, reported that partial recruitment was observable in cases of what they term "fixation" of the ossicular chain but not observable in cases of "interruption" (breakage) of the chain. Otosclerosis is a major fixation-type conductive disorder, and Anderson and Barr diagnosed this condition in 18 of their 24 fixation cases. This result of course is contrary to Fowler's (1936) hypothesis, and furthermore, Anderson and Barr found increasing partial recruitment with increasing severity of the fixation effect. An earlier and comprehensive report by Lansberg (1954), which seems to have been overlooked by both Anderson and Barr and other authors in this field, devotes considerable space to consideration of partial recruitment in conductive disorders of a type akin to Anderson and Barr's fixation category. Lansberg's theory of conductive recruitment invokes abnormal impedance–intensity relations to explain the effect. His explanation is beyond the present author's understanding; it is mentioned merely to cue the curious who would pursue the issue. Anderson and Barr (1966) offer no specific theory to account for their findings.

The purpose in referring to documented evidence regarding conductive (partial) recruitment relates more to arguments about the alleged way recruitment interferes with auditory perception. It is worth bearing in mind that partial recruitment reportedly manifests in some types of conductive disorder.

Explanatory Hypotheses

Harris (1953) gives a comprehensive account of the early development of interest in the recruitment phenomenon, as well as brief notes on the various theories which have emerged to account for it. I will elaborate on only two of the traditional theories, as these have had most support from authors in the field. A recent model of recruitment is also described on pages 206–208.

Loudness Units

This traditional account is based on the mechanism of summation of neural activity as the basis of loudness coding—which summation is in terms of increasing numbers of activated cochlear units with increasing input to the cochlea and increasing rates of discharge of units with rising input. The account that superseded this, which relies on differential unit sensitivity, is based on the hypothesis that the outermost row of cochlear hair cells has the lowest threshold, the second and third rows have respectively higher thresholds, and hair cells in the single inner row are activated at levels well above baseline threshold.

The summation account is neatly argued by Steinberg and Gardner (1937). From an earlier study of loudness, Fletcher and Munson (1933) developed the concept of arbitrary loudness units and showed by various methods the relation between intensity of a 1 kHz reference tone and loudness of matching tones (the basis of the sone scale). If loudness units correspond to numbers–rates of activity of cochlear neurons, then a cochlear disorder will presumably render some fixed number of such units inactive. Subtracting a fixed number of loudness units as a hypothetical model of cochlear disorder means that loudness in the disordered ear begins at a higher intensity level than it does in the reference ear (i.e., there is an elevation of threshold). However, since loudness increases in a logarithmic relation to sound level, the loss of a fixed number of units becomes proportionately of diminishing importance with rising intensity above threshold, and the growth of loudness curve in the disordered cochlea climbs to meet the loudness curve in the normal ear. By contrast, in an ear with attenuative disorder prior to the cochlea, a constant proportional reduction of sound level into the cochlea is occurring, not a fixed loss of active neurons in a population otherwise stimulated by sound of the *same* intensity as in a normal ear. Loudness growth in a conductive disorder simply mirrors loudness growth in the normal ear but originates at a higher intensity level.

Steinberg and Gardner (1937) went on to demonstrate experimentally the analogy given at the beginning of this chapter. In a normal ear masked by white noise, the growth in loudness of a tone shows precisely the effect of a disordered cochlea. Anderson and Barr (1966) showed the other effect, namely of plugging a normal ear. This expedient produces an increase in level at threshold but no recruitment. Masking has the effect of negating activity in a fixed number of cochlear neurons (by maintaining their activity). An earplug has the effect of reducing the intensity, in constant proportion, of a sound prior to the cochlea.

A variant of the "loudness units" account is given by von Békésy

(1970), based on actual modeling of the cochlea using vibration of the human forearm. When the arm is vibrated with a large frame, the self-recording threshold trace (threshold of detection of vibration) shows wide excursions from "signal absent" to "signal present." When a vibrating needle is used, the threshold level increases—i.e., more current is required for detection—and the trace width diminishes. Von Békésy argues that in the first case we have an analog of the normally functioning cochlea, where a large number of units can summate at low input levels to allow detection, but by the same principle of combined discharge, the growth of sensation is gradual. In the needle condition, only one or two units are stimulated, hence summation cannot occur and threshold of detection is higher. However, once the single unit is activated, it obeys the all-or-none principle of neural discharge; and so the transition from signal absent to signal present is almost instantaneous. In the disordered cochlea, reduction of functioning units will produce this sort of effect, especially at the basal end of Corti's organ where the number of stimulated units is small to begin with. This will result in marked "threshold recruitment" at higher frequencies.

On pages 210–212 we consider the relation of changes in loudness growth to changes in the pattern of threshold of detection, for it seems these are by no means measures of the same phenomenon.

Differential Cell Sensitivity

The "place" theory of loudness, based on differential sensitivity of hair cells depending on their location, has become the more favored hypothesis to account for recruitment. Until very recent times, it held prime position as regards both loudness coding and hence, by implication, loudness disorder. Davis, Morgan, Hawkins, Galambos, and Smith (1950) developed the explanatory concept of recruitment, at least regarding noise-induced cochlear disorder. The "place" theory of loudness as a basis for explaining noise disorder has anatomical evidence in its favor (Schuknecht, 1953). A typical cochlear picture of noise injury shows greater destruction of outer hair cells than of inner. Hence if the "place" theory of loudness coding is accurate, an explanation of disordered loudness growth is straightforward. The low threshold (outermost) cells can no longer be activated; but as input intensity increases, there is a rapid return to normal loudness experience as the higher threshold and intact inner hair cells begin to respond. Electrocochleographic recording by Portmann, Aran, and Lagourge (1973) apparently bears out this picture. A "place" explanation of recruitment is harder to sustain in Ménière's syndrome, where anatomical changes are not selective but instead metabolic changes affecting the whole of the end organ seem to occur. Schuknecht (1970) tries to reconcile these different types of disorder by an explanation that partly passes over the selectivity principle and relies on the occurrence of disproportionate destruction or disturbance of hair cells rather than fibers innervating the hair cells, irrespective of location. His explanation is obscure, however, and notable only inasmuch as it seems to beg an interaction between fibers innervating inner and outer hair cells, a concept that defies the "place" hypothesis.

Tuning Curves

In recent times, the state of understanding as regards cochlear coding systems for both loudness and pitch has undergone radical revision. Coding of loudness is now as theoretically problematic as coding of frequency (Simmons, 1970). However, a recent review by E. F. Evans (1975), which provides a fair overview of current understanding, is of special interest because quite a new model of recruitment is offered on the basis of that review. From the work with cats and guinea pigs of various researchers, including Evans, it emerges that individual cochlear nerve fibers exhibit highly specific tuning characteristics. That is to say, individual neural units fire at low input levels in response to signals of specific audio frequency. The frequency at which response is elicited at the lowest input level is known as the unit's "characteristic frequency." With increasing input level, these same units behave like tuning circuits by showing responses to neighboring audio frequencies. Especially in the 2–20 kHz region, the frequency threshold curves or "tuning curves" of these units spread out with increasing signal level, and around 40–50 dB above threshold they show a dramatic unilateral broadening of response. They are thus activated by signals throughout the audio-frequency range lower than the characteristic frequency. These effects are shown in Figure 8.2 for a variety of individual units having different characteristic frequencies.

As E. F. Evans (1975) points out, one very important feature to emerge from the growing body of data of the kind shown, is that recordings from cochlear fibers are most likely to be from neurons innervating *inner* hair cells. This is because at least 90% of such fibers terminate in these cells. Despite the greater population of outer hair cells, innervation of these is relatively sparse (Spoendlin, 1972). The work of Dallos, Billone, Durrant, Wang, and Raynor (1972) nonetheless shows marked reduction of the gross cochlear microphonic in response to selective destruction of outer hair cells; and Kiang, Moxon, and Levine's work (1970) showed abnormal threshold responses from *inner* hair cell fibers following *outer* hair cell destruction. The necessity then is for some process of interaction between inner and outer hair cells. The study by Zwislocki and Sokolich (1973) provides evidence, and the more general review by Zwislocki (1975) provides a plausible model for such interaction based on the concept of outer and inner hair cells operating in phase opposi-

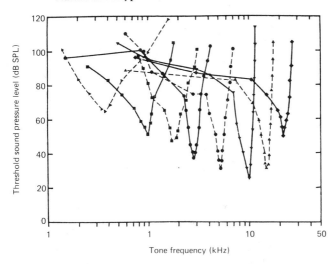

Figure 8.2. Frequency threshold curves ("tuning" curves) of eight individual cochlear nerve fibers from six guinea pigs, showing lower-level, sharply tuned segment and unilateral broadening of frequency sensitivity with increasing signal level. From E. F. Evans (1975), © S. Karger, A. G., and reproduced with permission of publisher and author.

tion. Zwislocki's (1975) model in effect solves E. F. Evans' (1975) interaction problem.

Of more immediate practical import is the effect of disruptive events within the cochlea. Characteristically, the result of selective destruction and of chemical interference (anoxia, hypoxia) is disappearance of the lower-input, sharply tuned segment of the frequency tuning curve, leaving only the higher-input, broadly tuned segment intact. Such an outcome, incidentally, is predictable from Zwislocki's interactive model. The outcome suggests a new model of recruitment based not on missing units affecting loudness growth but on missing segments of units' tuning curves. A schematization of Evans' model is shown in Figure 8.3. Normally a single-frequency tone will activate only a small group of units at threshold, but with increasing input level other units will respond as the tone invades their broadening frequency tuning curves. At higher levels still, a large proportion of cells will respond. In the damaged cochlea, with the lower-input, sharply tuned segments missing, initial response threshold will be elevated, but beyond threshold the number of units responding will increase rapidly rather than gradually. Assuming loudness is at some level coded as total amount of electrical activity from the cochlea, this picture of recruitment is highly plausible. In particular, the model can account for recruitment arising from various forms of assault upon end-organ receptors.

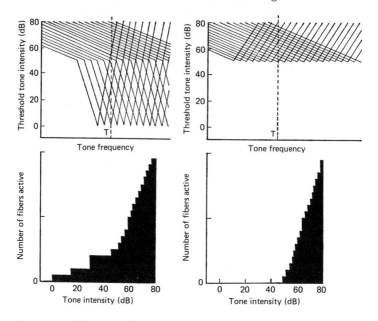

Figure 8.3. Evans' (1975) model of recruitment based on disappearance of lower-level, sharply tuned segments of FTCs following injury or toxic assault upon the cochlea. In the upper diagrams, schema of the responses of normal and disordered cochlear fibers are shown. In the lower diagrams, the summed loudness functions resulting from these two states are shown. In the normal cochlea, with sharp tuning characteristic intact, the engagement of neighboring cells as signal level rises is gradual. In the damaged cochlea, initial threshold is at a higher level because of the missing lower-level segments, and the engagement of neighboring cells is rapid with increasing signal level because of the remaining broadly tuned segments. From E. F. Evans (1975), © S. Karger, A. G., and reproduced with permission of publisher and author.

THE MEASUREMENT OF RECRUITMENT

The treatment in this section is cursory. Its purpose is not to give a technical guide to the estimation of recruitment; any standard audiological handbook can provide that information. Its function is merely to remind readers of certain ways that recruitment is expressed and of certain clinical characteristics that limit the ways open to its determination. I also refer to some critical work by Jerger emerging from his comparison of different techniques.

Alternate Binaural and Monaural Balancing

Fowler's original clinical groups (1936, 1937) were of people with unilateral auditory disorders. Recruitment was assessed by loudness matching across the two ears to provide the sort of diagram shown in Figure 8.1. The alternate binaural loudness balance (ABLB) test was

Fowler's important development in 1936, and it is a technique administered to this day to people with unilateral disorder. There are problems with the ABLB technique, insofar as the shape of the interaural loudness growth function may not show the nice regularity depicted in our schematic figure. Harris, Haines, and Myers (1952) distinguished four basic functions: straight line, asymptotic curve, biphasic ("dogleg"), and biphasic–asymptotic. They found no regularity of type against diagnosis. Hallpike and Hood (1959) on the other hand, report finding mainly straight-line functions in listeners with unilateral Ménière's disease. The latter authors concluded that a reliable scheme to describe degree of recruitment depicts it in terms of the angle subtended by the interaural equal-loudness line as a function of increasing intensity. When interaural loudness is equivalent, then at equal intensities from threshold to the upper intensity limit, that angle will be 45° when each ear's responses are plotted on an $x-y$ graph. When a straight-line recruitment manifests in one pathological ear, the line will originate somewhere along the x or y axis and meet the 45° (theoretically normal) line at some point. Hence a more obtuse angle will be made by the equal-loudness line and the x or y axis. The greater the degree of recruitment, the larger that angle will be. Clearly this scheme can only function validly for straight-line relationships.

The ABLB technique can only be used in cases of unilateral pathology, and even then there is always the problem of the loudness growth function in the contralateral ("normal") ear. Greven and Oosterveld (1975) addressed themselves to a question which bears on this point. In a group of 292 people with Ménière's disease, 70% showed signs of sensorineural disorders of the "better" ear, 26% showed recruitment "signs" by self-recording threshold trace. If these data are generalizable, they suggest that use of ABLB has to be severely restricted, in Ménière's cases at least; for otherwise, "observations" of partial or complete recruitment could be made which are mere artefacts generated by interaural balancing of *two* disordered ears. This sort of limitation suggests that the use of ABLB is an occasional luxury and not an everyday clinical routine. That the research group (Dix, Hallpike, Hood, & colleagues) at National Hospital, London has been able to apply the technique repeatedly can presumably be ascribed to the special clientele arriving on their doorstep, making large sample selection more feasible than it would be in a general clinical population.

Monaural techniques for estimating recruitment have been developed by a number of researchers, and clinical tests of what Jerger (1961) has termed "allied phenomena" have also emerged. This latter point is crucial in discussion of recruitment "detection" or estimation. We return to it in a moment. Monaural alternate loudness balancing relies upon the equal loudness contour concept and in effect gets the listener to reenact

Fletcher and Munson's (1933) experiments. Naturally, results are often equivocal. Inexperienced listeners find it hard to provide equal loudness estimates across frequency. The purpose of the test being to see whether loudness is "compressed" at any point, it requires that recruitment be restricted to a particular bandwidth. Pathologies of different kinds do not happily go along with this demand, although noise-induced disorder would be the most likely exception. AMLB testing is probably a valid indicator of recruitment in such cases, and of course it is usually the only equal-loudness technique applicable in such cases, since they are typically bilateral.

Short Increment Sensitivity Index (SISI) and Békésy "Types"

The tests which have emerged as capable of monaural application are the SISI test of Jerger, Shedd, and Harford (1959) and von Békésy's (1947) self-recording tonal threshold technique. The latter's rationale has already been discussed, narrowing of trace width being the sign that von Békésy attributes to "recruitment." The SISI test is a development of the differential loudness threshold concept (difference limen). In a recruiting case, the difference limen will be reduced, hence very small changes in input level should be more readily detectable, on average, in the recruiting ear than in the nonrecruiting.

Palva (1957) showed the von Békésy phenomenon to hold at higher frequencies but not in the .25 to 3 kHz range. A certain amount of overlap in distributions of trace width between recruiting and nonrecruiting ears was also observable at higher frequencies. Jerger (1960) reported on different categories of self-recording tonal threshold traces, especially different patterns of response among different listeners, when an interrupted tone was used as stimulus rather than a continuous tone. The "Type I" audiogram, in which the continuous and interrupted traces are fairly consistently matched, typically was found in people with conductive disorder. The "Type II" audiogram—showing higher level at threshold beyond .5 to 1 kHz for continuous rather than interrupted tone combined with a narrowing of trace width—was consistently manifest in people with cochlear disorder. "Types III and IV" audiograms—showing "tone decay" for a continuous stimulus ("Type III") and higher level at threshold for a continuous stimulus throughout the audiofrequency range ("Type IV")—were found in people with retrocochlear disorder.

Attack on the Concept

In 1961, Jerger published a report of both empirical and conceptual importance. He argued that "recruitment" had become reified as the diagnostic sign *sur tout*, search for its presence or absence being taken as an end in itself. Furthermore, the ABLB test was seen to be the criterion measure of recruitment so that other tests such as the SISI or self-recording types were to be judged by their ability to coincide with the ABLB measure. The flaw in this line of approach, Jerger points out, is that the aim of the exercise is to pinpoint the site of the disorder in a person's auditory system reliably, not to find out whether that system manifests recruitment or not. While Dix *et al.* (1948) showed recruitment to be always present in their cases of Ménière's disease by the ABLB test, the reverse did not obtain. That is to say, the presence of recruitment as determined by the ABLB method did *not* always signify Ménière's disease. Recall here that recruitment was noted by Dix *et al.* (1948) in retrocochlear disorders, and partial recruitment has been noted in conductive disorders (Anderson & Barr, 1966; Lansberg, 1954). The ABLB test then may be the only valid measure of *recruitment*, but recruitment may not be as useful a diagnostic weapon as other "allied phenomena."

To explore this contention, Jerger compared test results in groups of people, all with independently verified unilateral disorders. Three clinical samples were studied: conductive ($N = 21$); cochlear (Ménière's, $N = 20$); and retrocochlear (acoustic neuronoma, $N = 11$). Each group was tested with the ABLB technique, and individual listeners were classified as showing "no recruitment," "partial recruitment," or "complete recruitment." In the conductive group, all were classified as showing "no recruitment"; in the cochlear group, however, only 10 were classified as showing "complete recruitment"; 5 showed "partial recruitment" and 5, most surprisingly, showed none at all. In the retrocochlear group, 9 showed "no recruitment" and 2 showed "partial recruitment."

The SISI test was negative in 15 of the 21 conductive cases, doubtful in 4 and positive in 2; the SISI test was positive in all 20 cochlear cases and negative in 10 of the 11 retrocochlear cases. "Type I" audiograms were noted in 19 of the conductive cases ("Type II" in the remaining 2); "Type II" audiograms were noted in 19 of the cochlear cases ("Type I" in the remaining 1); and "Types III and IV" were noted in all 11 of the retrocochlear cases.

It is obvious from this study that the self-recording "types" emerged as the most useful diagnostic tool, missing only 3 of 52 differential diagnoses. Of equal concern and more immediate present interest, the lack of agreement between the tests is quite marked. This was demonstrated even more forcefully in a further group of 75 listeners with unilateral sensorineural disorder of unknown etiology. Whereas 54 of them provided "Type II" audiograms and 12 provided "Types III and IV," only 16 showed complete recruitment, and 37 showed none at all. Evidently the various tests used in diagnosis are tapping different signs of auditory disorder. The fact that the audiogram "types" cannot predict ABLB results ("recruitment") or vice versa makes this conclusion inevitable. Equally important, the ABLB test is quite unreliable in diagnosis in comparison with the audiogram "types." Recruitment then, from the above analysis, is an elusive phenomenon. The major flaw in Jerger's (1961) report, it should be pointed out, is absence of detail regarding classification procedures for diagnosis on the one hand, and performance test results on the other. It is not stated whether these were done by independent observers.

ALLEGED EFFECT OF LOUDNESS DISTORTION ON HEARING

Jerger's (1961) concern is to identify the tests that reliably aid in differential diagnosis. Nowhere does he discuss the meaning of this or that diagnostic sign in relation to the nature of hearing disturbance. His results support a conclusion that whatever the mechanism(s) underlying the special problem of (for example) disturbed speech discrimination ability in sensorineural disorder, recruitment, or at least its signs in the ABLB test, can be only partly or occasionally responsible. Of course such a conclusion cannot firmly emerge from his data as no speech discrimination testing was undertaken, hence any variation in that ability could not be compared with variations in each diagnostic test. It is unfortunate, but to my knowledge no such systematic study has ever been done. A few data sets are available to let us examine the interrelation between recruitment assessed by various methods and speech discrimination ability; But as far as I am aware, there are no data from a systematic study on relations between the latter and either SISI or von Békésy audiogram "types."

Résumé of Work Reviewed in Chapter 6

We have already considered studies in which loudness compression measured by various methods was compared with speech discrimination ability as part of more general studies among people with sensorineural disorder. It is useful to gather these results together here as a reminder that in clinical sensorineural samples as a general category, and in people with noise-induced disorder in particular, no evidence was forthcoming to demonstrate a relation between the two measures. Palva's (1955) data were analyzed to show that in people manifesting recruitment, measured by ABLB or AMLB, no lesser speech discrimination ability was observable than in people not so manifesting. In addition, only a marginally greater correlation was noted between speech discrimination and tonal threshold average at 1, 2, and 4 kHz in people who showed recruitment compared with those who did not. Mullins and Bangs (1957) assessed loudness compression by observing the intensity range between lower tonal threshold and the threshold of discomfort at .5, 1, 2, 3, and 4 kHz in a group of veterans. Correlation (r) between this measure and discrimination score ranged from $-.113$ to .084. Ward *et al.* (1961) measured loudness compression by AMLB in two groups of noise-deafened workers, and my analysis of their data showed that this measure correlated (r_s) with discrimination score at .079 in one sample of listeners and at .015 in the other. Finally, Ross *et al.* (1965) measured loudness compression by the difference-limen-for-loudness method in a clinical sample. Correlation with discrimination score was $-.01$ in the right ear and $-.1$ in the left.

All in all, results examined so far support a conclusion that recruitment or loudness compression is quite unrelated to problems of discrimination. However, before closing the case one should look in more detail at the literature that sets out to make such a case. There is a suggestion that if speech discrimination is differently approached the recruitment–discrimination pattern of interrelation may be emergent.

Reorientation to pro-Loudness Distortion Literature

The main contemporary protagonist of recruitment of loudness as a cause of the discrimination difficulty experienced by people with cochlear disorder is Hood of the United Kingdom National Hospital group. He has never ventured an explanatory mechanism for the causal effect, but he has produced one item of evidence to support the claim (Hood, 1968). The initial impetus for the loudness recruitment–speech discrimination interaction can probably be traced to Huizing (1949) and Huizing and Reyntjes (1952). Huizing (1949) provides no evidence of an effect on speech discrimination ability that can be attributed to loudness distortion but presents a theory to the effect that compression of loudness is problematic in that the amplitude modulations of speech will be distortedly received and hence affect intelligibility. This problem will be especially exacerbated if an ordinary hearing aid is used. Huizing and Reyntjes (1952) reiterate this theoretical point, but once again evidence is not forthcoming to back it up. However, in their 1952 paper the authors present an idealized picture of the articulation function of a typical person with recruitment of loudness. They claim that in such a case intelligibility of speech may increase up to a point with increasing signal intensity and then deteriorate again with further energy increase. This picture is contrasted with the more usual articulation function. The phenomenon is schematized in Figure 8.4.

More substantial evidence of this configuration comes first from Dix,

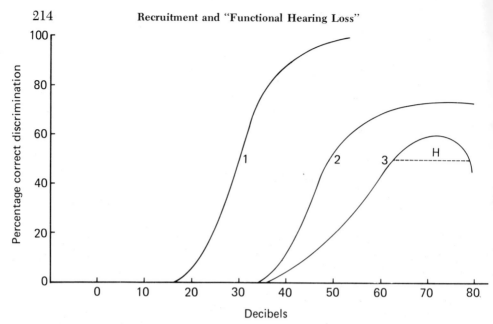

Figure 8.4 Articulation functions in various conditions. The lines represent (1) typical normal articulation function; (2) articulation function in a sensorineural case showing nonmaximum asymptote; (3) articulation function allegedly typical of people with recruitment, showing "rollover." The dashed line (H), suggested as a measure of discrimination difficulty by Huizing and Reyntjes (1952), is an expression of the signal width throughout which 50% articulation is possible. The measure is a suggested improvement over single-score expressions of discrimination ability in that more of the information in a "rollover" articulation curve is utilized. Schema from Huizing and Reyntjes (1952), reproduced by permission of *The Laryngoscope*.

Hallpike, and Hood (1949), who demonstrated relatively uniform articulation functions in people with conductive and retrocochlear disorder but found a picture of the articulation function in people with Ménière's disease consistent with the scheme given by Huizing and Reyntjes (1952). The result of Dix *et al.* (1949) was confirmed by Eby and Williams (1951) and by Cawthorne and Harvey (1953).

Three points for consideration emerge from this literature. First, there is the theory put forward by Huizing (1949) regarding disturbed amplitude modulation; second, there is the peculiar shape of the articulation function in cases of Ménière's disease; and third, there is the common feature of presence of both recruitment and distorted articulation in the case of Ménière's and the absence of both recruitment and distorted articulation in the case of conductive and retrocochlear disorder. Actually, as regards these cases we have already noted that partial recruitment may be observed in conductive disorder and complete recruitment in retrocochlear disorder. We have also observed that recruitment as assessed by ABLB may be undetected in cases of Ménière's disease. Leaving aside these anomalies, the discussion can center on the general fact that recruitment by ABLB measurement more often than not occurs in Ménière's but does not occur to the same degree in the other pathological categories. We should note, however, that there has been opportunity to test the speech discrimination–recruitment relationship *across* pathologies by virtue of these anomalies, but this has never, to my knowledge, been attempted.

Returning to the first point, the important challenge to Huizing's (1949) theory comes from Licklider and Pollack's (1948) study of the effect of infinite peak clipping on speech intelligibility. The latter has already been discussed in Chapter 6. The point to be made here is that infinite peak clipping entirely removes amplitude modulation information from the speech signal; and while this affects intelligibility, it does not negate it; and furthermore, listeners can improve their performance with practice, thus retrieving the speech information. It should be the case, therefore, that if amplitude modulation disturbance is the root of the intelligibility problem for people manifesting recruitment, it should not be as profound as it appears to be, and it should meliorate with the passage of time.

As regards the peculiar shape of the articulation function in those with Ménière's disease (and/or recruitment), the practical import is that a single measure of discrimination ability like that used by the various authors mentioned in pages 212–213 may be an inadequate gauge with which to compare degree of recruitment. Huizing and Reyntjes (1952) in fact suggest the measure of discrimination shown and explained in Figure 8.4, and Hood (1968) adopts a similar approach for similar reasons. We will come to the latter work presently.

The last of the three points is scientifically the most troublesome. Gross discrimination problems are observable in people with Ménière's disease, and recruitment is also found in such people. The contrary is the case in other pathologies. On the other hand, recruitment is present in noise-induced disorder (a cochlear disorder like Ménière's) but its relation to discrimination problems is nondemonstrable. By contrast, tonal threshold level and audiogram shape in such cases can be shown to link with speech reception–discrimination ability (MacRae & Brigden, 1973). By further contrast, audiogram shape at least cannot be invoked for Ménière's sufferers because it is as often akin to a conductive audiogram shape as to any other pathology.

But the important point is that as regards threshold level and profile there is an a priori explanatory mechanism to be tested. No such satisfactory state of affairs exists regarding recruitment. Mere coincidence or lack of coincidence of the kind already described is taken by authors such as Dix *et al.* (1949), Cawthorne and Harvey (1953), and Hood and Poole (1971) as sufficient explanation for a *causal* connection between recruitment and speech discrimination loss. Scientifically, this is unacceptable for the straightforward reason that no theoretical guide can be given to the conduct of empirical studies.

Hood (1968) has gone somewhat further than previous authors by attempting to show a relationship between degree of recruitment and extent of discrimination difficulty, though unfortunately only in people with Ménière's disease. There is another unfortunate feature of Hood's (1968) report which we mention presently; but his study, as far as I know, is the only one to have made this small step toward empirical verification, so it is worth considering in detail.

Following Huizing and Reyntjes' (1952) point that the whole articulation function needs to be expressed, Hood (1968) devised a scheme to integrate the area of articulation that is lost in reversed or asymptotic articulation functions. On the assumption that a normally shaped sigmoid represents 100% discrimination ability, any deviation from that shape, irrespective of intensity required to achieve it, means a loss of articulation. This measure is similar to maximum articulation score but has the advantage of utilizing more of the available data in the articulation curve. Hood shows a scattergram of recruitment angle (Hallpike & Hood, 1959; Hood, 1960) and percentage of loss according to the discrimination index in 27 listeners. Discrimination test material is not described, but it was probably the United Kingdom Medical Research Council recorded lists of PB words. No correlation analysis was actually made, but the data points are given. Hence by application of a transparent matrix to the scattergram, a consistent set of values can be read off from both axes. Correlation (Spearman) then calculated gave a value of .46 ($N = 27$). This is certainly an improvement on the correlations summarized in pages 212–213, but it is not remarkable nor is it a convincing datum in support of the supposed causal link between recruitment (as measured by ABLB) and speech discrimination difficulty. Such a degree of association is in fact on a par with the findings of Harris (1965) about the relation between discrimination score and higher frequency tonal threshold. As in previous literature in this area, no explanatory mechanism is invoked to account for the recruitment effect.

In addition to these data, Hood (1968) reports data from an individual case. These consist of tonal threshold, speech discrimination function, and recruitment records of a person in stages of recovery from unilateral deafness associated with disseminated sclerosis. Whereas the audiogram shows a minor departure from normality in the worst phase of the disorder (as indexed by the articulation function) and apparently total normality at a stage where the disorder is still slightly apparent, the loudness recruitment record parallels the articulation record. Thus the recruitment record more accurately reflects the state of disturbance. The baffling feature in this instance is that the disordered loudness function shows "recruitment reversal"—that is to say, a *retarded* growth of loudness with increasing intensity in the affected ear. We are invited then to accept not only that *compression* of the loudness–intensity function affects speech perception (as in the correlational study) but also that decompression of that function has an *identical* effect. Whatever may be the mechanism of recruitment on speech discrimination, the issue is quite clouded by this example of Hood's. The reason for that cloudiness is precisely that no a priori case has been made and substantiated regarding cause and effect.

On the evidence to this point it may be concluded that loudness distortion is a sign of disorder and hence perhaps of disturbance, but there is just no evidence that loudness distortion *of itself* is the cause of that disturbance. There may be a case for suggesting that recruitment has a larger role to play in Ménière's disease and hence contributes to the greater discrimination problems suffered by people with that disorder. Such can only be a suggestion, however, since no systematic study has been done of various other contributory factors. In the final event, to have observed such a contributory effect in one disorder is to have said nothing about other disorders. In regard to Carhart's (1946b) work, I complained that a mechanism (audiogram shape) was being invoked to compare with speech hearing ability with no control for the interaction of pathological type. In the case of research on recruitment and speech hearing, we witness the contrary shortcoming: a mechanism being invoked with no *disregard* for pathological type.

One minor point to be noted in concluding this section is in regard to compression–amplification hearing aids. If loudness compression in and of itself were really the basic problem, then it should be overcome by use of such aids. These devices function to reduce the dynamic range of incoming signals and hence to match their modulations to the operational dynamics of the "recruiting" ear. Vargo (1974), after reviewing a number of evaluative projects (including his own) that used such devices, concluded that, "the assumption that the hearing-impaired listener possessing recruitment, can effectively utilize compression amplification for speech discrimination enhancement has not been clearly supported [p. 7]."

Conclusion

Compared with the evidence presented in support of a frequency-filtering effect as causal in the speech discrimination problem in cochlear disorder, the evidence supporting recruitment (at least as assessed by ABLB) is weak. An absence of mechanism, combined with paucity and tenuousness of data, makes it difficult to perceive the link between ABLB loudness distortion and poor speech intelligibility.

In the final event, I do not think the frequency-filtering effect as a causal mechanism has a great deal going for it either. What we are dealing with in gazing at either of these phenomena (high-tone hearing loss; loudness distortion), are signs of disorder in the cochlear system. We are a long way yet from unraveling this (these) disorder(s) and understanding their disruptive effect(s). The high frequency threshold effect may just represent a more reliable index of the pathological condition of the cochlea than does the loudness distortion effect.

It seems to me, however, that in E. F. Evans' (1975) model, presented at the beginning of this chapter, we have the outline at least of a more rational explanation of speech discrimination disturbance. Evans is careful in fact to discuss separately the recruitment effect and other effects arising from fine-tuning degradation. It emerges as a clear possibility that if the cochlea, once damaged by whatever agent, is capable of only gross frequency discrimination, the features and modulations in that domain which seem to be vital in discrimination of speech sounds (see Chapter 1) will no longer be so readily detectable. Of course, we still need to find out why discrimination decreases in many cases rather than merely reaches an asymptote (as in many others) with increasing intensity. Such a task is beyond the present scope, however.

"FUNCTIONAL HEARING LOSS"

Aims of the Present Discussion

The two tasks I have set myself in this part of the chapter are (a) to show where the uncertainties lie in detection and assessment of "functional hearing loss" ("FHL") and (b) to put a case for scrapping the current definitional approach to the problem by introducing the concept of *fakability*. The definitional problem must take paramount position because use of a term like "functional hearing loss" draws attention to the person as though the person were presenting a clinical disorder. Once that perceptual act has occurred, once the person is seen as a potential clinical case, signs that supposedly confirm the clinical disorder are taken as proof that the person is indeed presenting this "type of hearing loss." Such a diagnosis can then be used, in circular fashion, to explain the presenting signs. I will "unpack" these contentions on pages 228–229.

I said at the beginning of this chapter that "recruitment" and "FHL" are unrelated. That is correct, I think, but there is an underlying connection at the conceptual level. Writers have assumed that "recruitment" causes a certain hearing disturbance and taken evidence of its presence or absence, along with evidence of the presence or absence of the disturbance, as proof of the cause–effect relation. That is to say, the presentation of deviant loudness growth is taken as a *clinical symptom* of disturbance rather than a *psychoacoustical sign* of disorder. In analogous fashion, a certain pattern of audiometric response is taken as a *clinical symptom* of "FHL" rather than a sign that the test is being faked or that the test is unreliable. I do not want to try to squash these issues into parallel juxtaposition, but I do want to argue that a common feature of both is that they direct attention in certain ways as a result of a previous definitional exercise whose nature is questionable.

Let me be clear also about the fact of fake test results. It is undoubtedly the case that people will fake on a test if the result improves their chances of gaining some sought-for reward or sanction that cannot be gained *except* by means of these tests.

In my view, however, it is shortsighted (or perhaps narrowsighted) to see this situation as a clinical problem residing in the person and in no way as a problem generated by administrative procedure which involves use of unreliable (fakable, insensitive, or inadequate) tests.

Definition and Problems of Definition

"Functional hearing loss" is the term put forward by Ventry and Chaiklin (1962) as the least ambiguous and (it is hoped) least judgmental label for loss of hearing that is suspected to be feigned or exaggerated. At the same time, these authors suggest that the term "psychogenic hearing loss" should be reserved to describe "actual" deafness or partial deafness of "apparent psychological origin." It seems fairly clear from this distinction that "FHL" is to do the semantic job that the word *malingering* used to do. Ventry and Chaiklin provide many good reasons why *malingering* should be dropped from the medicolegal vocabulary. One reason is that *malingering,* having such pejorative connotations, is damaging in its effect not only to the person so labeled but also to the *labeler,* who can be sued as a libeler if his "accusation" is not backed up by an admission on the malingerer's part. It is just as critical, in the view of Ventry and Chaiklin (1962), that "malingering" cannot be differentiated from other forms of "FHL" and therefore has no useful medicolegal status.

This last point is interesting because it suggests that "FHL" is taken to be different from "malingering"; but the only difference I can make out is a difference of intent on the physician's or audiologist's part when "FHL" rather than "malingering" is applied as a "diagnosis." "Malingering" has a willful connotation, a criminal quality; "FHL" is more clinical and sterile and lacks the same accusatory flavor. A person may present "FHL" rather than "psychogenic hearing loss" yet not be seen in the same contemptuous light as he would had he been "malingering." "Malingering" is something wrong that a person *does;* "FHL" is something wrong that a person *has*. The one is a "criminal" or at least a "delinquent" act; the other is a "clinical" disorder. The replacement of "malingering" by "FHL" thus takes the moral sting out of the situation. I want to show what happens to people (both physicians and "patients") as a result of this transformation; to show that it is an unsatisfactory state of affairs, scientifically and morally; and to suggest a fresh approach that could help clear away the muddle that presently interferes with straight thinking about the issue.

Where did "malingering" get its awful quality? The answer is clear from a remark by Collie (1913) that "not many years ago it was practically only in naval and military circles that one heard the term used [p. 1]." My dictionary definition of the verb *malinger* is "to feign sickness in order to avoid duty." To do such a thing, of course, would carry criminal penalties, for in societies like ours which conscript (i.e., force) people to engage in mortal combat, fear and repugnance not unnaturally lead people to avoid such conscription. To counteract this move, the message from the state must be that avoidance is cowardly, unpatriotic, or otherwise reprehensible. Hence "malingering," a term with a bad odor in its very construction, will become associated with highly "antisocial" meanings.

In contrast to those in this military circumstance, some people in ordinary life present themselves to physicians or to family and friends as supposedly suffering a disorder. They may end up being classed as hypochondriacal, psychosomatic, hysterical, or whatever. These might be terms of abuse or terms to which psychotherapists turn in efforts to locate the origins of these problems. Although it may be that some function is served by illness that is acted-out (seeking affection, attention, seeking to inflict guilt in or to manipulate another), the tendency has never been to regard such manifestations as disgraceful or cowardly.

It is not unexpected that the term *malingering* has adhered to any feigning of sickness within military purview, including malingering for the purpose of gaining compensation. The term spread to nonmilitary medicolegal circles, assisted by such eminent figures as Sir John Collie, in a book entitled *Malingering* (1913), which deals in fact only with people seeking Workmen's Compensation. Collie made a stab at trying to fathom the "malingerer's" psyche, but the full-blooded medicalization of social deviance (Szasz, 1971) had only just got into gear in Collie's day, so not much space was given over to the attempt. Even 40 years later, the word is still used in reference to military people falsely seeking compensation (Glorig, 1954). Glorig's tone, however, is that of the thief catcher, and he sees the situation as a game of wits between the "malingerer" and the physician. Szasz (1956), more penetratingly, sees the physician as umpire in a game between the "malingerer" and the system. The system, however, has set the rules of play, so only the "malingerer" is interested in cheating.

I argue in various places throughout this book that the rules of the system can be seen as a form of cheating too and that scientists, as umpires, should watch both players with equal detachment.

The Clinical Transformation of "Malingering"

Ventry and Chaiklin's work (1965a) established once and for all the transformation of "malingering" into the clinical condition, "functional hearing loss." As I indicated earlier, this had the effect of negating any censorious attitude but replaced it with the "clinical gaze." That move is a miniature of the larger historical transformation detailed by Szasz (1971) in his book, *The Manufacture of Madness.* Szasz's thesis, abundantly supported by published work, is that institutional psychiatry (which he is careful to distinguish from contractual psychiatry) has replaced the Inquisition and that the person delivered up to institutional psychiatry (as opposed to the person who seeks the services of a psychiatrist in a contractual arrangement) is in the same social position as the person delivered up to the Inquisition as a heretic, Jew, or witch.

The image of identity between these two types of institutions is tellingly given in Kesey's (1962) novel, *One Flew over the Cuckoo's Nest.*

Szasz (1971) throughout his work shows how the "mental patient" is never treated at the hands of institutional psychiatry in the way a patient as "client" is treated within contractual psychiatry, yet all the terminology and procedure of medicine is used in treatment of the former patients as well as the latter. This similitude of clinical approach masks differences in attitude. All manner of intrusive and punishing procedures can be visited upon the mental "patient" in the name of psychiatric treatment. The removal of moral disapprobation cuts two ways: While it frees the person from criminal conviction (for example, in an "insanity" plea at law), it also frees the psychiatrist from reflection upon the morality of his procedures—because these can no longer be regarded as punishments visited on the wicked, simply as treatments visited on the sick.

The transformation of "malingering" into "FHL" is a model of the movement Szasz identifies, and the treatments meted out to "malingerer" and "FHL" sufferer are similarly a model. These treatments are further down "the scale" of treatments Szasz is concerned with, but their form is identical.

The Ventry and Chaiklin (1965a) report is of a multidisciplinary inquiry into "FHL," an inquiry whose research participants included physicians, psychologists, and psychiatrists. The first point of interest is that the study was conducted under the aegis of the Veterans Administration and that the persons studied were former servicemen presenting for suspected "FHL." Thus we already have an institutional framework for the conduct of this study. The population to be examined is made up not of clients seeking help but of former soldiers seeking money from the army. These people have been delivered up to the researchers by the system within which they all (veterans and researchers) operate.

The "imprisonment" of people in what Goffman (1961) terms a "total institution," such as the army, helps explain why the subjects for this study could be coerced and intruded on in ways that would never be acceptable in society at large. Two groups, one showing "signs" of "FHL" (i.e., discrepancies in test results not supposedly explicable by error or known organic disorder), the other not showing this discrepant pattern, were selected at random from the male veteran population referred to San Francisco Veterans Administration hospital for assessment for compensation. Without being told that they were to be participants in an intensive research study, the persons selected were required to be hospitalized for 3 to 4 days. In the "FHL" group, this was explained as necessary because test discrepancies entailed more thorough examination. "A great amount of persuasion was required to convince many subjects of the need for the required period of hospitalization [Ventry & Chaiklin, 1965a, pp. 182–183]." Of the men originally selected to be in the "FHL" group, 5 refused to be hospitalized. The final number in this group was 64. Of the men originally selected to be in the non-"FHL" group, 3 refused. The final number in this group was 36.

It is not stated what reason was given to the non-"FHL" control subjects for their hospitalization; but it should be obvious that since veterans are no longer in the armed forces, the obligation to be interned in a hospital is even more grossly intrusive that it would be were they "prisoners" of the system. It is only conceivable that these people could be forced, without their informed consent about their participation in the research study, because of the compensation context. That context consisted in this instance of the interaction between subject as claimant and researcher as examiner.

This feature of the research design alone belies any claim to its being akin to some other research inquiry that might involve hospitalization. Furthermore, if one is told that there are "discrepancies" in test results and this requires 3 to 4 days in an army hospital for more thorough examination, the threat element in quite unmistakable.

On presenting at the hospital, non-"FHL" control subjects were interviewed and told that the examiners (researchers) *had been requested* to engage in a thorough inquiry of persons with hearing disorder. Thus, the examiners exonerated themselves by making it seem that they were "under orders" to carry out this task. Subjects in the "FHL" group were given a blunter (and more truthful) explanation, namely that they showed "unacceptable differences" between results on the earlier tests and that this needed a thorough investigation. These subjects were asked, before being told this, if they knew why they had been hospitalized; and the whole interview was designed "to provide a possible stimulus for resolution of their functional hearing loss [Ventry & Chaiklin, 1965a, p. 189]." By "resolution" the authors mean presentation of nondiscrepant test results. Now a most interesting outcome of the whole program is that despite masses of tests and interviews, including considerable shots of GSR (electric-shock) audiometry, 20 of the 64 men in the "FHL" group remained "unresolved" or "persisted" in presentation of discrepant results; 19 "resolved" as a result of the hospitalization; and the remaining 25 had "resolved" by the time they got to the hospital.

The unresolved group, as mentioned, were given extra sessions of GSR testing, cajoled by further interviews ("counseling"), and in general punished for the discrepant "signs" they "persisted" in showing. But persist they did, and sustained an "unresolved" label at the end of 3 to 4 days of hospital "treatment." Various psychiatric measures were made of resolved and unresolved cases, but nothing showed up to account for the differences in behavior (Ventry, Trier, & Chaiklin, 1965).

Much more significant, the major difference between "FHL" and non-"FHL" groups as a whole (Trier & Levy, 1965) was an average $2000 per annum greater family income enjoyed by the latter group. That was the only reliable difference, in fact, between the two groups in a psychiatric and psychological study that involved examination of personal records and data of each person, close inquiry into personal history and background, assessment of IQ, and a vast battery of other tests. This extraordinarily intrusive procedure, for purposes unknown to the participants, again belies any claim that the research program was like any other investigation of *hearing* disorder.

The vital purpose of the study was to find a performance measure that would reliably indicate the presence of "FHL." The critical index against which any test could be judged was GSR audiometry. We discuss GSR testing presently, but the question to be answered here is, "why bother finding another test if GSR was considered adequate to the task?" One might entertain the notion that the Veterans Administration was humanely interested in avoiding electric shock as a means of testing a person's hearing. However, much more germane is that the research was funded partly by the Veterans Administration but mainly by the United States Public Health Service. The reason given by the author–editors for so massively engaging in research into the issue is that the incidence of "FHL" was increasing because of increased numbers of people seeking compensation for industrial hearing loss. GSR testing would just be unacceptable in a purely civilian population, hence a reliable but benign measure was needed. Nowadays, of course, the GSR technique has been superseded by evoked response audiometry, and we consider that test presently. In view of this more recent development, there is little point in detailing results of Ventry and Chaiklin's program. However, it was found that speech reception threshold–1 kHz tonal threshold discrepancy was the most reliable performance measure in comparison with GSR (Ventry & Chaiklin, 1965b). Data of my own from an industrial sample of listeners, which bear upon this outcome, are discussed in the ensuing section.

THE "MEASUREMENT" OF "FUNCTIONAL HEARING LOSS"

Like the section on the measurement of "recruitment," this section is not meant to contain a textbook listing of all the ingenious methods people have devised over the past 100 years to pick out the "malingerer" or the "FHL sufferer." Any standard clinical work can provide that information, and of course Ventry and Chaiklin's (1965b) study can provide details of how the more widely used tests fare in comparison with an objective test. My purpose rather is to seek out evidence that bears upon the validity of objective tests and upon the one voluntary performance measure that Ventry and Chaiklin found to be a reliable guide.

Tests for "Functional Hearing Loss"
(Galvanic Skin Response) (GSR) Audiometry

Doerfler and McClure (1954) published one of the earliest accounts of this test applied to adults in a clinical setting. The authors do not say how listeners were persuaded to engage in this study, only that they were selected from hospital files. The technique of the test, as conducted by Doerfler and McClure, is as follows: Tones of various intensities at 1 kHz are paired, as unconditioned stimuli, with an "unpleasant" electric shock to the fingers of one hand, and a continual 60% reinforcement (shock) schedule is followed. A conditioned GSR recorded from the opposite hand is noted in response to the tone alone once that has become the CS. A more than usually barbaric feature is that shock is continual and random. Shock occurs on 60% of the trials, to sustain the conditioned GSR, hence it will at times be "paired" even with genuinely *undetectable* tones.

The monumental flaw in Doerfler and McClure's study is that voluntary thresholds *for the same tones* were always obtained *after* the conditioning session. It is not altogether surprising therefore that volunteer thresholds were very closely related to GSR thresholds. Subjects in this study were 30 people with pure conductive disorders. Burk (1958) confirmed Doerfler and McClure's findings in a group of normally hearing listeners, and Chaiklin, Ventry, and Barrett (1961) found GSR thresholds to be within ±5 dB in both normally hearing listeners and listeners with otosclerosis. These are the validation data on which Ventry and Chaiklin (1965b) rely in using GSR on veterans (i.e., people with largely cochlear or other sensorineural disorder). There are therefore no data apart from those presented by Ventry and Chaiklin (1965b) on the latter sort of group, so the generalizability of the earlier work is quite unknown.

But let us suppose that "FHL" was an incorrect "diagnosis" in at least some of the people studied by Ventry and Chaiklin (1965a, b). The result obtained would then suggest that GSR–voluntary threshold relations in *sensorineural* disorder are not so close, hence the GSR test is not valid in such a group. Logically, this conclusion is as inevitable as any other. We will return to this point later.

Stapedius Reflex Threshold Audiometry

I mention at the beginning of this chapter that a fortuitous link exists between "recruitment" and "FHL." That link is the stapedius reflex threshold (confusingly abbreviated in some reports to "SRT." We will avoid such a mixup here). The muscles of the middle ear, stapedial and tympanic, reflexly contract in both ears when a sound is about 70 to 85 dB above threshold in *either* ear. By use of an impedance bridge or some other device to assess admittance to the middle ear in the contralateral external ear, this reflex can be detected. Given that the reflex usually bears a constant relation to threshold, it has been suggested by Lamb and Peterson (1967) that the measure could serve as an objective indicator, by inference, of lower threshold in a listener. These authors acknowledge that in cases of cochlear disorder recruitment of loudness would interfere with the usual lower threshold–reflex threshold relation. This very feature of the stapedius reflex was exploited by Anderson and Barr (1966) to determine the presence of recruitment in people with conductive disorder; for this reason, the stapedius reflex is apparently not a valid guide to threshold in the people most likely to present themselves for compensation.

However, Niemeyer and Sesterhenn (1974) found a fairly regular relationship between observed tonal threshold and the difference between average stapedius reflex threshold for tones and for white noise. The reflex threshold for white noise is at a lower intensity level than the average reflex threshold for tones (reflex thresholds averaged across .5 to 4 kHz). As a white-noise reflex threshold gets closer to the tonal reflex threshold, the elevation in *lower* tonal threshold becomes greater. Calculated and observed average (.5 to 4 kHz) lower thresholds in 125 people with sensorineural disorder showed agreement within ±10 dB in 73% of cases; ±15 dB in 17% and ±20 dB in 10%. Hence the technique, while overcoming the barrier thrown up by recruitment, is a fairly rough approximation. Niemeyer and Sesterhenn did not look specifically at noise-induced cases. They note, however, that in cases where the audiogram is unsymmetrical their calculation is less reliable. An approximation to the unsymmetrical audiogram can be obtained, they claim, by use of high- and low-pass filtered noise in place of white noise, but no data relating to that modified calculation are presented.

Sesterhenn and Breuninger (1977) have since refined the stapedius reflex threshold technique by using a loudness subtraction procedure that permits estimation of lower tonal threshold at individual audio frequencies. In listeners with higher frequency threshold elevation, and diagnoses of sensorineural disorder, about 70% of tonal threshold estimates by the reflex threshold procedure were within ±10 dB of measured tonal threshold in the .125 to 4 kHz range. The bulk of remaining estimates were within ±20 dB of actual levels and about 6% were within ±30 dB.

Clearly the reflex threshold approach holds some promise of practical utility though its accuracy is still in need of improvement.

Average Evoked Response Audiometry

This technique has become widely used and celebrated as an objective method of threshold determination. It is based on the technique of summing evoked responses of the central auditory system to trains of signals. An individual evoked response cannot be abstracted from an EEG record because it is "buried" in the mass of other electrical activity going on simultaneously and picked up by surface electrodes; but a repeated signal will produce a time-locked repeated response, and summing of total potential activity shows this time-locked response to emerge gradually as a signal over noise.

Davis (1965) showed a relatively close correspondence between evoked response and voluntary threshold in a group of deaf young people (10 to 16 years old). Typically, evoked response threshold was at the same or a slightly higher acoustic level than voluntary threshold. In a few cases, it was at a lower level. Roeser and Rose (1968) showed that evoked response threshold at 4 kHz was within −5 to +15 dB of voluntary threshold (mean difference = +6.5 dB) in 10 hearing listeners (aged 18 to 25 years) and within −10 to +10 dB (mean difference = −5 dB) in 10 listeners with cochlear pathology of an unstated type (aged 17 to 23 years). McCandless and Lentz (1968) also found that whereas voluntary threshold was typically at a lower level than evoked response threshold in hearing listeners, the opposite was the case in listeners with disorder of hearing.

Rose, Keating, Hedgecock, Miller, and Schreurs (1972) reported data from a group of 50 typical clinic outpatients assessed by evoked response audiometry following voluntary threshold determination. The important feature of this study is that the audiologists involved in assessing threshold by evoked response did not know the level at voluntary threshold in any of the cases. This is the first study to control for expectancy effects. It is important to have such control because the "sign" of a response at or around evoked response threshold is subject to considerable variability. Controlling for this factor produced results that showed differences between voluntary and ERA thresholds (.5 and 2 kHz) of between −20 and +100 dB. The authors, on the basis of this and related data (Rose et al., 1971) stated, "We question the generalization that the ERA procedure can be used routinely to accurately measure hearing level [p. 242]." One highly provocative feature of this and the other study (Rose et al., 1971) was that between 12 and 24% of control (no signal) runs were judged as showing signs of an evoked response. It should be emphasized that massive discrepancies were observed in the judgments of both highly experienced and novice audiologists.

On the specific matter of evoked response lower than voluntary threshold levels in disordered ears, a study by Pugh et al. (1974) can throw some light. They found lower thresholds by cochlear action potential recording than by (operant) conditioning in monkeys with temporary threshold shift, but not in preexposure or postrecovery conditions. Pugh et al. (1974) considered that physiological noise generated at the cochlea following overstimulation could have masked a signal centrally, hence behaviorally, which would still show electrically by virtue of the summing technique.

Results to date, then, do not support the conclusion that a reliable and painless (therefore acceptable) method of objective threshold determination is to hand. Despite this, I have witnessed evoked response audiometry used in the United Kingdom in assessment-for-compensation cases, and I have no doubt its use will continue. Urgently required is a study along the lines of those of Rose et al. (1971, 1972) in which listeners with noise-induced hearing disorder are tested using evoked response by researchers ignorant of the listeners' voluntary thresholds so that the variability of the test, in those who may be subjected to its whimsical character, can be unearthed.

Speech–Tone Threshold Relations

Ventry and Chaiklin (1965b) found that speech–tone threshold discrepancy was most effective in picking out "FHL" cases, and Ventry

(1976) spelled out in detail the underlying nature of this sign. The level at speech reception threshold is typically about 12 dB SPL higher than the level at 1 kHz tonal threshold. However, people who present "FHL" typically show lower levels at SRT than at 1 kHz tonal threshold. Speech audiometers are calibrated to a biological zero, hence 1 kHz tonal and speech reception thresholds should match. In simulation studies, Ventry (1976) reports that listeners use comfortable listening level for both tones and speech to provide a reasonably reliable "fake" threshold. But the comfortable listening level for speech is at about the *same SPL* as the comfortable level for tones. However, in *audiometric* terms, use of comfortable listening level produces a lower level at (fake) threshold for speech than for a 1 kHz tone.

This, then, is the likely reason why tonal threshold is higher than speech threshold in "FHL" cases. Of course, the viability of tone–speech discrepancy relies on establishment of the initial relationship in nonfaking listeners with noise-induced hearing disorder. The data reviewed in Chapter 6 are hardly likely to back up that requirement, however. To explore the issue a little further, I went back to unpublished data (Noble, 1969) collected from 44 volunteer listeners with various degrees of noise deafness. The SPL difference of about 12 dB in levels at 1 kHz tonal and speech reception thresholds is apparent in the group result (right ears only). Individual pairs of results did not fall in with this overall picture, however. In 6 of the 44 cases, 1 kHz threshold (SPL) was *higher* than SRT (SPL) by 1 to 21 dB, and in a further 5 cases it was identical or only a few decibels lower. Right ears were tested second in both tests, hence data in most cases are likely to be reliable.

What are we to make of these results? I have already (Chapter 6, pp. 122–123) produced an explanation for the effect. The "FHL" fancier would of course conclude that the results show evidence of that condition. I reserve comment on this point until the next section, but I would say simply enough that "FHL" could only be one hypothesis among others to account for this result obtained in a noncompensation setting.

The "Categorical" Error of "Functional Hearing Loss"

The fundamental conceptual flaw regarding "functional hearing loss" is that of putting a mere pattern of results into a diagnostic category. Through this approach, a nonexistent quality is regarded as a real thing. When authors speak of "FHL" they take it that they speak about an actual type of hearing loss; but in fact *if* what they are observing is real, its essential quality is precisely that it is *not* a hearing loss. This is a categorical error, and it leads to a further and more drastic error. By the fact that "FHL" has been given an identity even though it is nothing more than a pattern of audiometric response—its existence cannot be located except within that pattern—a very dangerous scientific step is taken. The pattern becomes the "sign" of the "disorder," and the "disorder" is reified each time the pattern occurs. But because *nothing but the pattern* is the quality being investigated, then no instance of the pattern can be taken to be *anything but the quality.* But that is an error: The fact that all xs are ys does not prove that all ys are xs. Because all suspected cases of "FHL" show pattern x, it does not follow that pattern x shows "FHL." Yet because FHL does not exist apart from the inconsistent audiometric pattern, because its independent existence cannot be demonstrated, therefore, neither can anything else be taken to explain the pattern. In Ventry and Chaiklin's (1965a) study, there were 20 cases of "unresolved FHL"; in my data there are at least 6 cases of "suspected FHL." Neither of these conclusions is at all justified, because the existence of "disorder" cannot be revealed in any other form than via the audiometric pattern.

If the reader complains that I labor this particular point regarding categorical error, let it be remembered that 20 people were punished with extensive electric-shock audiometry precisely because of that error.

FAKABILITY: A RESOLUTION OF THE PROBLEM

In discussion of audiometric reliability, I showed how the term spilled over from consideration of the test to that of the person being tested. I argued then that variability of the quality being assessed must be separated from variability of the measure being used to test it. The same issue is at hand here: Functional hearing loss may exist in the case of a person who pretends inability to hear for some purpose or other. A pretended inability to hear, however, requires that the person take on a partially deaf role and play it out. If we wish to distinguish pretended deafness of this kind from phenomenally experienced but nonorganic deafness (caused, say, by some emotional trauma), then I am sure we are free so to do.

But if we do not want that distinction, no harm will come about. The distinction that must be made, however, is the distinction between a person who pretends to be deaf and a person who is faking on a test. I submit that the traditional audiological outlook cannot see that any distinction exists here. What is deafness but that which shows up on a test? Similarly, what is normal hearing but that which does not show up on a test? Clearly, the answer to both of these questions is that hearing and deafness are conditions experienced by people in their everyday lives. A client does not become deaf on entering the clinic and listening to tones. The client is there in the first place because of experienced difficulty. The distinction now becomes a little clearer. Let us assume that as a not-too-well-off veteran I wish to maximize my pension and elect (perhaps in desperation, perhaps with great coolness) to fake on a hearing test. I have no psychiatric problem, I just do not have very much money. I have no intention of *pretending to be a deaf person,* I simply intend to fake on the test. I cannot get a decent-sized pension any other way, so this is my only choice. In making it, I may be revealing a larcenous stripe, but it is a relatively narrow one.

Such a person is not suffering from anything (apart from lack of money). He does not have a diagnosable condition, he is merely engaging in a dishonest action of a quite minor kind. And it should be added that ripping-off the system (as Australians put it) is a game all persons play, including, I am quite sure, academic researchers into "FHL," psychiatrists, and even, occasionally writers of books.

I have tried to show throughout this part of the chapter what happens to people, both examined and examiner, when a diagnostic attitude is adopted toward actions that at most can only be described as dishonest. To abandon a moral stance in favor of a so-called scientific one cannot work to the melioration of either morals or science. That people may be punishable for dishonesty is one thing, but that they should be punished outside the law for dishonesty is itself unlawful. It is time that we abandoned such approaches to our endeavors and looked afresh.

The problem, and it is one I freely acknowledge, is that tests can be faked. The seat of the problem, then, is the test. Faking as an activity is beyond the purview of scientific audiology, whose province is the construction, along scientific lines, of reliable and robust tests. If it is thought that the only way a test can be made fakeproof is to turn it into an inquisitorial device, then science here has joined company with the jailers. Other tests of a nonpunitive kind can reveal in the bulk of cases whether the person being tested is faking. That is known, and it should be enough that it is known to all parties in the test situation. If such revelation is insufficient to change the behaviors of the person being tested, that is not an audiological issue. A scientific attitude can only strive to find better, less fakable instruments and continue to make sure its attitude is one of perpetual doubt about its own findings.

If a test can be faked, it is unreliable and should be replaced, if possible, by one that cannot be faked, or faked so readily. If that is impossible, then it is unfortunate but unavoidable if testing is the route chosen by the system for people who lay claim upon it. In my view, if it is impossible to find a nonfakable test, even if the problem of faking is so gross that the system is crumbling under its pressure, then radical rethinking that still ensures fairness and humanity to all must take place. In any case, faking is justifiable so long as the system which sets up the tests is also operating dishonestly. We have had ample evidence presented throughout this book to show that most systems in operation, especially that of the AAOO–AMA, are scientifically groundless and erected upon sheer economic interest. It is an instance of bad faith for researchers to produce "functional hearing loss" and to berate and degrade claimants under that label while remaining silent about the ill treatment claimants receive at the hands of the system even when they act honestly.

In Chapter 12, I consider possibilities that may allow the whole issue to be circumvented.

PART III

A REDIRECTION IN HEARING LOSS AND HANDICAP ASSESSMENT

This final section (Chapters 9–12) begins with a summary of the problems and inadequacies of existing mechanical hearing tests and the systems derived from them. With reference to the descriptions given in Chapter 1 of the auditory world and the nature of hearing in that world, a preliminary attempt os made to reorient our approach to hearing assessment. It is evident that adoption of self-report is a necessary first step in this redirection. Review of self-report methods leads up to a detailed description of the author's own questionnaire, The Hearing Mesaurement Scale.

In Chapter 10 is a review of comparative studies between self-report and mechanical tests and between different self-report scales. Again, a detailed analysis of the Hearing Measurement Scale is made. The theoretical and practical properties of self-report are discussed in Chapter 11, and the final chapter is a broader excursion into hearing impairment, handicap assessment, and the possibilities for social change.

9

Development of Self-Report Scales for Hearing Assessment

OVERVIEW OF PRESENT PRACTICE

The first two tasks of this work are now complete. Historical features of hearing loss assessment were uncovered in Part I to show the quality of contest between claimant and institution claimed against in the medicolegal context. While it requires little by way of argument to show that this contestlike quality exists—it is a legal issue after all—more extensive review and discussion is needed to show that science has not been a disinterested arm in the battle over legal defence and prosecution. Systems have been devised that are shown to serve the interest of the defending institution and to harm the interest of claimants. While such a state of affairs is not altogether astonishing, what needs to be emphasized is that "experts," scientific and medical persons, have attached the imprimatur of science to these systems by claiming their validity in assessment.

The portrait of science as a practice in this field, which is quite thoroughly identified with the interest of the defending institution, is more than sufficiently drawn in the question of so-called "functional hearing loss." Bending scientific inquiry, however unwittingly, toward a particular interest can only result in poor-quality work. More far reaching than that, it helps to undermine the status of science in the perception of the contestants at law. On the one hand, science is seen as a malleable and convenient device with which to minimize certain consequences of harmful action; on the other, it is seen as a trustless institution in its own right which cannot be relied upon to provide the means for a fair appraisal of damage.

This is not to claim that the whole of the scientific enterprise in this field of inquiry has necessarily been corrupted. Quite the contrary, sufficient information is publicly available to allow evidence regarding the validity of assessment systems to be appraised. In spite of the biased ideological penetration of the scientific endeavor, the practice of that enterprise cannot help but reveal its own areas of uncertainty, overstatement, and faulty conclusion.

One reason why false conclusions can be drawn in this field lies in the very way in which the issues are approached in the first place. Because the devices used for assessment, not only in the medicolegal but also in the clinical sector, are off target as regards everyday hearing experience, then semimythical accounts of that experience can be made which arise without even the knowledge of those making the accounts. It is only in very recent times that anyone has stopped to inquire just what is involved in hearing in the day-to-day world and what is involved in impairment of hearing in the day-to-day world. The still prevailing approach to hearing and deafness is made through the constructs of mechanical testing. Given that such tests are misleading at worst and inadequate at best, it is not so surprising that there has been room for manipulation of the assessment system to make it operate in a one-sided fashion without anyone quite realizing what has been going on. If the tests themselves, no matter how disinterestedly used, cannot properly describe the nature of the individual's difficulty, when they are used wrongly, their misleading character will remain covert.

There is, at this stage of discussion, no empirical evidence to support the assertion that existing tests cannot measure everyday hearing loss and handicap. That empirical evidence will emerge in this and the following chapters. But a priori a strong case can be made in support of the above assertion.

We need first to reconsider the description of hearing acts given in the first chapter of this book. There it was pointed out that hearing in the world involves the active search for information in an ongoing communicative relation between oneself and others. It involves attention to a wide range of acoustic features of the behavior and actions of people, other animals, and objects. These features are not only linguistic, and one's attention to them is not at the punctate level but at the level of higher-order structure. While there must be a broad relation between sheer auditory sensitivity and ability to operate effectively within the everyday audible world, the relation is not simple and direct because different people do different things, act differently in similar circumstances, have varying repertoires of behavior.

We saw empirically verified instances of this variability in connection with the studies by Quist-Hanssen and Steen (1960) and by Ward *et al.* (1961). These authors found consistent differences in speech hearing performance between different groups of listeners unaccounted for by sheer sensitivity or some other audiological factor. Rather, the differences were more plausibly attributable to the different occupational styles of the various groups of listeners in question. Such features of people's lifestyles and the interaction between these features and auditory processing skill are unexplored by conventional tests, whose character consists solely in the assessment of sensitivity or discrimination ability. The tests do not represent the world of everyday hearing although they may represent analogs of that world.

I suggest in Chapter 6 that SRT, for example, may be a fairer analog for everyday hearing than its surface content suggests. Results presented in the next chapter bear upon that possibility. It emerges that disyllable SRT relates at the same level of association as discrimination score to self-reported hearing ability. The a posteriori hypothesis one may produce to account for this equivalency of association entails consideration of the listener's task in undertaking each of these tests. Despite the unpromising face and content validity of the disyllable SRT test, the actual task may represent a parallel with aspects of everyday hearing for someone with hearing difficulty. Everyday speech is highly redundant, and a good proportion of the physical signal can be missed while the information in the speech train is still picked up. In the SRT test, listening conditions are unfavorable—the level for 50% correct detection is being sought—but redundancy is very high. Thus there is an analogy with certain everyday hearing conditions.

The discrimination test, on the other hand, is analogous to a different everyday hearing circumstance, one in which the acoustics are favorable but redundancy (predictability) is low. In talking with a stranger or listening to a public speaker or to a TV or radio program, one may encounter analogous conditions. The additional quality of discrimination testing is that it takes more account of the whole auditory threshold profile. The discrimination score can thus be used to represent something of the problem associated with unsymmetrical higher frequency threshold elevation. This latter phenomenon, as is argued in Chapters 6 and 8, may be a reliable guide to the extent of disorder in an injured or diseased cochlea, and as such may have reasonable predictive validity as regards problems of auditory information processing. Data in Chapter 10 bear out this contention.

But analogs and operational predictors are not *measures* of hearing handicap. The content and theoretical construct validity of these kinds of tests is the problem remaining. The following section describes the form of redirection that is seen as necessary in the field of hearing loss and handicap assessment if fair and valid appraisal in both clinical and medicolegal settings is to be achieved.

A REDIRECTION IN HEARING ASSESSMENT

It is clear from the foregoing that while performance tests of hearing have many advantages as regards ease of administration, scoring, and so forth, they are at best inadequate guides to hearing function. It could be said indeed that the very striving after easier procedure has compromised their value. For in seeking universality of application, test constructors have had to pare down meaning and content so that local idiosyncrasies would not confound results. For example, as soon as meaning comes too forcefully into the picture, a test of hearing using speech is jeopardized. As a result, the tonal test, stripped of virtually all meaning, is the favorite. Although this is perfectly reasonable for certain purposes, the problem arises when the tonal test, because of its very universality, is taken to be somehow intrinsically valid as a measure of hearing ability. Authors are obviously torn between acceptance and rejection of such a position. On the one hand, the tonal test offers a great deal by way of standardization and even at times in the realm of predictive validity. On the other, it is so obviously unrelated to everyday hearing experience, so unexpressive of the multifarious aspects of that experience, as to be barren in its measurement.

The same ambivalence is found in speech tests. Those that can be relied upon are so corseted in terms of content and style that they are freakish forms of speech as it is heard in the world at large. Conversely, those that try to emulate everyday conditions provide such widely variable results that no firm outcome emerges from their use.

On top of these problems is the evident fact that speech hearing ability in actual everyday conditions has never been systematically related in any research considered so far to performance tests using speech. Thus, a formula may be derived that allows tonal testing to be used with equanimity in regard to performance on some seemingly realistic speech test, but no evidence is available to show that the speech test itself bears any relation to actual performance at listening or communicating in everyday conditions.

And were that not enough, there is the problem that hearing as an everyday activity involves more than listening to speech. In the same way that the visual system functions to pick up features of the world other than written symbolic information, so the auditory system picks up information apart from vocal symbols. The pickup of symbolic vocalized information may be a paramount function of man's auditory capability, especially in technological society, but it is not an exclusive function

If all this is now becoming clearer to the reader than it may have been before approaching this book, the question that needs facing is: How *do* you assess hearing loss and handicap? There is no answer to that question. The next three chapters explore the features of a radical alternative to mechanical tests, but I do not pretend that this method—self-report—provides a lasting, satisfactory answer. Indeed I would like to take space here to consider two other possible answers. In so doing, I argue, however, that these other alternatives are not independent of self-report. In fact I argue that self-report is a necessary preceding step to both of them. Self-report hence emerges both as a starting place for the emergence of new forms of hearing assessment and as a viable assessment method in its own right.

Testing of Hearing

The testing of hearing as such should not be discarded; it can be retained but fundamentally remodeled. It is my intention not to try to think up a new range of performance tests but rather to put up guidelines for their design. Given a more thorough understanding of hearing acts of the sort described in Chapter 1, we could design tests to examine a person's strategies and successfulness in undertaking these acts. Such tests would be in effect experimental observational vignettes of real-world hearing situations. Irrespective of the degree of impairment revealed by functional tests, different people have different coping strategies. They may act with variable success in everyday listening and communicating, depending on their strategic repertoires and the variable constraints upon use of these strategies.

Partially deaf people and those who work with partially deaf people know very well what actions can be taken to retrieve communicated messages in difficult listening circumstances. Rehabilitation is concerned with imparting skills that allow more successful pickup of auditory information. The testing of hearing approached from this sort of orientation would look to the amount of compensatory effort the person engages in to optimize or at least improve the pickup of information. And of course the amount of information can be quantified as well as the effort required to get it. Equally important is to index what are adequate levels of information received: Can the person act appropriately on the basis of the amount and quality of information he is typically able to obtain? Take a very simple but not trivial everyday situation—finding the right amount of money to exchange for goods over the counter: How much effort is involved in hearing what amount is required? Can the person successfully retrieve the message from the often noisy ambient background? A simple way for all parties to know this is behaviorally displayed by the amount proffered. If it is usually the right amount, then the effort involved has led to success; if not, then it has not. A test in this situation has metric possibilities over and beyond acoustics and functional threshold levels.

The analog of this sort of approach is found in speech tests using questions in which only one answer to each question is appropriate if all information has been received. In a redesign of such tests, *conversation*, as an ongoing communication loop, would be involved, so that the exploratory strategies of the partially hearing participant, which must affect the behavior of the other participant, can be witnessed.

In regard to auditory spatial perception, work at our laboratory is directed to experimental inquiry into the strategies used by people in judging the whereabouts of an unseen source. The preliminary step in this design is to construct an auditory environment in which the listener is free to adopt search strategies by movement of head and body so that unseen sources of sound can be pinpointed. The data in such an experiment are the observed actions a listener undertakes to optimize search time and effort. Concern, therefore, is with the modus operandi of spatial location, not with error rate as a function of spatial position. The traditional approach to auditory localization "locks" the listener passively in a prestructured environment. There is no opportunity for him to explore the features of the auditory microworld in which he is placed. The new approach we are presently designing has quite far-reaching assessment possibilities when it comes to examining the problems people with disordered hearing have in locating sound sources.

It emerges that the testing of hearing along lines like these cannot proceed until we have more thoroughly observed, in a purely experimental way, what goes on within and between persons when hearing acts are undertaken. Current tests have all emerged from experimental backgrounds in which the subject is treated as a passive receiver of stimuli. We know enough to know that hearing is not passive. We do not take action without being reasonably sure of our grounds for so doing. In the face of degraded or ambiguous information, we take steps either to avoid action or to upgrade or clarify the information. In this way, our actions can be appropriate to the circumstances. In other words, we constantly rely on feedback, both from ourselves to the source, by way of signals indicating uncertainty or a need for greater clarity, and back from the source to provide us with additional data.

Tests of hearing of the sort I am advocating will only result from different sorts of laboratory experiments. The knowledge we have now, while sufficient to tell us that hearing is an active process, is insufficient for us to plan appropriate tests of hearing acts. In sum, the laboratory experiment is another instance of the necessary feedback loop required before appropriate action (assessment of hearing) can take place.

Observation

Before any experiments can be set up, more straightforward observation is needed "in the field," for it is unclear at this stage what constitutes the hearing repertoire or the frequency of performance of different acts within that repertoire. The current assumption that "hearing handicap" refers to problems in hearing speech in the everyday world has already been questioned as to its sufficiency, given all the other functions of everyday hearing. It is assumed that speech hearing is man's primary auditory function. That may be so, but no specific observation has ever been made to support the truth of it. Speech is not only spoken but accompanied by visual signs. How adequately would a person operate if the vocal features of speech were degraded or even absent? This varies from one deaf person to another as we know. But more important, is vocal speech a universally critical source of information? This is unknown. The very question appears odd. People talk to each other all the time, so it must be universally critical. One may except hermits and those taking Trappist vows from this condition; and that being so, the universality of the rule does not hold. A better picture may be that vocal speech is variably critical depending on social circumstances. It is highly critical to the urban middle class, the group from which most "universal" observations about the everyday world emanate. But it may not be so critical for people whose communication relies heavily on gesture. I am not saying here that vocal language is unimportant for such groups of people. I am merely pointing to the possibility of variable levels of importance depending on social circumstance.

Within the range of vocalized linguistic events, moreover, what proportion are participatory, what proportion of a mere listening character? Given the increased possibilities for feedback in the former situation, are there critical differences in the way people manage when engaged in conversation as opposed to auditing a conversation? These are vital issues in the process of coming to understand everyday speech hearing.

It needs to be observed how much reliance people place on hearing as a monitor of events around them. To what extent are audible signals critical in safe orientation to different parts of the daily environment? To be sure, there are many circumstances where listening is only an alternative to looking; but there must be situations in which listening is the only means available to detect important events. The speeding automobile out of sight around a bend in the road or the (nonproverbial) snake in the grass may be detectable solely by the auditory information they broadcast. To what extent must we rely on auditory information of this nonlinguistic sort to sustain a safe existence?

Just as important, though less dramatic, is the question of sheer interpersonal contact through the nonlinguistic auditory world. To what degree is communication with the environment dependent on the registering of transient auditory events? The typical instances cited of this quality are the bird call and the dog bark. For some people, these would be important as routine and reliable events in their lives. But the sounds of less "lyrical" occurrences—people and cars in the street, household noise—may have vital significance in the maintenance of social identity for some people. Very little is known of this aspect of hearing beyond the opening pieties uttered in the "psychology of deafness" chapters of outmoded textbooks. No observation of hearing at this level has been done, to my knowledge.

My colleague, John MacRae, pointed out that we do not know over what distance communications can and typically do take place. For instance, in face-to-face situations there must be an interaction between personal lifespace and auditory capability, but no one knows what it is. Nor is it known what distance separates us from the sounds we attend to in our auditory world. These can be vastly variable, and the important question is what happens to the person as that distance is attenuated? One may be able to hear what is going on up to 20 feet away, but beyond that not at all. What handicap is associated with this kind of loss, a loss not so much of "hearing," as of the auditory horizon?

The reader must appreciate by now that we really are quite ignorant with regard to ecological acoustics and real-word hearing and listening.

Inquiry: Self-Report

A prior step that is necessary before intelligent observation can take place is inquiry of people with various degrees of acquired partial deafness about the ways they are limited and the effects they notice as a result of this change in hearing. Only by this means can some clues be derived about hearing acts and the impairment of these acts. The author's own investigations of this kind were not in fact intended to furnish information with this goal in view. The intention was to put together a scale for assessing hearing loss based on self-report, but the aims of that kind of exercise must coincide with the aim of realistic observation if the job is to be done properly. Thus it turns out that some statements can be made about everyday hearing as a result of inquiry based on a self-report scale.

Self-report is the oldest device known to man, I presume, whereby information about one's condition is transmitted to the world at large. It is not an invention of twentieth-century social science. Even its formalization as a set of questions designed to elicit self-assessment reports is not the property of contemporary inquiry. The "clinical interview" has been a key feature of medical investigation since the beginnings of that discipline as a rational science.

Social and human sciences such as psychology and sociology, in striving to be scientific, have paid as much attention to their assumptive frameworks, their methodologies, as to the objects viewed through these frameworks. In contrast, the medical purpose in using the "clinical interview" is directed more toward specifically medical questions. Its content is dictated by the understanding prevalent in the *medical* world.

What this means is that the worldview of the person being interviewed is ignored as irrelevant, the clinical interviewer simply uses certain statements of the person as diagnostic clues, that is as part of the medical structure. The interview, as used by social science, is for the purpose of coming to understand and typify, in this case, the nature of the disturbance under scrutiny. I am aware of the problems surrounding that sort of purpose and elaborate on them in Chapter 11. These problems notwithstanding, the aim of social science is to find ways of objectively portraying and, where appropriate, quantifying features of human function. With respect to a question like impairment of hearing, its precise and valid assessment is the concern of psychology, since that science deals with individual function. The role of sociology is to attend more to the treatment of hearing impairment as a social construct and to the fate of people with hearing impairment as members of societies. While I operate as a psychologist in being concerned with the valid assessment of disturbance of function in the individual, I freely engage in a sociological approach to the concept of "impaired hearing" as it is manifest at a social level. These two kinds of approach are evident in the first chapter of this work.

In point of fact, a social-science approach has been made to self-assessed hearing ability on only two occasions and, I would argue, has only approached the issue with approximate reliability and validity on one occasion. Other efforts to obtain reports from individuals about their ability to hear have mainly been made by physical scientists or physicians. Hence first of all, the technical problems of measurement by means of self-report have not been realized and second, the style of questioning has been along "medical–diagnostic" lines. Nevertheless, these rudimentary efforts at self-reported hearing assessment are worth examining.

SELF-REPORT QUESTIONNAIRES

Scaled and Nonscaled Questionnaires

There is an important difference between a scaled questionnaire and a nonscaled. In a nonscaled questionnaire, no more than a nominal assessment is made: namely, a checklist of instances which evoke a positive response. The questionnaire devised by a group in Dundee, Scotland is a good example of this type. A scaled questionnaire tries to assess not only incidence but degree by asking people to rate the extent to which they experience some phenomenon or other. A scaled questionnaire of hearing loss quantifies the degree of manifestation of that loss in the individual; a nonscaled questionnaire can only quantitatively describe the population response to the list of questions. A nonscaled questionnaire is not trying to do anything other than add a somewhat human touch to the "real" data. A scale, if it is properly put together, is a new source of data to be pitted against data from other tests.

Early Inventories

The 1935–1936 United States Public Health Survey Scale

It is curious that the inquiry made of respondents in the 1935–1936 USPHS survey (USPHS, 1938) tried to do the work of both a scaled and nonscaled questionnaire. That is to say, the checklist of questions had a rank order so that supposedly the more questions checked by a respondent the more severe the partial deafness. This kind of scaling, formally developed by Guttman (1944), was used again in the 1960–1963 USPHS survey (Schein, Gentile, & Haase, 1970), which we consider later. Reference has already been made to aspects of the 1935–1936 self-report questionnaire in Chapter 7. In summary, there were five major categories of response, separately applied to each ear:

1. No noticeable difficulty in hearing
2. Inability to understand speech in an auditorium or group conversation
3. Inability to understand speech in face-to-face conversation
4. Inability to understand speech on telephone
5. Inability to understand speech in any circumstance

As noted in Chapter 7, considerable overlap occurred in the threshold levels for tones of people reporting different degrees of difficulty according to this scale. In particular, the separation of threshold distributions between categories 3 and 4 is not very distinct except in thresholds at 1 kHz. This is an expectable outcome: The audio-frequency characteristic of telephone systems gives maximum output in the 1 kHz region. Despite the expectation built into these categories, namely, that difficulty should be experienced in face-to-face conversation before difficulty is experienced in telephone conversation, it would not be surprising to find the opposite report, given that factors beyond the listener's control can interfere with telephone transmission. This is probably the reason for the considerable overlap between categories 3 and 4. In regard to the other categories, threshold testing showed fairly distinct modal differences at .5, 1, and 2 kHz, demonstrating that the items were ranked in increasing order of difficulty.

Very little can be said beyond that. The knowledge that on average people who cannot hear tones at very high levels also cannot hear any other sounds, whereas on average people who cannot hear tones at moderate level also cannot hear some other sounds is not the most penetrating discovery. Much more concern should be assigned to the fact of quite vast variability in measure X when measure Y is constant. That finding shows people's abilities are affected by all sorts of contingencies which remain covert in this kind of investigation. The same conclusion can be drawn from virtually all subsequent studies.

The St. Louis Scale

The work of Silverman, Thurlow, Walsh, and Davis (1948) is concerned with the relationship between self-assessment of hearing and various test results in a group of people having undergone the fenestration operation for otosclerosis. These people were sent a scaled questionnaire after the operation, and they were asked to rate their remembered ability to hear in various situations prior to and at various times following the operation. The situations listed were akin to those listed in the USPHS survey questionnaire, except that listening in an auditorium was separated from conversation in a group, and group and face-to-face conversation were considered in quiet and in noisy conditions. There were thus six circumstances, abbreviated here, all relating to speech hearing:

1. Face-to-face conversation (quiet)
2. Face-to-face conversation (noise)
3. Group conversation (quiet)
4. Group conversation (noise)
5. Auditorium
6. Telephone

Respondents were asked to apply a code number from 1 to 5 to each situation depending on whether they

1. Understood perfectly
2. Understood with slight difficulty
3. Understood with considerable difficulty
4. Could hear but not understand
5. Could not hear

The demand on respondents was quite considerable in that people, aided no doubt by their families, had to try to remember how well or badly they fared in each circumstance on 6 different occasions in the past; namely, prior to the fenestration operation, then 1 month, 3 months, 6 months, 9 months, and 1 year after the operation. A rather low-level correlation ($r = -.50$) was noted between self-report and the "social adequacy index" (see Chapter 3). The self-rating scale was nonetheless used to identify quite specific loci on the social adequacy index, representing "thresholds" of social adequacy and inadequacy.

Several procedural problems attend this study—not least of which is the lead-time between self-report and life circumstance to be reported upon. The expectation of clients would introduce unnecessary bias to the picture when they were asked up to a year later to rate what they thought their hearing ability had been prior to and following an expensive and hazardous operation. Finally, the few situations listed all refer to certain speech hearing occurrences so that, as with the USPHS survey questionnaire, there is no adequate sampling of self-reported ability.

The 1960–1963 United States Public Health Service Survey Scale

The USPHS survey of 1960–1963 included a self-report questionnaire designed similarly to the one used in the 1935–1936 survey but using different questions. An expanded version of the rather limited 1960–1963 scale, designed on Guttman-type principles, was later drawn up (Schein *et al.*, 1970) and took the following form:

Four items, requiring yes–no answers, asked if the respondent could "usually hear and understand what a person says without seeing his face" when he

1. Whispers across a room
2. Talks normally across a room
3. Shouts from across a room
4. Talks loudly into one's better ear

A further three questions asked whether the respondent could distinguish speech from nonspeech sound, distinguish one sort of nonspeech sound from another, or hear any sort of loud noise. In addition, people were asked to rate their hearing on a 4-point scale from "good" to "deaf" in each ear.

This questionnaire was administered to clients attending several audiology clinics. Of 1815 people responding to the questionnaire, data of 1345 were usable—the data from the others being inconsistent. That is to say, 88 people neglected to answer certain questions, 39 filled the thing out "improperly" (giving multiple or graded answers), and 343 answered in a nonscaled fashion—that is, negatively to certain items following a positive response to a lower-scaled item. This last feature is interesting: A not inconsiderable number of respondents failed to treat the items according to the compilers' perception of their rank order of decreasing demand on hearing.

It was found that the bulk of inconsistency arose from responses to two items: the one on distinguishing speech from nonspeech and the one on distinguishing one noise from another. This is hardly a surprising outcome as these items are rather difficult to understand (What do they mean?). The first four items provided a neat scaling of responses in the vast majority of cases, and this is hardly surprising either. Anyone could see that to answer "yes" to Question 1 (*can* hear a whisper) and then "no" to Questions 2, 3, or 4 (*can't* hear ordinary to shouted voice) would be downright silly. Taken in conjunction with the fact that the items cannot be said to represent typical everyday situations for the respondents but rather owe more to the scaling desires of the authors, it is not difficult to see that people would respond in a manner which they figured was expected of them rather than according to their actual experience. What the questionnaire uncovers about the condition of partial hearing or about a person's self-rating of that condition is quite unknown.

More Recent Questionnaires on Older Lines

Lindeman (1969) mentions use of a seven-item questionnaire covering situations much like those listed in Silverman *et al.* (1948) and scored according to the number of positive responses to the item-list. Lindeman made no attempt to scale the items, but simply counted positive responses. Again because of the narrowness and brevity of the questionnaire, little is gained from its use.

In the USPHS 1960–1963 survey, the aim was to find items that best predicted .5 to 2 kHz tonal threshold average. In Lindeman's study, the aim was to note whether self-reported speech hearing ability in noisy circumstances related to a test of discrimination in noise. The point to note is that the questionnaires were designed to give some content validity to mechanical tests. Their content is therefore closely bound in with the perceived content of the mechanical tests. Whether or not they represent everyday hearing acts, even speech hearing acts, is not part of the researchers' interest.

Taylor, Pearson, Kell, and Mair (1967) and Kell, Pearson, Acton, and Taylor (1971) had a somewhat different aim in compiling a nonscaled questionnaire to assess the "social effects" of hearing loss due to occupational noise disorder. In their studies, positive responses were noted to items inquiring about difficulty in hearing at public meetings, during encounters with strangers, during encounters with friends, in using a telephone, and in listening to radio and television. Results were presented as incidence statistics showing thereby the areas in which difficulty was most manifest in a group of textile workers. Their results extend somewhat the data presented by Barr (1886). In a later analysis (Pearson, Kell, & Taylor, 1973), self-report results were related to results on performance tests. These are discussed in the next chapter.

While the above authors could not be said to have exhaustively inquired into the hearing experience of people with disorder of hearing, their aim is at least to find out something of the experienced difficulty. Their studies are of particular interest in that results come from people with occupational noise-induced hearing disorder.

We turn now to scaled questionnaires on which a certain amount of analytical work was done to estimate the performance of the instruments themselves. That is to say, to this point no technical development of the questionnaire as a measurement device akin to any other test has been undertaken. Authors have for the most part been content to think up some items and apply them without considering whether they have special significance, relevance, or representativeness. Taylor et al. (1967) report piloting a large number of questions as a first approach to the problem and using only those identified by their pilot group as ones which referred to important areas of everyday auditory experience. They give no details of this initial exercise. We do not know what the item pool comprised, nor do we know on what basis items were identified as showing consistency and as revealing handicap.

The Hearing Handicap Scale

High, Fairbanks, and Glorig (1964) produced a questionnaire, the Hearing Handicap Scale, whose development has certain of the features necessary for the production of reliable assessment.

The aim of the High et al. study was to devise a self-report scale that would directly measure hearing handicap in order to gain better evaluations of people about to undergo treatment and reacting to that treatment. Even so, the paper is introduced with a reference to the medicolegal definition of *handicap* as disadvantage in daily life resulting from hearing impairment, and care is taken to distinguish *handicap* from *disability*. However, the authors make no claim about their scale in the context of assessment for compensation. They do mention that the self-report method is highly susceptible to exaggeration and that its utility is therefore limited to cooperative respondents. The inference one may draw is that the Hearing Handicap Scale is unsuitable for assessment-for-compensation purposes.

The scale is a parallel forms design, comprising two sets of 20 items each. The items in the two forms do not necessarily coincide as regards content but rather provide (or at least provided in the original sample) quite highly consistent total scores. Items were in fact randomly assigned from the pool of 40 to each parallel 20-item form. This was possible because of the high internal consistency of responses to the items as a whole, so that scores on half-lists (Forms A and B) drawn from random sampling of the original item pool provided a reliability coefficient of $r_{A,B} = .96$.

Because of the stated aim of the Hearing Handicap Scale in context of clinical treatment, respondents ($N = 50$) in the experimental trial were people with largely conductive hearing disorder. The items in the scale are almost all concerned with speech hearing ability in various everyday circumstances—conversation with individuals in face-to-face and more distant encounters, in groups, in noisy surroundings, in auditoriums, on the telephone, and from radio or television. In other words, the content is very much like the content of all previous questionnaires taken together. Items were scored on a 5-point scale, and all were positively worded so that a response of "almost always" carried the lowest score. Other response categories were "usually," "sometimes," "rarely," and "almost never."

Content validity of the Hearing Handicap Scale was tested by drawing up 45 questions and distributing them to a large number of otologists and audiologists throughout the United States. The original item list is not given, but it is described as containing items not only on reception of speech but also on localization of sound, occupational problems, and emotional response to hearing impairment. About half the professional people asked to comment on the items responded to the request. They had been asked to comment on the preliminary list of items from the viewpoint of relevance to handicap assessment. Items other than those dealing with speech perception were ruled out by many respondents and dropped from the inventory. More items on speech perception were added.

Fifty items were then administered en bloc to the clinical group described earlier in this section. Inspection of item-total coefficients and dispersion of scores allowed the final 40 items to be abstracted. The two 20-item forms were then derived from that pool. Results from the scale were correlated with performance test data, and this analysis is discussed in the next chapter.

Though much effort was clearly expended on development of the Hearing Handicap Scale, certain weaknesses are apparent in the procedures involved. Relying on professional opinion only to secure valid content is a self-sustaining exercise. The outlook of otologists and audiologists toward the nature of "hearing handicap" would undoubtedly coincide with that of the audiologist–otologist authors of the questionnaire. The issues these people consider important may not coincide with what clients find important; and even though professional workers would have knowledge of problems facing partially deaf people, they would never have actually made systematic study of the partial deafness experience. Clients seeking such professional services also limit their narrative to what is deemed important in the clinical setting. The important fact of hearing as far as professionals are concerned, as has always been evident, is hearing of speech.

Hearing handicap, by this procedure, is defined for the hearing-impaired person by those who set up as experts in the area. But such experts are not much less ignorant than the population at large, also being people with normal hearing, when it comes to knowing the experienced world of the partially deaf person. This observation is not confined to the content of the Hearing Handicap Scale. Most other scales and questionnaires are even more removed from the repondents' reality. But it is important to stress the point in this context, precisely because the procedure of High *et al.* might be regarded as somehow a major step forward in content validation.

Another more technical weakness in this research is the reliability-estimating method. Respondents answered 50 questions in one sitting. From these responses, 40 items with favorable characteristics were extracted, and split-half reliability was estimated. However, no further application was made of these forms. The split-half reliability technique is usually the first step in a program, followed by readministration of the forms to an independent sample to discover the performance reliability of the new forms themselves. The consistency of response to 50 somewhat homogeneous items is bound to be fairly high. Consistency on 40 of these will not be so high when that 40-item list is administered (Anastasi, 1961). And the actual consistency of two forms administered separately needs to be observed afresh simply because the test is now in a form different from that of the original. High *et al.* did not do this, nor has it subsequently been done. However, Blumenfeld, Bergman, and Millner (1969) found that each form of the scale provided inconsistent relational results when compared with functional test performance.

Despite these shortcomings, the Hearing Handicap Scale is important as a landmark in the history of assessment of adult hearing. For the first time, a self-report inventory of questions was treated with some seriousness of purpose, and this departure from traditional practice has pointed the way to more thorough research effort in the area.

The Social Hearing Handicap Index

Ewertsen and Birk-Nielsen (1973) reported results using the Social Hearing Handicap Index. In terms of content, this questionnaire is not much different from the Hearing Handicap Scale, but it is differently structured. Items demand a yes–no answer although there is provision for uncertain responses. It is difficult fully to evaluate the Social Hearing Handicap Index because it is a Danish instrument, and as its authors say, translation to English may not completely capture its nuances. One thing that can be said: 10 of the 21 items are negatively worded ("Do you have difficulty . . . ?"), and 11 are positively worded ("Can you hear . . . ?"). The authors claim this expedient gets around the problem of response bias, people tending to answer "yes" or "no" because they prefer to give yes-type or no-type replies. Items are supposedly balanced within the positive–negative categories so that split-half consistency can be calculated. But, of course, the items cannot be balanced completely, and respondents could answer "yes" to an item worded negatively ("Yes I do have difficulty") and "yes" again to the same item worded positively ("Yes I can hear") because the meaning is different in the two cases ("Yes I can hear in spite of the fact that; Yes I have difficulty"). It is for this reason, I believe, that split-half consistency is so poor in this scale. No statistic is given, but the scattergram (Figure 1, p. 184), from visual inspection, suggests a coefficient of about .7 at the most.

The positive and negative items are interspersed in the Social Hearing Handicap Index. Given that respondents will want to be consistent in their replies and hence check how they answered other items, the task becomes quite confusing as negative answers to both negative and positive questions are matched or unmatched with the opposite occurrences. The impression a respondent might have of the questionnaire is that it is deliberately designed to catch people out and frustrate them. It would be worthwhile testing differently worded and constructed versions of this questionnaire to see whether it could be improved.

If Ewertsen and Birk-Nielsen have not managed successfully to get around the problem of response bias, they have at least raised it as an issue. There is no evidence one way or the other, however, to say if it is a critical issue or not.

An important feature of both the foregoing scales is their length. Because they both concentrate on speech hearing, the items in each inventory sample a good number of everyday speech hearing acts. In comparison with questionnaires that ask only for a few responses, these instruments are bound to provide more accurate assessment in the individual case of degree of experienced difficulty simply because respondents are questioned on a variety of situations. No single situation will have the same significance or meaning for different respondents, but a range of situations allows these differences to be evened out so that the questionnaire portrays the aggregate experience of each person.

The Hearing Handicap Scale is a more advanced device than the Social Hearing Handicap Index. Its response categories allow more subtle differentiation in regard to each question so that a more accurate and reliable overall response is likely to emerge. Ewertsen and Birk-Nielsen avoided multiple-category responses because they felt that respondents would take insufficient care to check off the most appropriate alternatives. Reducing responses to yes or no they felt gives a more reliable score. That may be so, but the structure of their questionnaire does not optimize that strategy. Were some inherent Guttman-type scaling built into their instrument, then the yes-or-no response requirement could certainly pay off. As it is, given the somewhat inconsistent item content, respondents will not be likely to provide answers that reflect their experience in every case.

I return to this important aspect of self-report when discussing the development of the Hearing Measurement Scale.

Finally, despite the improved sampling of experience in the content of both of these scales, the issue of "representativeness" and the related issue of "relevance" are not touched on. This brings us back to the opening of this chapter. Because we do not know what constitutes the repertoire of hearing acts, the first problem in construction of a questionnaire is to find out what its main content should be. The face validity of the Hearing Handicap Scale and the Social Hearing Handicap Index is fairly good. The items all refer to everyday familiar acts. But is the balance of content representative of the balance of different everyday speech hearing acts? Are there areas not covered or covered too densely? Are the questions meaningful in the way they are asked? Are the questions all equally relevant to each respondent? None of these questions has an answer within the programs of these authors; and of course these scales virtually cover no more than speech hearing.

THE HEARING MEASUREMENT SCALE

Development

This scale, compiled by the author (Noble, 1969; Noble & Atherley, 1970), goes some considerable way beyond any previous scale. Its content and construction are the result of extensive inquiry among partially deaf people. The scale has in fact been revised since its original publication, and the new version is presented in an appendix to this chapter.

The Hearing Measurement Scale itself is a development of various prototypes, the earliest of which is presented in Noble (1968). This consists of a 13-item questionnaire for use in an interview setting. The items cover speech hearing in the usual circumstances described by previous questionnaires and problems resulting from impairment of speech hearing ability (reduction in social contact; problems at work). Most items are scored on a 5-point scale (always; nearly always; sometimes; hardly ever; never). Because the device was intended as an interview rather than a paper-and-pencil form, the labels on the scoring categories are nonproblematic as regards meaning. They are arbitrary ordinal points. The tactic in interview is to ask each question, and to follow that up with questions seeking clarification of the response. In this way, the specific nuance that the respondent desires is "negotiated" between interviewer and respondent. The interviewer then selects the response category that best fits the respondent's meaning. For instance, estimates by respondents that difficulty is experienced, "about half the time" or that "about half of what was said is missed" or that "some difficulty is experienced, not a lot but more than a little" are all scored at the midscale point ("sometimes"). This procedure was checked by applying a pilot version of the original scale (Noble, 1968) to 17 people with sensorineural disorder attending an audiology clinic. Two researchers were involved, alternating as interviewer and observer with each new respondent. Both people scored responses on all interviews. Subsequent examination of the two sets of scores showed three instances of disagreement between the two researchers, all varying by only 1 point. The procedure could therefore be taken as reliable.

This sort of procedure is time consuming, as indeed is the interview method in general. But the interview, allowing open-ended response, controls for two major sources of uncertainty that the paper-and-pencil method does not. The first and more critical control is over response style. Three types of scaled response have been used in questionnaires: binary, temporal, and intensitive. The first (binary) is "yes–no," used by various authors, and demands that the wording of items be susceptible to unambiguous responding. All questionnaires could be designed this way if all shades of experienced hearing difficulty were known. Thus a Guttman-type scale could be adopted wherein graded degrees of severity are presented in different questions and the approximate changeover point from one response to the other in a two-alternative design would mark the level of handicap experienced.

Temporal scaling is used in the Hearing Handicap Scale, the respondent being asked to report the proportion of time that difficulty is experienced in different situations. Intensitive scaling is used by Silverman *et al.* (1948), and respondents are asked to report the *degree* of difficulty they experience in different situations. The temporal approach assumes that people integrate their experience over time and come up with an aggregate. The underlying assumption is that because experience in a given situation will vary from time to time an overall appraisal across experience will give a subjective average of proportional difficulty. Intensitive scaling assumes that experience is the same from time to time in a given situation and varies only with different situations. Thus people can report that they have a given amount of trouble when they are in a certain situation; another given amount in another situation. Although neither of these assumptions has been empirically fortified by previous authors, the temporal integration concept has more going for it a priori than the intensitive concept.

An interview avoids the assumptive problems embodied in these approaches by allowing respondents to put their own constructs on the matter and describe their experience according to an appropriate scale type. Of course, the way that questions are asked of people implies a framework for answering, and in the original interviews of Noble (1968), a temporal framework was implied. Most people, it turns out, prefer to think in temporal rather than intensive terms, but there are circumstances in which the latter provide a more appropriate response style. This is typically the case in listening situations where the output, say from a controllable source like a radio, and the listening conditions are fairly fixed.

The other variable that is controlled for in interview is relevance. It immediately becomes apparent that some listening situations are not engaged in by everyone. It is important to know what are and what are not universal daily hearing experiences. In the first place, if a situation is rarely experienced, the respondent's knowledge of his capability in that situation is incomplete and answers are likely to be uncertain. In the second place, a situation may be rarely encountered because the person deliberately avoids it, knowing how difficult it is. This latter sort of information is at the heart of hearing handicap assessment. Handicap is defined as *disadvantage* in daily life, and there could be no more eloquent sign of disadvantage than restriction on activity previously enjoyed.

Principally for these reasons, an interview was originally seen as the appropriate method of self-report. An interview is the best way of coming to know the problems experienced by the individual, precisely because it sidetracks and is repetitive. A paper-and-pencil test remains fairly fixed in structure and content so that ramifications of impaired hearing not considered by the authors in originally compiling it may remain unknown.

The original prototype of the Hearing Measurement Scale (Noble, 1968) was an inadequate instrument as it stood, but by reason of subsequent interviews with people attending an audiology clinic, the problems and difficulties not previously realized were unearthed. As a result of the initial exercise, it became clear that the reaction of the person to hearing disturbance was a vital ingredient of everyday handicap. It was also apparent that disturbance of the monitoring role of the auditory system was a critical element in self-rated ability. Additional dysfunction like tinnitus could also present major problems for a person, irrespective of the degree of impairment of hearing. This picture did not emerge all at once. Further lengthy and partially structured interviews at the homes of people who had presented themselves in the audiology clinic filled out impressions gained from the initial research.

The aim of the program as a whole was to devise a valid and reliable method for assessing the hearing impairment and handicap suffered by people as a result of hearing disorder caused by occupational noise. Whatever the peculiar disturbances to hearing wrought by that disorder, the main aim was to find the important circumstances and events in the lives of these and other people with sensorineural disease in which they experienced difficulty in hearing. One major effect of cochlear sensorineural disorder, as we have seen, is reduction of discrimination ability. There is no doubt that this problem is a major contributor to difficulty in hearing, but the primary task in assessing hearing handicap is to inquire into that difficulty rather than into the discrimination problem per se. To be sure, items in the Hearing Measurement Scale on distortion of speech produce a positive response from people with noise disorder. But such people are conscious, in conversational and listening situations, sheerly of the amount of trouble experienced in catching on to what is happening. Because the discrimination problem interacts with the circumstance of listening, it is important to cover, with as fair a balance as possible, all the circumstances where difficulty is encountered or noticed and affects the individual's well-being and activity. It is less important, from a hearing handicap point of view, accurately to assess the extent of the discrimination problem, for it is only a problem once it interferes with important daily hearing acts.

A prototype of the Hearing Measurement Scale was derived from the extensive home interviews of people with sensorineural disorder attending the clinic. It was applied as an interview to a group of 27 iron-foundry workers in the United Kingdom who had a wide range of hearing impairment. Item analysis was performed from these results; and items which gave null responses or responses inconsistent with apparently related items were discarded or modified. Items were added to the section on spatial localization since this emerged as an important area of disturbance according to these men, and the section on emotional response was recast to inquire more specifically into the effect on social relations of impaired hearing (Noble & Atherley, 1970).

Reliability and Sensitivity

The questionnaire form that emerged was then applied to an independent group of foundrymen working in various departments within the one organization. From scrutiny of employment records, the names of 30 men were selected, and they were approached individually to take part in the study. In all, 27 of the men were able to do so: 13 molders, 8 grinders, and 6 chippers. The jobs of each subgroup are in increasing order of noisiness, with roughly 10 dB(A) overall difference between each of them.

In developing the original scale (Noble, 1968), we had conducted interviews with groups of people from different and increasingly noisy trades (busdrivers, cotton mill carders, weavers, and boilermakers). Results with the questionnaire showed clear and significant differences between the groups. Self-report was obviously sensitive, therefore, to differences in degree of impairment. It was of value to check the sensitivity of the new scale under more controlled conditions. The men from the various departments of the foundry had similar backgrounds, residence, interests, and so forth. Differences emerging on self-report between these groups would more certainly be attributable to differences in level of noise to which they were exposed.

The study had a second purpose of equal developmental importance: The men were asked if they would undergo tonal threshold testing and interview with the scale on two occasions separated by a 6-month interval. Repeat testing allowed the stability reliability of both the tonal test and the scale to be calculated and compared. Repeat testing over an interval long enough to eradicate familiarity effects is by far the most demanding trial for any human measurement device. If the questionnaire is ambiguous or lacking in representativeness, responses are likely to vary considerably from one occasion to the next, there being no fixity of understanding on the respondent's part about what the questions mean. Consistency of a response to similar items on a scale during a single test can provide some information in this direction, but there is risk that the particular way the person perceives the questions, together with knowledge as to how similar questions have just been answered, may allow a spurious consistency to emerge because of the single test occasion. Repeated testing demands that the items continue to have stability of meaning even though they may be differently perceived on a repeat trial.

Interviews with the men were tape-recorded as well as scored, though technical problems prevented complete recording of the two series. All recordings were independently analyzed and scored and then compared with the scores made at the time of interview. Where disagreement occurred (and it was again of the order noted with reference to the earlier comparative test), the tape was checked by both the original interviewer and the independent scorer to find out whether an error of scoring on either part had occurred. On only a very few occasions was the recorded response sufficiently muffled or unclear to prevent disagreements from being resolved. In those cases, the interview score was taken as probably more correct.

From responses on the original test and the repeat test 6 months later, scores were computed for each man. A high level coefficient ($r_s = .928$) emerged between total scale scores on the two test occasions. The reliability of average 1–6 kHz tonal threshold levels was $r_s = .846$.

Prior to the reliability study, the items of the questionnaire were subjected to a weighting process which was based on the judgments of a panel of five people who had various different interests in the area of hearing loss assessment plus advice from an audiology technician, a man who was partially deaf and worked at an audiology clinic. This weighting procedure assigned items to nine categories of importance, with increasing scores attached to responses depending on item weight. Interjudge agreement was high, even prior to the meeting of the panel, and the consensus of the panel accorded with the independent ratings of the clinic technician.

These weighted scores were used in computing the reliability coefficient and in examining the scale's sensitivity. Data from the first series of tests for the three subgroups of foundry workers were compared. The mean scale score of the molders was 17.8, of the grinders 34., and of the chippers 75. These scores are significantly different from each other (Kruskal-Wallis variance analysis: $H = 10.28$; $df = 2$; $p < .01$).

Description

The foregoing results allowed the conclusion that the scale was as reasonably developed as need be in terms of stability and sensitivity and that no further modification was required. This form thus became the Hearing Measurement Scale. The scale consists of 42 questions on various aspects of hearing difficulty and reaction to that difficulty. These are arranged in seven sections:

1. Speech hearing (11 items)
2. Nonspeech hearing (8 items)
3. Spatial location (7 items)
4. Emotional response to impairment (7 items)
5. Distortion of speech (3 items)
6. Tinnitus (3 items)
7. Personal opinion of hearing ability (3 items)

In the original form, there were several additional nonscoring items which inquired into features of fluctuating hearing and tinnitus. These are omitted from the published versions of the scale (Atherley & Noble, 1971; Noble & Atherley, 1970). Most items are scored on a 5-point scale, but some are 3-point and some are 2-point. This variety of scaling is in conformity with the way respondents typically answered the questions. In addition, some items in Section 4 (emotional response) seek kinds of answers quite different from the binary–temporal–intensive type. Because the Hearing Measurement Scale in its original form is intended for interview, scaling terms once again are not critical. The actual procedure for interviewing requires considerable experience of that method, and detailed instructions are given in a test manual available from the author (Noble, 1971).

A more recent revision of the Hearing Measurement Scale has been undertaken as a first step in production of the scale in paper-and-pencil form. This is seen as necessary because use of the scale is restricted in view of the time and skill needed for interviews. The experience gained from interviews has allowed most of the qualifications regarding relevance to be built into the revised form. Even so, the wording of items has had to be changed because there is no opportunity for negotiation of meaning in a paper-and-pencil administration. The paper-and-pencil form is undergoing test at the present time; and assuming that the form can be satisfactorily developed, it will be published and available commercially. The interview version will of course continue to be freely available. The new version of the scale, currently under test, is given in the appendix to this chapter.

Validity

The validity of the Hearing Measurement Scale is primarily given in its content; the balance of content, and the differential weighting of items. All that has been said in this book about hearing in the everyday world makes it obvious that a questionnaire that concentrates only on speech hearing (and on that act within a fairly narrow compass) is an unrepresentative instrument. Hearing in the world involves more than hearing of speech, and hearing of speech itself has two major components: listening and conversing. The strategies available in each of these situations to optimize the signal are different. Both aspects need to be represented equally in an inventory. One obvious problem in conversation is communication breakdown, where the information flow between participants is discontinuous. The result of this can be a severe emotional disturbance as the hearing-impaired person operates with lessening effectiveness in social situations. The response of the person himself and the behavior of others around him are crucial elements of experienced handicap. People cope with varying degrees of success, but all persons manifesting hearing loss for speech also reveal a measure of emotional disturbance. This and other patterns of interrelationship are observable from the values given in Table 9.1. Results are taken from interviews with 73 foundry workers: 27 from the reliability study already described and 46 from a study described in Chapter 10.

Because different Hearing Measurement Scale sections have different numbers of items, scores on the smaller sections (2, 5, 6, and 7) are not sufficiently well distributed to allow correlation analysis, either among them or between them and larger sections (1, 3, and 4) and the total score. The mean-square contingency coefficient (C) can be adopted in these circumstances, provided the number of cells in the calculation matrix is constant for each comparison. Even with this provision, the values observed for C are only comparable within themselves and are not comparable with the correlation coefficient. With that caution, it is still possible to examine the pattern of interrelationship in Table 9.1.

An important feature, immediately apparent, is that scores on the first section—speech hearing—relate to all other section scores except that on

TABLE 9.1

Inter-Section and Section-Total Analysis of the Hearing Measurement Scale from Results in 73 Listeners with Various Degrees of Noise-Induced Disorder [a]

	\multicolumn{7}{c}{Section}	
	Speech 1	Non-speech 2	Local-ization 3	Emotional response 4	Distortion 5	Tinnitus 6	Personal opinion 7	Total
1	—	.622*	.440*	.740*	.619*	.419	.649*	.880*
2		—	.583**	.583**	.444	.464	.400	.619*
3			—	.538*	.567**	.407	.492	.681*
4				—	.575**	.286	.674*	.861*
5					—	.449	.600*	.620*
6						—	.489	.364
7							—	.701*
Total								—

* $p < .001$.
** $p < .01$.
Values in italics are Pearson correlation coefficients; values in roman type are Pearson mean square contingency coefficients.
[a] Adapted from Noble and Atherley, 1970.

tinnitus. This is expectable: People often suffer tinnitus as a disturbance independent of any other, and conversely many suffer impaired hearing without the problem of tinnitus. The further proof of that observation is shown by the lack of significant relation between scores on the section on tinnitus and scores on any other section.

The high correlation between the section on speech and that on emotional response (Section 4) plus the high correlations between each of these and the total score bears out the earlier point. Increasing difficulty with speech hearing is associated with increasing emotional disturbance, and these two factors are bound in with the overall hearing impairment and handicap the person sustains. The high correlations between each of these sections and the total, of course, also reflect the fact that the total score is often primarily composed of scores in these sections. This point is borne out in Table 9.2, which shows the distribution of scores found in the composite group of 73 people whose results went to make up the values given in Table 9.1. A striking feature of the results shown in Table 9.2 is the virtual absence of response to items in Section 2 (hearing for sounds other than speech). It is evident from this outcome that reduction of sensitivity is not so noticeable as increase in unintelligibility. The minimal scoring rate in response to Section 2 means that interrelations between scores on that section and other sections will be somewhat depressed. Even so, as seen in Table 9.1, the

TABLE 9.2

Median and Quartile Total Scale Score Values and Values on Each Section of the Hearing Measurement Scale (N = 73), Range of Scores Observed, and Maximum Possible Scores

	Total	Section						
		1	2	3	4	5	6	7
First quartile	11	3	0	1	1	0	0	0
Median	23	9	0	2	5	1	1	0
Third quartile	47	18	3	6	12	3	2	2
Interquartile range	36	15	3	5	11	3	2	2
Range	0–127	0–52	0–15	0–24	0–39	0–12	0–14	0–9
Maximum possible	226	76	28	28	45	20	16	13

highly significant C value (.622) between Section 1 (speech) and Section 2 suggests that a part of the problem with speech is attributable to reduced sensitivity. It is a neat outcome that the above C value of .622 is almost identical with the value of C = .619 between speech hearing scores and speech distortion (Section 5) scores. This suggests that while distortion may be more noticeable than reduced sensitivity, each is equally associated with difficulty in handling speech.

The significant association tabulated in Table 9.1 between hearing for nonspeech sound and both localization (Section 3) and emotional response (Section 4) is also an interesting pattern. Given the medium-level correlation between the latter two, it suggests a multiple interaction among the features of hearing measured by these three sections. This in turn supports a conclusion that localization difficulty and reduced sensitivity for everyday nonspeech sounds have a contributory effect on the experienced handicap resulting from hearing loss. It is interesting to note, however, that while the person's own opinion of his state of hearing (Section 7) relates to his speech hearing score (Sections 1 and 5) and to his emotional response to hearing difficulty (Section 4), problems with localizing and detection do not figure much in that appraisal. It suggests that at least within the interview setting the individual is more conscious of the effect of disorder on the major hearing function (speech reception) than on other functions. Yet these other functions, by virtue of their relatedness to emotional response, are important facets of overall handicap. Furthermore, while speech distortion (Section 5) relates to speech hearing (Section 1), it is not related to hearing for nonspeech sound, suggesting that response to the latter is partially independent of response to speech hearing items per se.

The fact that response to localization items (Section 3) *is* related to speech distortion but not closely related to speech hearing reveals potential support for the observation made in Chapter 1, namely, that localization breakdown may make it difficult to "unravel" a speech signal. It further suggests that localization breakdown may be partly caused by the same mechanism as that which produces distortion of speech—detuning of the cochlea—so that frequency modulations are less easily handled by the auditory nervous system.

With the exception of the tinnitus score, all section scores are significantly associated with the total, the pattern of that association being a faithful reflection of the internal relationships already described.

It is evident from Table 9.2 that hearing for speech and emotional response to hearing disturbance dominate scoring on the scale, so one should be cautious in drawing conclusions about other patterns of relationship simply because these may be yoked to the major scoring components. Nonetheless, the foregoing analysis does not overstretch the data provided in Table 9.1. While it is beyond the present purpose to undertake the task, a factor analysis of response patterns to the Hearing Measurement Scale could usefully be made to discover whether there are genuinely separate factors within Sections 2 and 3 as against Section 1, as I have suggested here.

It is worthwhile analyzing aspects of the finer structure of scoring patterns since items within sections were by no means interrelated. The most striking of these discrepancies occurred in Section 1. Whereas all the items on communication (Items 1 to 6 in the Appendix) were significantly interrelated and most of the items on listening were significantly interrelated (Items 7 to 11), there was little association between individual item scores on these two types. Listening to television and radio was easier for these respondents than communicating or listening at a public gathering. This result presumably is attributable to the greater controllability of the signals from electronic sources, but the lack of association between the two major speech reception settings is not explicable by reduced range-of-scores effect in listening as against communicating, because the interrelationships of scores within the listening items were generally close. Rather, the pattern suggests a difference in speech processing across the two situations.

An additional interesting feature is that listening at a public gathering was related to both communication and listening items, suggesting that this circumstance has elements of both situations. Two interpretations suggest themselves: (a) that in some public gatherings there is a communication element—questions to the speaker, etc.—that might explain the link between face-to-face and audience situations; (b) the live-voice feature of some public gatherings may be an important feature in common with daily conversation voice quality. At the same time, there are enough elements in common between listening in an audience and listening to a TV or radio broadcast to allow an association to emerge between responses to items about these two types of situations.

Separate summing of the scores on Items 1 to 6 and Items 6 to 11 allows scrutiny of the overall interrelationship of each type of speech hearing and of each type to the other functions assessed in different scale sections. Inclusion of item-6 score in both sums makes sense, in view of the commonality of that item to both item sets. The correlation between scores on Items 1 to 6 and 6 to 11 is $r = .67$ ($N = 73$). This shows that the two sets of scores are related, which is quite expectable, but not by any means closely. The correlation value is also affected by the inclusion of the item-6 score in each data set.

Separate correlation of the score on Items 1 to 6 and on 6 to 11 with selected other scores on the scale shows that for the most part these two sets are equally associated with other results. The actual analysis took account of the following features: A within-sections analysis, not reported here, showed that scores on items in Section 2 and also in Section 3 were fairly well interrelated; scores on items within each of Sections 4, 5, and 7 were, in contrast, not all closely associated. The best strategy, therefore, was to calculate the correlations between scores on Items 1 to 6 and 6 to 11 and scores on Sections 2 and 3 and to calculate the contingency coefficients between the two sets of speech items and scores on selected items from the other sections. The restricted range of scores on Section 2 rules out a correlation analysis, however, so a contingency coefficient has been used for that comparison. Also, Section 4 scores are well enough distributed to allow the overall correlation between the separate speech items and emotional response items to be observed. Correlations are presented therefore, in addition to contingency coefficients using individual items from Section 4. These results are all shown in Table 9.3.

It is immediately apparent that responses on the separate speech items relate fairly equivalently to responses on other parts of the scale with the notable exception of relations between subaspects of speech and Section 3 scores. We return to that outcome presently. Occasional other differences are observable between the relationships. Item 31, which concerns emotional response to inability to follow conversation, relates somewhat more closely to the communication items than to the listening items. It is curious that Item 35, which inquires about lack of clarity of speech on TV, does not show a marked closer association with listening items as against communication items.

These results taken generally suggest that listening and communicating are of equivalent status in the hearing repertoire of these respondents. Neither type of activity shows a greater degree of association with items concerning distortion of speech, loss of sensitivity for other sound,

TABLE 9.3

Correlation and Mean Square Contingency Coefficients between Communication Items (1 to 6), Listening Items (6 to 11), and Selected Other Scores on the Hearing Measurement Scale ($N = 73$)

	Communication items (1–6)	$r_{1-6,6-11}$ .67	Listening items (6–11)
Section 3	*.409*		*.292*
Section 4	*.690*		*.680*
Section 2	*.497*		*.50*
item 27	.582		.589
29	.482		.503
31	.652		.586
33	.562		.552
34[a]	.262		.275
35	.482		.490
36	.570		.549
42	.575		.604

Values in italics are Pearson correlation coefficients; values in roman type are mean square contingency coefficients.

[a] In this item, restricted range of scoring entailed use of 3 × 3 rather than 5 × 5 contingency table. Maximum possible coefficient is thus reduced from .8 to .66.

emotional disturbance caused by hearing difficulty, or feelings of personal handicap. The one markedly different correlational outcome is that between each subsection of speech items and the localization score. The communication items are somewhat associated with localization; the listening items barely so.

Such an outcome is in line with the point made earlier that localization and speech processing may interact. Localization only figures in relation to *communication*. This in turn typically means speech heard from different directions in a real setting. Localization is not related to *listening*, and this in turn usually means speech from fixed sources, hence not requiring to be located. No firm conclusion can be drawn, of course, from these results, but they are not inimical to this interpretation.

These analyses serve to show that people's responses to a detailed inventory of questions about difficulty they experience in hearing can be used to gain some insights into hearing disturbance per se and also to obtain some clues about the repertoire of hearing acts. The Hearing Measurement Scale by no means represents an exhaustive form of inquiry, but there can be no doubt that it provides a fuller picture of hearing loss and handicap than other questionnaires. It remains in the following two chapters to examine the interrelations between self-report and other test performance and to consider advantages, disadvantages, and applications of self-report in the assessment of hearing.

APPENDIX

The Hearing Measurement Scale

The form of the scale given here is a revised version of previously published forms. This revision is seen as necessary for development of a paper-and-pencil form, currently under test. The scaling of items will be simplified in this version, though the actual scores attaching to responses will remain as given in Noble and Atherley (1970) and in detail by Noble (1971). The purpose in presenting this new wording of the scale is to allow those intending to use the device in interviews to adopt this wording as probably a less ambiguous form of presentation to respondents. Actual procedure for an interview still requires reference to the test manual (Noble, 1971) accompanying the original version. The section headings, which do not appear in the actual revision of the scale, are given here simply as a reference aid for textual purposes. The scoring categories are omitted as they are still being developed for the paper-and-pencil version.

Section 1. Hearing for Speech

1. Do you have difficulty hearing in a conversation with *one* other person when you're at home?
2. Do you have difficulty hearing in *group* conversation at home?
3. Do you have difficulty hearing in a conversation when you're with *one* other person *outside*? (By "outside" I mean some place outside the house where you would be talking to others.)
4. Do you have difficulty hearing in *group* conversation outside?
5. At work do you have difficulty hearing in a conversation?
   (If yes) Is this due to your hearing, due to noise at work or a bit of both?
   Circle 1, 2, or 3
   1. Due to hearing
   2. Due to noise
   3. A bit of both
6. Do you have difficulty hearing the speaker at a public gathering (assuming that you are standing or sitting in a place that makes it possible to hear properly)?
   If you generally don't attend public gatherings, mark "X" here. Tell me, however, whether that is because hearing difficulty makes it pointless to attend, and/or for other reasons, circle whichever applies (both if appropriate)
   1. Hearing difficulty
   2. Other reason
7. Do you have difficulty hearing what is said on the *news* on

television (assuming in this and in the next three questions that the 'volume' is up at its *usual* level in your household)?

8. Do you have difficulty hearing what is said on TV programs *apart from* the news?
9. Do you have difficulty hearing the *radio* news?
10. Do you have difficulty hearing radio programs *apart from* the news?

If you generally don't watch TV news, mark "X" here.
If you generally don't watch TV apart from the news, mark "X" here.
If you generally don't listen to the radio news, mark "X" here.
If you generally don't listen to the radio apart from the news, mark "X" here.
If you have marked X anywhere above please tell me whether you generally don't watch or listen because of hearing difficulty and/or other reasons.

Don't watch		Don't listen to	
TV news	Other TV programs	Radio news	Other radio programs
1. Hearing difficulty	1. Hearing difficulty	1. Hearing difficulty	1. Hearing difficulty
2. Other reason	2. Other reason	2. Other reason	2. Other reason

11. Do you have difficulty hearing what's said in a film at the cinema? If you generally don't go to the cinema, mark "X" here and tell me why by circling 1 and/or 2
    1. Hearing difficulty
    2. Other reason

Section 2. Hearing for Nonspeech Sound

12. Are you surprised by the arrival of someone at the house because you did not hear their footsteps?
13. If you have a cat or dog or bird as a pet, *can you hear it* when it mews or barks or chirps?
    (What type of pet?)
14. If someone calls at the house, can you hear them ring the doorbell or knock on the door?
15. When you're in the street, can you hear the sound of a car horn?
16. When you are in a room facing away from the door, can you hear it when someone opens the door to come into that room?
17. Can you hear the clock ticking in the room?
    (Assuming you have a ticking clock; if not, mark 'X' here.)

18. Can you hear the water running when you turn a tap on?
19. Can you hear the water boiling in a pan when you are in the kitchen?

The next seven questions ask about a different aspect of your hearing. They are all concerned with how you get on in telling *whereabouts* a person or an object is that you can *hear* but cannot see.

Section 3. Spatial Location

20. When you can hear the sound of people talking outside the room you are in, do you have difficulty telling whereabouts this sound is coming from?
21. If you are with a group of people and someone behind you starts to speak, do you have difficulty telling whereabouts that person *is* behind you?
22. If you hear a car horn or a bell and you can't see it, do you have difficulty telling which direction it's coming from?
23. Do you turn your head the wrong way when someone you can't see calls out to you?
24. Do you have difficulty judging how far away that person is, just from the sound?
25. Do you notice that cars you can *hear* but not *see* turn out to be much closer than you thought?
26. Do you tend to move the *wrong* way to try to get out of the path of someone or something coming up from behind you?

The next seven questions are about effects on you as a person of any hearing difficulty you have. The questions are mainly relevant in fact to people who have difficulty in hearing. If you do not have difficulty in hearing, then the questions may not be relevant.

Section 4. Emotional Response

27. Do you give the wrong answer to people because you've *misheard* them? Some people don't tend to do this if they mishear what another person says, but rather ask the other person to *repeat* what they said. If you tend to do this rather than give the wrong answer, treat the question as: Do you have to ask people to repeat what they've said because you have misheard them?
28. If you give the wrong answer *or* ask people to repeat what they said, do *you* treat this lightly or do you get upset?
29. Do other people get irritated by your wrong answers or by you asking them to repeat what they said?

30. Do you think other people are tolerant about any difficulty in hearing you have or do they make fun of you?
31. Do you get bothered or upset if you are unable to follow a conversation?
32. Do you think you are generally more irritable than other people, about the same, or less irritable?
33. Do you get a feeling of being cut off from things because of difficulty in hearing?
    If yes, does this feeling upset you?

These final questions cover various features of your experience—they are relevant to everyone completing the questionnaire.

Section 5. Speech Distortion

34. Do you find that people fail to speak clearly?
35. Do you find that announcers on TV/radio fail to speak clearly?
36. In everyday conversation with friends or family, do you find you cannot unravel the words being said even though you can *hear* what is being said?

Section 6. Tinnitus

37. Do you get buzzing or ringing noises inside your head or ears?
    If "occasionally" or more often in answer to question 37:
38. Does this head noise prevent you from getting to sleep?
    If "occasionally" or more often in answer to question 37:
39. Does this noise upset you?

Section 7. Personal Opinion

40. Do you think your hearing is normal?
41. Do you think any difficulty in your hearing is particularly serious?
42. Does any difficulty in hearing restrict your social or personal life?

Nonscoring and Followup Items

43. Do you rely on lipreading to help you understand what other people are saying?
44. Do you think you rely on your eyesight more than others do?
45. Are there any questions that have been asked here which you found hard to understand or to answer? If so, please list them and say why they were hard to understand and/or to answer.

46. Please describe any situations in your everyday experience in which you have difficulty in hearing that have not been considered in this questionnaire.

If you are uncertain of answers you have marked to any question, check over the questionnaire and make any notes on it that would clarify where you are uncertain.

10

Relations between Self-Report and Hearing Test Performance

PURPOSE AND SCOPE OF RESEARCH

For the reader committed to traditional hearing assessment methods, this chapter will represent a crucial point in the present work: The research discussed will be taken to bear critically upon the validity of the self-report technique. For the reader (and there may be only one) committed to the self-report approach, this chapter must represent a retrograde step in an otherwise progressive program. For the majority of readers, I hope that the subject matter of the chapter represents an interesting analysis of performance–self-report relations out of which can emerge a better understanding of the likely assessment function of some, at least, of the different mechanical tests. For my own part, I see the comparison of self-report with performance test results as necessary in achieving such an understanding, and I acknowledge a vestigial alignment with the first attitude and a rudimentary alignment with the second.

Different authors have examined self-report for various purposes, as noted in the last chapter. In earlier times, the sole concern was to find a way of giving some verbal label to different tonal threshold level ranges. Later, with more sophisticated systems of performance testing, self-report was used to try to anchor and validate various tests and systems. Only recently has self-report been seen as an alternative assessment method in its own right. It follows, therefore, that in the main, authors have been concerned to use tests of performance and self-report to "prop each other up." The validity of either system has seemingly been substantiated by reference to the other. Since my attitude from the start has been one of skepticism toward existing tests from the viewpoint of hearing handicap assessment, it was never the aim of the program leading to the Hearing Measurement Scale to give substance to the self-report or to any other method by means of concurrent validity.

The first kind of attitude has meant that authors have either deliberately designed questionnaires which are likely in their content to reflect only what performance tests provide or modified their questionnaires the better to do that job. Hence we would expect good agreement between the two types of assessment. The second kind of attitude, not having this aim in mind, leads to the construction of questionnaires whose content may or may not reflect that of performance measures. Hence one cannot expect agreement between the two types of assessment. Certain agreements might be expected between different performance tests and certain sections of the Hearing Measurement Scale, but one is unlikely to observe agreement between results from the scale as a whole and any single performance measure.

All this should be borne in mind, therefore, as we approach the research literature on this topic.

RESULTS FROM EARLIER STUDIES

1935–1936 United States Public Health Service Survey

We have already examined results from the United States Public Health Service survey (1938) in connection with the issue of so-called normal hearing. In that survey, a stratified sample of people in the United States were questioned about difficult speech listening–communication circumstances, and self-report results were compared with tonal threshold levels at octaves from 62.5 Hz to 8 kHz. These data were used, and have been subsequently relied upon, to provide descriptive statements attaching to various ranges of tonal threshold levels.

In the previous discussions of the USPHS data, the point was made that the overlap was not inconsiderable between thresholds of persons reporting different degrees of impairment. It is worthwhile taking a more extensive look at the USPHS (1938) data, particularly with reference to the various degrees of self-reported difficulty and the relation between them and tonal threshold at .25, .5, 1, 2, and 4 kHz. It is unfortunate that individual average threshold values cannot be retrieved from the original data source, so the pattern of self-report and threshold relations can only be looked at by single audio frequencies.

Figures 10.1 through 10.5 are plots, at .25, .5, 1, 2, and 4 kHz, of the proportions at each threshold level of persons reporting different degrees of impairment. The stages of self-reported state of hearing as shown in these figures correspond to the following descriptions:

Stages	Descriptions
"Normal"	No noticeable difficulty in hearing
"Stage 1"	Inability to understand speech in an auditorium or group conversation
"Stage 2"	Inability to understand speech in face-to-face conversation
"Stage 3"	Inability to understand speech on telephone
"Deaf"	Inability to understand speech in any circumstances

The overlapping of thresholds associated with these different stages is evident, especially at 2 and 4 kHz. This latter outcome has no doubt been taken to demonstrate not only that threshold levels at .5 and 1 kHz are a more reliable guide to everyday hearing difficulty but also that thresholds at frequencies above 2 kHz are quite unrelated to everyday self-reported difficulty. However, as I stated earlier, the questionnaire used in this survey was a very crude measuring instrument. Specific patterns of individual difference could never be revealed by such a device. People providing apparently similar self-reports would undoubtedly have shown quite different types and degrees of problem if they had been questioned at greater length in regard to each situation represented by the items in that inventory.

The result shows that self-report and tested performance are broadly in direct relation to each other. Some additional features of interest are revealed in the depicted distributions in Figures 10.1 through 10.5. Whereas at .25, .5, and 1 kHz there are distinct end points at the upper tail of each distribution associated with different degrees of impairment, this is not evident in the distributions at 2 and 4 kHz. On the contrary, whereas at .25 and .5 kHz and to a lesser extent at 1 kHz the *lower* limits of the distributions are less distinct, lower limits are clearly different in the 2 and 4 kHz distributions as a function of self-reported impairment. This picture shows that there are upper bounds of sensitivity associated with different degrees of impairment at lower frequencies and lower bounds at higher frequencies. Conversely there are less noticeable lower bounds at lower frequencies and less noticeable upper bounds at higher frequencies. What this in turn suggests is a differential involvement of lower and higher frequencies in everyday hearing. It says, in other words, that the characteristic feature of a person with *mildly* to *moderately* impaired hearing is one of mild loss of sensitivity at lower frequencies and either mild or severe lack of sensitivity at higher frequencies. On the other hand, the typical picture of a person with marked to severely impaired hearing is one of severe lack of sensitivity at higher frequencies and moderate to severe lack of sensitivity at lower frequencies. In sum, one may find a person with mild hearing impairment showing severe high frequency loss of sensitivity, but it is next to impossible to find someone with severe impairment who does *not* show severe high frequency loss of sensitivity.

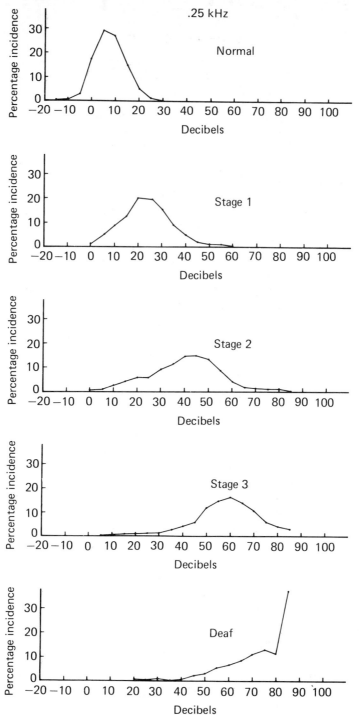

Figure 10.1. Distributions of .25 kHz tonal threshold levels in the "better" and "equal" ears of persons reporting various degrees of hearing impairment. Details of "stages" in text. Data here and in Figures 10.2 to 10.5 from the 1935–1936 USPHS Survey. "Normal" N = 7439; "Stage 1" N = 2454; "Stage 2" N = 1697; "Stage 3" N = 1384; "Deaf" N = 667. Reference zero level = 39.3 dB (SPL) as given by Fletcher (1953, p. 122).

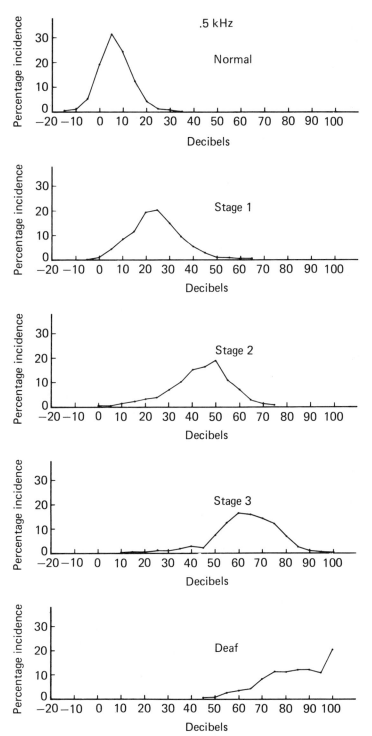

Figure 10.2. Distributions of .5 kHz tonal threshold levels as a function of self-reported ability. "Normal" $N = 7310$; other numbers as in Figure 10.1. Reference zero level = 39 dB (SPL) as given by Fletcher (1953).

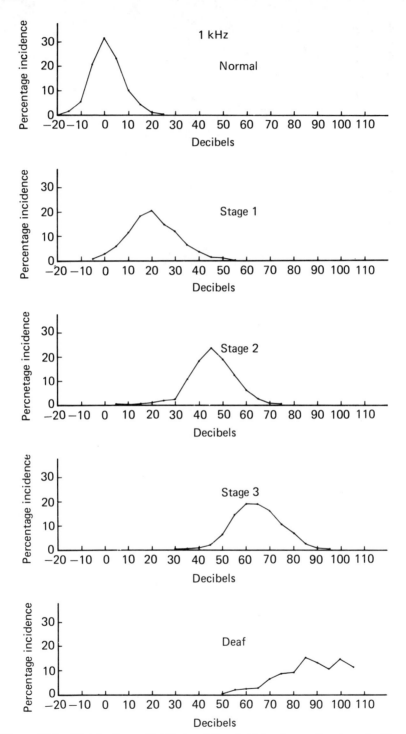

Figure 10.3. Distributions of 1 kHz tonal threshold levels as a function of self-reported ability. "Normal" $N = 7416$; other numbers as in Figure 10.1. Reference zero level = 22.6 dB (SPL) as given by Fletcher (1953).

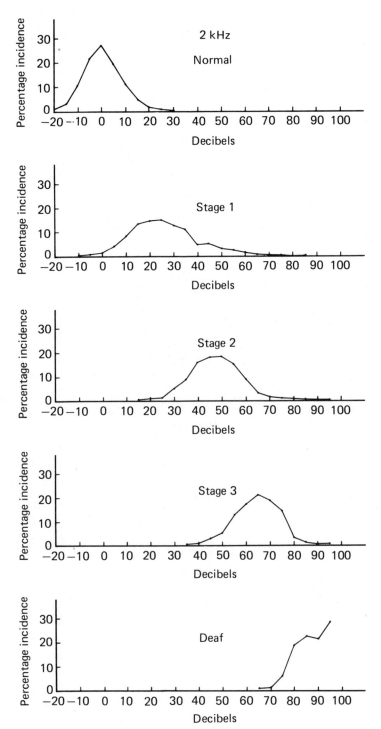

Figure 10.4. Distributions of 2 kHz tonal threshold levels as a function of self-reported ability. "Normal" $N = 7130$; other numbers as in Figure 10.1. Reference zero level = 23.6 dB (SPL) as given by Fletcher (1953).

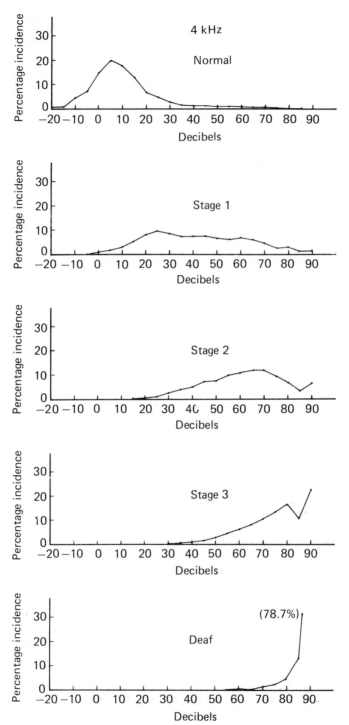

Figure 10.5. Distributions of 4 kHz tonal threshold levels as a function of self-reported ability. "Normal" $N = 6868$; other numbers as in Figure 10.1. Reference zero level = 20.7 dB (SPL) as given by Fletcher (1953).

1960–1963 United States Public Health Service Survey

Schein *et al.* (1970) reported on a revision of the questionnaire used in the 1960–1963 United States National Health Survey. The aim of their endeavors was to develop a shorthand verbal system for evaluating hearing, one that would do the job of a tonal threshold screening test. To this end, they examined the relations between responses to their questionnaire and levels at threshold averaged across .5, 1, and 2 kHz. The self-report component consisted of the person's rating of his or her hearing in each ear, as either

1. My hearing is good
2. I have a little trouble hearing
3. I have a lot of trouble hearing
4. I am deaf

In addition, respondents answered the questions given in Chapter 9 concerning ability to hear whispered, spoken, and shouted speech. Five degrees of difficulty were identified on the basis of these latter questions. Analysis was made of the "better" ear .5 to 2 kHz threshold average (whichever ear showed the lower average level) as a function of rating on the 4-point scale of each ear, and as a further function of score (from 1 to 5) on the questions about speech hearing. Thus respondents might claim that their hearing in one ear was in line with one of the four statements above, further claim their hearing was similar or different in the other ear according to that scheme, and then provide a score anywhere between 1 and 5 on the questionnaire. Ideally, of course, the authors hoped that some kind of regular interaction would emerge between rating on the 4-point scale, self-report on the 5-point questionnaire, and average level at threshold.

While a broad picture of that kind emerges from the rather convoluted analyses performed, the large spread of threshold data at each self-report interval and the inconsistent relationship between self-report and even average threshold suggests that certain confoundings were operative in the initial study. The major confounding can, of course, be traced to the questionnaire itself. Overall rating (opinion) of hearing ability and self-report of degree of difficulty experienced in different hearing situations are related, but not closely. This was shown in Chapter 9 in considering the interrelations between different aspects of the Hearing Measurement Scale and respondents' personal opinions about their hearing. These are two separate aspects of self-report which do not necessarily coincide.

Another source of confounding is in the Schein *et al.* (1970) analysis itself. By selecting only "better" ear threshold levels for comparison with self-rating and self-report, the authors made the assumption that irrespective of the person's differential rating of each ear, or even similar rating, the actual level at threshold in the "better" ear is a valid performance guide to the person's auditory ability. It is not surprising, then, that inconsistent relations emerged between "better" ear thresholds and self-reported difficulty regarding speech hearing in those cases where there was a reported major discrepancy between the two ears. This occurs because the degree of experienced difficulty would be importantly governed by the extent of impairment in the poorer ear.

The Hearing Handicap Scale

Since this was the first substantial study of self-report, the authors of the Hearing Handicap Scale (High et al., 1964) were concerned to assess its performance in relation to a number of audiometric tests. However, the major problem with this aspect of their study is that listeners were people with predominantly conductive disorders. The authors acknowledge that this factor helps to account for the higher correlations between scale scores and both .5 to 2 kHz tonal threshold and SRT than between scale scores and tests of discrimination. However, they tend to discount discrimination problems as contributing to hearing handicap (p. 228). On what evidential basis they can do so is unknown. Be that as it may, Hearing Handicap Scale scores correlated at $r = .65$ with "better"-ear threshold at .5 to 2 kHz and at $r = .7$ with "better"-ear SRT. "Better" ear was determined as the ear showing lower .5 to 2 kHz tonal threshold average. Correlations between either better or poorer ear discrimination score (W-22 and Fairbanks' test of phonemic differentiation, 1958) and scale score were in the .04 to .24 range. The authors concluded that, "better-ear hearing sensitivity . . . is probably the major determinant of hearing handicap as measured here [p. 227]."

On their own data base, that conclusion is certainly justified, but it should be generalized with caution. The first, more obvious reason for such restraint is because of the sample of people involved. There being little by way of disturbance to their hearing except loss of sensitivity, other factors would necessarily play a minor role. Whether the same picture would emerge in a sample of people with predominantly sensorineural disorder is unknown to the authors. Subsequent investigators have looked at this question, and we will consider their results presently. The second reason for caution is that the disparities between "better" and "poorer" ears were about 15 dB on average. With such a small interaural difference, poorer ear influence on overall hearing difficulty would be negligible. But, as shown by the results of Schein et al. (1970), major discrepancies between two ears can be associated with major problems, even when the better ear shows a relatively low threshold level. A different picture might therefore emerge from results obtained in people with marked interaural threshold differences. To my knowledge, this question has not received subsequent attention. My own investigation of the issue is at an early stage, but results so far suggest that marked unilateral disorder can have a much more handicapping effect than would be predicted from "better" ear threshold levels.

Blumenfeld et al. (1969) applied the Hearing Handicap Scale to a group of 55 people, half of whom were aged at least 65 years. We have already remarked one curious outcome of this study, namely, the inconsistent interrelations between each "parallel" form of the Hearing Handicap Scale and results on Fairbanks' (1958) test. Not enough detail of procedure is given by Blumenfeld et al. (1969) to allow a firm conclusion regarding this outcome, so one cannot say whether the result is attributable to an order-of-test effect or shows a genuine lack of equivalency of the two forms: It is certainly a problematic finding in view of their supposed equivalency (High et al., 1964).

The diagnostic composition of the Blumenfeld et al. (1969) sample is unstated. Composite audiograms suggest the presence of no specific pathology in the group. Rather it appears as though "presbycusis" is the factor which gives rise to the elevated higher frequency tonal threshold levels observed. Details of scale scores and discrimination test scores are not given, and all in all it is hard to weigh up the result of this study. Nevertheless, the finding of interest is that negative correlations of between .31 and .55 were noted between Hearing Handicap Scale and left ear discrimination test scores. While these are hardly close, they are higher than the values found by High et al. (1964) for the same tests in a group with predominantly conductive disorder. This suggests that diagnostic composition does have a part to play in everyday speech hearing. Such a finding will surprise no one in view of what has long been understood about the different disturbances of hearing associated with these different disorders. Yet another unfortunate feature of the Blumenfeld et al. study is the absence of comparison between scale scores and tonal threshold. That exercise would have allowed appraisal of the relative contributions of sensitivity and discrimination ability in their sample.

In a somewhat more penetrating analysis of the issue, Speaks, Jerger, and Trammell (1970) compared relationships between Form A only of the Hearing Handicap Scale and measures of both tonal and speech reception threshold and speech discrimination. All tests were of one ear only of each listener—selection being on the basis of the ear showing lower .5 to 2 kHz threshold level. Tonal threshold was taken as the average in the "better" ear at .5, 1, and 2 kHz. SRT was the level for 50% correct responses using half-lists of PAL monosyllables and the level for 50% correct recognition of synthetic sentences (Speaks & Jerger, 1965) in quiet and in competing speech conditions. Speech discrimination for monosyllables and sentences in competing conditions was measured at various intensities. The indices used for analysis were discrimination score for monosyllables at 40 dB re: 1 kHz tonal threshold; maximum score on monosyllables (PB-max); monosyllable score at 110 dB (SPL); maximum score on sentences; and sentence score at 110 dB (SPL). In addition, the area under the articulation function for both monosyllables and sentences was computed (an index similar to that used by Hood, 1968; see Chapter 8). Finally, an arbitrary index combining speech threshold and discrimination values was computed.

Listeners were 60 men and women attending an audiology clinic. Of these, 49 had diagnoses of sensorineural disorder; 6 had mixed disorder; and 5 had conductive disorder. Ages ranged from 19 to 78 years (average, 59). The performance of this group on tests and their responses to the Hearing Handicap Scale were distributed widely. A fair picture of the correlation between each measure and the scale is thus guaranteed from results in these listeners. The highest correlation (.72) was obtained between .5 to 2 kHz tonal threshold and Hearing Handicap Scale score, and the other three speech reception threshold indices correlated at levels ranging from .6 to .7. By contrast, the highest correlation between scale and discrimination score (PB-max) was −.52, the other discrimination measures ranging from −.11 to −.43. However, the area under the articulation function for monosyllables correlated at $r = -.68$ and that for sentences at −.58. Speaks et al. (1970) categorized the latter indices as combining sensitivity and discrimination. This follows, since these areas will be partly governed by threshold, partly by articulation (it is akin to the social adequacy index computation). The other 2 arbitrary sensitivity–discrimination indices correlated with scale score at $r = -.65$ and $r = -.49$.

It is thus clear that while discrimination ability plays a role in contributing to everyday hearing difficulty (at least as assessed by the Hearing Handicap Scale), sheer loss of sensitivity is a more dominant factor even in people with sensorineural disorder. An additional analysis was carried out by Speaks et al. (1970) of results from people whose audiograms showed greater high frequency levels at threshold. Eighteen people showed this as a marked characteristic, 17 of whom had diagnoses of sensorineural disorder. All the correlation values dropped to a range of .12 to .49, the threshold test results still showing the closer associations with scale score.

Speaks et al. (1970) were clearly dissatisfied with this outcome because it did not seem to make much sense. Discrimination, particularly for sentences, is surely a more valid indicator of everyday speech hearing problems than tonal threshold. But the only way they could rationalize the result was to suggest that the Hearing Handicap Scale is more concerned with sensitivity than with discrimination. They assert that "Our analysis of the 20 items on Form A . . . suggests that 12 of the

20 items are clearly sensitivity oriented. The remaining 8 seem to reflect both sensitivity and discrimination [p. 772]." They do not say on what criterial base this differentiation was achieved nor which items clearly show "sensitivity" content. My own scrutiny of Form A leads me nevertheless to go part of the way with Speaks *et al.* (1970). About half the items refer more to an ability simply to detect conversational or other speech rather than to comprehend what is going on. But about half the items use terms like "understand" or "follow without difficulty," thus inquiring about comprehension as much as about detection. I think, therefore, that Speaks *et al.* (1970) have the makings of an argument, but a more thorough content analysis of the Hearing Handicap Scale would be required before any final conclusion were arrived at.

It is more profitable, in my view, to question the validity of all the procedures used in assessment and not to assume that a discrimination test using synthetic sentences is related a priori to everyday speech hearing conditions. A worthwhile endeavor would be to look at subaspects of the Hearing Handicap Scale in relation to performance test outcomes and verify, where possible, content features of its items. The critical issue remaining is whether the Hearing Handicap Scale, irrespective of its relation to performance tests, is a valid measure of hearing loss and handicap. I have already argued that it is at best a limited measurement device.

Berkowitz and Hochberg (1971) reported a study that combines certain aspects of both the previous investigations. Listeners were 100 older people (aged 60 to 87 years; average, 70 years) and tests included monosyllable (W-22) and sentence (Silverman & Hirsh, 1955) discrimination score; SRT (W-1); and .5 to 2 kHz tonal threshold. Form A of the Hearing Handicap Scale was used. Performance test values, using the "better" ear, particularly for sentence discrimination, were somewhat restricted, so results are perhaps not so representative as those obtained by Speaks *et al.* (1970). Once again, threshold measures emerged as more consistently related to self-report than discrimination test results. The highest correlation value obtained was .64 (between .5 to 2 kHz threshold and scale score in female listeners). Curiously, a marked difference in test interrelationships between the sexes was noted. Male listeners' discrimination results showed almost zero correlation with self-report, whereas females' results correlated at around .4.

The pattern of test data from all these studies confirms that threshold measures and the Hearing Handicap Scale are related. I have already suggested that threshold, at least for speech, has an important assessment role. These results confirm that view. That .5 to 2 kHz tonal threshold should also emerge cannot be relied on too heavily at this stage. For one, the studies involving comparison of tonal threshold and self-report have not examined threshold levels at frequencies other than

.5 to 2 kHz, so the overall tonal test–handicap scale relationship is unknown. Second, the samples of listeners in question have comprised people with fairly widely distributed levels at .5 to 2 kHz threshold. The findings so far may not generalize to groups such as those with noise-induced disorder, in whom .5 to 2 kHz threshold is often unaffected.

The "Dundee Index"

Pearson *et al.* (1973) reported an analysis that serves as an excellent model for the use of self-report merely to provide concurrent validity for the tonal or speech audiogram. Results from their survey of factory jute weavers (Kell *et al.*, 1971) were scrutinized to find items within their questionnaire, responses to which most successfully discriminated people on the basis of tonal and speech thresholds (SRT for Fry's 1961 lists). Four items were isolated, concerning communication with family and friends, communication with strangers, telephone use, and audience listening. Three grades of difficulty in each of these situations were abstracted from response forms to provide a 12-point scale of "social handicap." By use of discriminant analysis, the tonal threshold pattern was identified that most effectively differentiated people scoring high from those scoring low on both the 12-point scale and the speech tests. The authors concluded that this formula: Threshold at 2 kHz minus one-half the level at threshold at 4 kHz plus one-half the level at threshold at 6 kHz—the "Dundee Index"—is a valid guide to social hearing handicap. Comparing it with a variety of more straightforward averaging techniques, the authors observed that the index misclassified fewer people in terms of the Pearson *et al.* questionnaire score.

The interesting feature of the Dundee Index is that tonal threshold at 6 kHz plays a significant role. Indeed, the one averaging method that included 6 kHz was closest to the index in terms of misclassification. This finding is especially interesting in view of the sample under study, namely, people with noise-induced disorder. The only flaw in the whole procedure is the assumption that performance tests hold the key to hearing loss and handicap assessment. On this assumption, the self-report aspect is tailored to conform with performance test results. Other non-conforming features of self-report were ignored. No independent proof was obtained that the situations isolated to provide the index's validity were themselves validly representative of everyday hearing difficulty.

The Social Hearing Handicap Index

Ewertsen and Birk-Nielsen (1973) compared responses on their questionnaire with SRT measured using recorded numerals. They found a lower-bound phenomenon such that handicap index scores varied from minimum to maximum in association with low SRT levels; but with increasing level at SRT, the range of self-report scores decreased so that no instances were observed of high level at SRT and low scale score. Listeners were 223 people, aged 21 to 92 years (average, 63 years), 198 of whom had some kind of hearing disorder. No details are given about these people, but presumably they represent a typical clinic sample. Ewertsen and Birk-Nielsen (1973) noted that people who gave high-level scale scores yet had low levels at SRT tended to be those with high frequency threshold rises.

No correlation analysis was done on the SRT–self-report data, nor were any other performance tests included. From the scattergram of scale scores as a function of SRT, the correlation looks meager. The content of Ewertsen and Birk-Nielsen's questionnaire does not appear to be much different from that of the Hearing Handicap Scale. Their result is in fact not unlike that of Speaks et al. (1970) when the latter isolated those listeners with elevation of higher frequency tonal thresholds. It is unfortunate that Ewertsen and Birk-Nielsen did not examine self-report and discrimination performance.

The state of things emerging from all of the foregoing is that in people with conductive disorder threshold at .5 to 2 kHz or SRT is associated, though not closely enough for predictive purposes, with self-reported hearing difficulty using the Hearing Handicap Scale. Discrimination score is not related to self-report in that kind of clinical group. In people with sensorineural disorder, relationships between self-report and performance are not so clear; discrimination score assumes somewhat greater importance than it does in people with conductive disorder, but threshold measures still provide a closer association.

In people with noise-induced disorder, high frequency threshold level has an important part to play in prediction of certain limited aspects of everyday hearing difficulty. And more generally, from the United States Public Health Service 1935–1936 survey data (1938), from the study by Pearson et al. (1973), and from that by Ewertsen and Birk-Nielsen (1973), high frequency threshold seems to be a critical variable in producing or at least signaling severe levels of handicap.

THE HEARING MEASUREMENT SCALE

Developmental Comparative Research

The picture is not necessarily to be clarified by reference to the comparative work carried out in connection with the development of the Hearing Measurement Scale. But one can look in some detail at the patterns of relationship between responses on that scale and a variety of performance tests.

The study to be described was conducted at the acoustical laboratory of the Department of Physics at Salford University in the United Kingdom. Listeners were men drawn from various trades in a number of local metal-founding and finishing works. Altogether 46 people were examined, aged 29 to 67 years (average 51), though not all were given every test in the battery. A summary of the findings is reported by Noble and Atherley (1970), and these will be reuttered here in a more detailed analysis.

A series of tests was presented monaurally through headphones, some of these were re-presented binaurally in the free-field conditions of an anechoic chamber, and yet other tests were conducted only in the latter conditions. The following is a list of performance tests used

1. Monaural self-recording tonal threshold at .5 to 6 kHz
2. Monaural SRT for prerecorded disyllables (W-1)
3. Monaural SRT for prerecorded continuous discourse
4. Monaural discrimination score for prerecorded monosyllables (W-22) at 25 dB re: SRT
5. Binaural SRT for disyllables in free field
6. Binaural SRT for discourse in free field
7. Binaural comfortable listening level for discourse in free field
8. Binaural threshold of discomfort for discourse in free field
9. Binaural localization of 1 kHz tone bursts in the horizontal plane in free field at 6 sensation levels

All 46 men were interviewed using the Hearing Measurement Scale, and almost all were given each monaural test.

The free-field testing set-up was not finalized until later in the study, so only about 20 to 30 of the 46 people were tested under these conditions. All tape-recording of speech test material was carried out by the present author according to the usual specifications for vocal production of disyllables, monosyllables, and discourse. The discourse consisted of an article on sport from a newspaper which these particular listeners were not likely to have read yet on a topic which interested them considerably. An exception to normal procedure is that no carrier phrases were used in the disyllable and monosyllable tests. It is unclear what, if any, affect this had on listeners' performance. With the exception of an unusual result in the monosyllable discrimination test, data conform with previously published results.

Tables 10.1 and 10.2 show the mean, standard deviation, median, and quartile levels at various thresholds (in dB SPL) and median and quartile error rates for discrimination and localization tests. Also shown are the different numbers of people tested on each performance measure. Table 10.1 gives results on monaural earphone tests; Table 10.2 results on binaural free-field tests. The unusual result (shown in Table 10.1) is a

TABLE 10.1

Means, Medians, Standard Deviations, and Quartiles of Results on Various Performance Tests (in dB SPL) and Percentage Error Rates on Discrimination Testing for People Tested Monaurally by Earphone Listening. Numbers of Listeners (N) Shown in Final Column[a]

	Test	Left ear						Right ear					
		Mean	SD	Quartiles			Mean	SD	Quartiles			N
				First	Second	Third			First	Second	Third	
1	.5 kHz	28.2	9.0	20.0	26.0	34.0	23.8	11.4	15.5	19.0	31.0	45
	1 kHz	21.7	13.3	10.5	18.0	28.5	22.6	14.9	9.5	16.0	33.5	
	2 kHz	32.7	22.6	14.5	24.5	40.5	38.1	23.4	18.0	28.5	65.0	
	3 kHz	44.2	24.8	20.0	33.5	64.5	49.7	22.5	28.0	48.5	68.5	
	4 kHz	57.5	28.3	36.5	55.0	77.0	57.1	23.3	37.5	55.5	76.0	
	6 kHz	71.6	22.3	53.5	72.5	91.0	72.9	20.1	52.0	68.0	91.5	
2		37.9	7.7	33.5	37.0	45.0	37.1	9.4	30.0	35.0	44.0	45
3		39.1	14.5	26.0	35.0	45.0	37.9	14.3	28.0	35.0	45.0	44
4		34%	20%	16%	28%	42%	27%	21%	12%	18%	38%	46

[a] Adapted from Noble and Atherley, 1970.
[b] Test 1: Tonal threshold at .5 to 6 kHz; Test 2: SRT for CID disyllables; Test 3: SRT for continuous discourse; Test 4: DS for CID monosyllables at 25 dB (SRT).

TABLE 10.2

Means, Medians, Standard Deviations, and Quartiles on Various Performance Tests (in dB SPL) and Percentage Error Rates on Localization Testing for People Tested Binaurally in Free-Field Listening. Numbers of Listeners (N) Shown in Final Column[a]

Test		Mean	SD	Quartiles			N
				First	Second	Third	
5		37.9	16.1	27	35	45	29
6		38.2	10.6	30	37	45	30
7		72.9	7.8	67	72	77	29
8		97.5	9.1	92	97	107	28
9	5 dB SL	48%	25%	25%	50%	67%	27
	10 dB SL	35%	26%	8%	33%	50%	29
	15 dB SL	24%	18%	0%	25%	42%	22
	20 dB SL	21%	21%	0%	17%	33%	28
	30 dB SL	19%	17%	0%	13%	33%	23
	40 dB SL	14%	14%	0%	8%	17%	21

[a] Adapted from Noble and Atherley, 1970.
[b] Test 5: SRT for CID disyllables; Test 6: SRT for continuous discourse; Test 7: Comfortable listening level for continuous discourse; Test 8: Threshold of discomfort for continuous discourse; Test 9: Horizontal plane localization of 1 kHz tone bursts at various sensation levels (SL).

marked difference between left and right ears in discrimination error level. In administration of the W-22 test lists, left ears were always tested first with list 1A, right ears then tested with list 2A. Responses were written rather than repeated vocally. Perhaps the omission of a carrier phrase, plus some unfamiliarity with the task, led to this difference in results between ears. It was noted that not only between the left and right ears but also between the first and second halves of the left ear test improvement occurred in correct identification rate. However, listeners had been given the disyllable test prior to the monosyllable test, so sheer familiarization cannot altogether account for the result. Rather, the absence of a carrier phrase presumably meant that listeners were unprepared for each word and had to become familiar with the 6-second interword interval used in order to acquire such preparedness. Data from the right ears showed no noticeable change between first and second halves of the test list, and therefore only the right ear data have been used in the present analysis.

The comfortable listening level–threshold of discomfort measure was included as a test of loudness–compression, hence of "recruitment." The localization test has been fully described by Atherley and Noble (1970). Six loudspeakers were used, set 60° apart in a circle around the listener and at the same height as his head when he was seated. The loudspeakers were acoustically balanced to within ±0.5 dB of one another. Signals were presented at various sensation levels relative to the listener's binaural free-field threshold level for a 1 kHz tone emitted from the loudspeaker judged by him to provide the quietest output. Obviously, loudspeakers behind the listener would provide less energy to the ears than those opposite or in front of the ears. By this means, all signals were bound to be audible at the lowest SL used (5 dB). All free-field speech testing employed a single loudspeaker placed directly in front of the seated listener at a distance of 2 meters. Output levels were continuously monitored by a microphone suspended above the listener's head.

Correlation and mean square contingency coefficients were calculated between each performance measure and the Hearing Measurement Scale total scores, section scores, and certain subaspects of section scores. These results are presented in five separate tables, Tables 10.3 to 10.7. In Table 10.3, correlations between total scale scores, Section 1 (speech hearing) scores, and monaural performance test results are shown. In Table 10.4, correlations between the same scale scores and binaural, free-field test results are given.

TABLE 10.3

Correlations (r_x) between Total Score on the Hearing Measurement Scale; Section 1 (Speech Hearing) Score; and Monaural, Earphone-Listening Performance Tests

Test[a]		Total score	Section 1
1 (L)	.5 kHz	−.01	−.03
	1 kHz	.24	.32
	2 kHz	.40**	.45**
	3 kHz	.50*	.55*
	4 kHz	.51*	.60*
	6 kHz	.48**	.50*
1 (R)	.5 kHz	.19	.10
	1 kHz	.06	.24
	2 kHz	.39**	.49**
	3 kHz	.50*	.58*
	4 kHz	.55*	.58*
	6 kHz	.42**	.50*
2 (L)		.58*	.56*
2 (R)		.41**	.43**
3 (L)		.38	.32
3 (R)		.49**	.42**
4 (R)		.56*	.50*

* $p < .001$.
** $p < .01$.

[a] 1 (L), 1 (R). Tonal threshold in left and right ears.
2 (L), 2 (R). Disyllable SRT in left and right ears.
3 (L), 3 (R). SRT for discourse in left and right ears.
4 (R). Discrimination score for monosyllables in right ear.

TABLE 10.4

Correlations (r_s) between Total Scale Score; Section 1 Score; and Binaural, Free-Field Performance Tests

Test[a]		Total score	Section 1
5		.63*	.47**
6		.45**	.35
7		.32	.23
8		.00	.09
9	5 dB SL	.30	.13
	10 dB SL	.13	.08
	15 dB SL	.03	−.03
	20 db SL	.11	.07
	30 dB SL	.25	.24
	40 dB SL	.37	.29

* $p < .001$.
** $p < .01$.
[a] 5. Disyllable SRT.
  6. SRT for discourse.
  7. Comfortable listening level for discourse.
  8. Threshold of discomfort *minus* comfortable listening level ("recruitment" index).
  9. Horizontal plane localization of 1 kHz tone bursts at various sensation levels.

In Table 10.3, results are from a least 44 listeners (see Table 10.1 for details of numbers). Results in Table 10.4 are from between 21 and 30 listeners (see Table 10.2 for details). Coefficient values in the two tables are not directly comparable, therefore, because it requires a larger r_s value to achieve the same level of significance when N is between 20 and 30 than when $N = 44$. The actual levels of correlation are comparable, however.

It can be seen from Table 10.3 that the tests which are at all related to the questionnaire as a whole are higher frequency tonal threshold (Test 1 at 2 to 6 kHz) and SRT for disyllables (Test 2). Discrimination score (Test 4) also relates to the questionnaire as a whole and at a level approaching that of SRT. Both types of speech test bear a slightly closer relation to the scale than the tonal test. Lower frequency tonal threshold, as is quite apparent, bears no relation to the total scale score and SRT for discourse (Test 3) is only loosely related. From Table 10.4 it is apparent that disyllable SRT (Test 5) and to a lesser extent SRT for discourse (Test 6) relate to total scale score. The comfortable listening level (Test 7) is very loosely related, while the recruitment index (Test 8) figures in no way at all. It is not surprising that the localization test (Test 9) is unrelated to total scale score.

These results tend to confirm the results of previous authors, though it is interesting that discrimination score is about as prominent in the pattern of relationships as SRT. Presumably this reflects the different content of the Hearing Measurement Scale as opposed to devices like the Hearing Handicap Scale. The role of higher frequency tonal threshold and the absence of a role for lower frequency tonal threshold is a result that conforms with previous studies in similar types of listeners. To some extent, these and previous results reflect the threshold audiogram profile, there being little obvious threshold reduction and a restricted range of values in the .5 to 1 kHz region. That does not, however, detract from a conclusion that no relationship is even emergent between .5 and 1 kHz threshold and overall self-reported everyday hearing difficulty. Even 2 kHz threshold, which shows no restricted range of values (see Table 10.1), bears only a slight association with total score.

A somewhat different picture is seen when scores on items in Section 1 (hearing for speech) are correlated with mechanical test performance. A broader tonal threshold involvement is observable (though the important frequencies are still 3 and 4 kHz), and the ascendant role of speech tests over tonal threshold is reversed. This suggests that the content of these speech tests is not *specifically* related to everyday speech hearing but rather more to overall hearing function. The tonal threshold–Section 1 relational pattern suggests that in everyday speech hearing sensitivity over the whole range of the speech spectrum is important. This result bears out MacRae and Brigden's (1973) finding as regards everyday sentence perception and the articulation index.

In Table 10.5, correlation analysis results are presented between the speech test values and items 1–6 (communication items) and 6–11 (listening items). The distinction of these two sets of items is made in Chapter 9. It is apparent that while communication items show stronger

TABLE 10.5

Correlations (r_s) between Communication Items (1–6), Listening Items (6–11), and Speech Performance Test Results[a]

Test	Items 1–6	Items 6–11
2 (L)	.58*	.40**
2 (R)	.43**	.32
3 (L)	.32	.43**
3 (R)	.44**	.51*
4 (R)	.50*	.44**
5[b]	.50**	.40
6[b]	.38	.29
7[b]	.27	.09

* $p < .001$.
** $p < .01$.
[a] See Tables 10.3 and 10.4 for key to tests.
[b] Tests 5, 6, and 7 had smaller numbers of listeners hence probability levels associated with r_s values are less extreme.

association than listening items with *disyllable* SRT (Test 2), the opposite is the case for SRT using *continuous discourse* (Test 3). The same pattern is not maintained in field listening conditions, and perhaps more surprising, the comfortable listening level (Test 7) does not relate at all to scores on listening items.

Free-field speech test results in general show a low level of association with self-report. The explanation I can suggest for the low association is that the listening conditions in an anechoic chamber using high fidelity broadcasting equipment in no way match the typical listening or communicating circumstances of the everyday world. Several of the men remarked, after the comfortable listening level test, that they wished they could hear conversation and TV shows with that kind of quality and lack of background interference in their own homes.

The earphone condition and the SRT task probably represent a better analog of everyday communication–listening than the freefield. And it is an expectable outcome that SRT for discourse should show a closer association with listening items than disyllable SRT. Furthermore, the closer association between disyllable SRT and *communication* items supports my contention in Chapter 9 that this test has features akin to everyday communication, namely, familiarity combined with a certain amount of redundancy, and yet at a level which is just comprehensible to the listener.

The complete absence of relationship between self-reported speech hearing ability and the "recruitment" index (Test 8) is not surprising given all the results previously discussed in Chapters 6 and 8. This measure of "recruitment" is not wholly satisfactory, but it did show a minor association with tonal threshold levels at 1, 4, and 6 kHz ($-.3$ to $-.4$) suggesting that it assessed the loudness distortion feature of this disorder to some extent. What this implies is that the absence of relationship with reported speech hearing difficulty cannot easily be dismissed on grounds that the "recruitment" test failed to measure anything of the dysfunction in question.

In Table 10.6 are presented correlations between all performance tests and scores on Section 3 (localization) and Section 4 (emotional response) of the scale. As regards the latter, there are no particular expectations about interrelationships since items in that section have little direct bearing on hearing performance. It is not surprising that the pattern simply reflects the Section 1 and total score associations since Section 4 scores are closely bound in with both of these other scores (see Chapter 9). Thus, whatever dependencies arise between performance and self-reported hearing difficulty will be most likely to dictate the interrelations between performance and emotional response to that difficulty.

Section 3 responses should obviously show some sort of relation to localization test performance as well as to other features of tested audi-

TABLE 10.6

Correlations between Scores on Section 4 (Emotional Response), Section 3 (Spatial Location), Items 20 to 23 (Directional Location), and All Performance Tests[a]

Test		Section 4	Section 3	Items 20–23
1 (L)	.5 kHz	−.08	.23	.05
	1 kHz	.17	.31	.18
	2 kHz	.28	.31	.19
	3 kHz	.46**	.40**	.35
	4 kHz	.50*	.34	.31
	6 kHz	.44**	.32	.25
1 (R)	.5 kHz	.17	.30	.19
	1 kHz	.12	.25	.15
	2 kHz	.18	.32	.23
	3 kHz	.38	.38	.34
	4 kHz	.48**	.46**	.36
	6 kHz	.44**	.56*	.37
2 (L)		.39**	.45**	.32
2 (R)		.26	.28	.24
3 (L)		.28	.34	.23
3 (R)		.34	.39	.24
4 (R)		.41**	.37	.17
		Binaural free-field tests		
5		.48**	.54**	.42
6		.37	.31	.28
7		.23	.38	.32
8		−.07	−.21	−.31
9	5 dB SL	.19	.43	.48**
	10 dB SL	.04	.01	−.04
	15 dB SL	.09	.03	.18
	20 dB SL	.01	.13	.19
	30 dB SL	.11	.26	.16
	40 dB SL	.25	.34	.34

* $p < .001$.
** $p < .01$.
[a] See Tables 10.3 and 10.4 for key to tests.

tory function. It is true that there is a slight relationship observable in the results. Also there is a concomitant absence of relationship between localization test results and other sections of the scale. But it is evident that Section 3 scores must be dealing with different and certainly more numerous features of auditory spatial behavior than the rather simplistic test of that function invoived in the developmental program.

In an effort to make the comparison a little more specific, scores on only those items (20 to 23) dealing with direction rather than distance have been compared with the localization test. As can be seen in Table 10.6, this expedient results in a slight increase at the lowest sensation level in association between tested ability and self-reported ability. That correlation is also higher than any other between scores on items 20 to 23 and performance. It is worth noting that higher frequency threshold level bears a somewhat consistent relation to general spatial perception as measured by self-report. This finding is consistent with the point made in Chapter 6 that higher frequency hearing loss, being a general sign of cochlear disorder, may thus be a sign of the deterioration that also affects locational ability (see Chapter 1).

In considering section-score–performance test comparisons for the remaining small sections of the Hearing Measurement Scale a somewhat different statistical approach is required. Given the varied content, scoring range, and types of scored value between the different tests, a uniform approach that does least violence to the data is nonparametric one-way analysis of variance. This is also the best way of handling the narrow range of scores on Sections 2, 5, 6, and 7 (see Table 9.2). By assigning ranked performance test values to different columns representing different scores on a given section, we can estimate the significance of the variance between performance and scale section scores using the Kruskal-Wallis test (Siegel, 1956). The probability levels associated with values of H, the statistic computed, are given in Table 10.7. Of course, quite a lot of information is lost in this approach, but the essential feature, namely the patterns of relationship, is still quite visible, and there is an improvement in uniformity within and between comparisons by this type of reduction.

The result is partly in line with expectation. There appears to be no relationship between test performance and Section 6 (tinnitus) scores, nor would any particular effects be anticipated. Section 2 (hearing for nonspeech sound) scores relate fairly consistently with tonal threshold but only in the 2 to 6 kHz range. This may be partly a function of a restricted range effect, or it could be that Section 2 scores are reflections of Section 1 scores. But it may also genuinely characterize the problem of detection of nonspeech sound in these particular listeners. Lack of higher frequency sensitivity may be sufficient at times to produce what in the final event is only a negligible detection problem for these men. Chances are high that any sound with a lower frequency component will always be noticed so that no association between lower frequency threshold and this aspect of the hearing repertoire emerges. I stress that this result is undoubtedly peculiar to these particular listeners, but it is important to note that if the result is not flawed or confounded (and there is no reason to suppose it is) then in this sample of people with noise disorder, .5 and 1 kHz threshold is irrelevant even to the detection problems they face in everyday life.

Section 5 (speech distortion) scores tend to relate to SRT for continuous discourse and to discrimination score (Tests 3 and 4), as would be

TABLE 10.7

Probability Levels ($p \leq$ the Value Shown) Associated with Values of H (Kruskal-Wallis One-Way Analysis of Variance) Derived from Comparison of Scores on Section 2 (Nonspeech Hearing), Section 5 (Speech Distortion), Section 6 (Tinnitus), Section 7 (Personal Opinion), and All Performance Tests[a]

Test		2	5	6	7
1 (L)	.5 kHz	.70	.20	.30	.80
	1 kHz	.50	.30	.90	.70
	2 kHz	.05	.20	.70	.02
	3 kHz	.02	.10	.70	.05
	4 kHz	.01	.10	.80	.02
	6 kHz	.01	.30	.50	.01
1 (R)	.5 kHz	.80	.20	.20	.70
	1 kHz	.50	.50	.50	.70
	2 kHz	.01	.20	.50	.20
	3 kHz	.05	.20	.30	.01
	4 kHz	.05	.30	.30	.50
	6 kHz	.20	.50	.10	.10
2 (L)		.02	.70	.30	.20
2 (R)		.02	.70	.70	.80
3 (L)		.10	.05	.50	.05
3 (R)		.05	.02	.20	.05
4 (R)		.01	.05	.50	.10
Binaural free-field tests					
5		.20	.50	.50	.05
6		.50	.90	.90	.20
7		.99	.80	.95	.50
8		.90	.90	.70	.95
9	5 dB SL	.70	.30	.90	.30
	10 dB SL	.20	.70	.70	.80
	15 dB SL	.95	.20	.10	.70
	20 dB SL	.55	.30	.30	.50
	30 dB SL	.70	.90	.50	.99
	40 dB SL	.50	.20	.05	.50

[a] See Tables 10.3 and 10.4 for key to tests.

anticipated. No other association is apparent. Finally, Section 7 score (personal opinion) tends to relate to various performance functions, though to none consistently. This suggests that personal opinion relies on a different sort of consciousness from that of self-reported experience, a point noted in Chapter 9. A not uncommon outcome of interviewing was for respondents to be themselves surprised at the extent (in terms of breadth rather than degree) of experienced difficulty in hearing when specific situations were pinpointed in each question. I have more to say on this issue in Chapter 11. It seems to be the case that when one is asked to produce an overall appraisal of one's hearing ability rather than assess difficulty in specific situations, whatever is important in one's consciousness at that moment guides the response rather than some accumulated, broad-spectrum synthesis of experience.

All in all, the interrelations between performance and self-report emerging from this study are medium level, insufficiently close to allow reasonable prediction yet fairly logically patterned. This suggests that the self-report method is sensitive to dimensions of auditory function also measured by mechanical procedures, but of course it is also sensitive to slices of reality to which the mechanical test cannot be. An excellent instance of this kind of additional sensitivity has been discussed by Noble (1974, 1975b) and is presented in the next chapter.

Subsequent Comparative Research

Study by Atherley and Noble

In the study by Atherley and Noble (1971), 18 drop-forge operators were interviewed with the Hearing Measurement Scale, and also underwent a self-recording tonal threshold test. The main feature of that report was a discussion of the inconsistency within individuals between self-report and tonal threshold level. A minor feature worth citing here was correlation of each section score with various tonal threshold averages. It is surprising that the .5 to 2 kHz average correlated with Section 1 score (speech hearing) at $r = .506$, whereas averages that included frequencies beyond 2 kHz showed slightly lower correlation levels. This result is contrary to the one from the original test group. None of the correlations in the follow-up study reached the .01 level of probability, which could mean that the variation in pattern of threshold–Section 1 score relationship is simply a result of sampling error. Nonetheless it suggests that the precise nature of association between Section 1 score and test performance is yet to be satisfactorily determined.

Higher and significant coefficients of correlation were calculated between Section 2 score (hearing for nonspeech sound) and threshold averages at .5 to 2 kHz ($r = .643$) and .5 to 3 kHz ($r = .583$). This result is partly in accord with the original findings. Section 3 scores (localization) correlated at a similar level as Section 2 scores with .5 to 2 kHz threshold and with .5 to 4 kHz threshold average. This result is again somewhat in accord with the original finding. Section 4 scores (emotional response) showed fairly consistent ($r = .502$ to $.559$) but nonsignificant correlation with all threshold averages. This outcome suggests that the close link between Section 1 and Section 4 is once again operative. Section 1 scores correlated nonsignificantly with threshold. Section 5 (speech distortion) scores correlated significantly with averages across .5 to 3 kHz, .5

to 4 kHz, and .5 to 6 kHz and with increasing levels of association as more high frequencies were included in the tonal average. This result entirely conforms with the earlier outcome.

Similarly with the remaining sections, those on tinnitus and personal opinion. The tinnitus section showed a complete absence of relation with any threshold average, and the personal opinion section showed variable association, none significant, with different averages—the highest correlation being .539 with average at .5 to 6 kHz.

The result of this follow-up study tends therefore to confirm previous findings with the exception of Section 1 scores. Further investigation is obviously required to clarify that aspect of the questionnaire in relation to tested function.

Study by McCartney et al. (1976)

A report by McCartney, Maurer, and Sorenson (1976) is illuminating in several ways. These authors applied the Hearing Measurement Scale as an interview to 36 people aged 60 to 89 years. This feature of their work allows one to gauge the viability of the instrument in a sample of people different from those among whom it was developed. A comparative study was also made of the Hearing Measurement and Hearing Handicap scales, so one is able to observe the relative performance of each device. Finally, various standard mechanical tests were administered to the group of listeners, so once again the relations between self-report and functional performance can be analyzed.

COMPARISON ACROSS SAMPLES

In regard to the first feature, Table 10.8 shows comparison of data (rounded to the nearest whole number) adapted from Table 9.2 in this book and selected data from the McCartney et al. (1976) report. Also shown are data from Noble (1969) obtained in 23 people with predominantly sensorineural disorders of hearing attending an audiology clinic. These people were selected to be as comparable as possible with occupational groups, hence their ages range from 42 to 66 years (average, 59).

It is evident from Table 10.8 that the two sets of data from Noble (1969) bracket that of McCartney et al. and that the varying patterns of response, while reflecting the different average degrees of difficulty between the groups, are nonetheless relatively similar across sections of the Hearing Measurement Scale. There are some anomalies even so. The occupational group shows a wider range of response than the older people in the McCartney et al. sample, but clearly the distribution of results is more skewed than the distribution in the older group toward the negative end of the scoring range. In part, these effects reflect the age range of the occupational group (29 to 67 years) and in part the highly variable amounts of noise to which different subgroups were typically

TABLE 10.8

Comparison of Total Scale and Section Scores on the Hearing Measurement Scale Observed by Noble (1969) and by McCartney et al. (1976)

	Total score	Section						
		1	2	3	4	5	6	7
Means								
Noble[a]	33	13	2	5	8	3	1	2
McCartney et al.[b]	70	29	6	9	13	6	1	5
Noble[c]	79	36	9	7	16	5	2	5
Ranges								
Noble[a]	0–127	0–52	0–15	0–24	0–39	0–12	0–14	0–9
McCartney et al.[b]	19–103	3–46	1–17	2–18	3–25	2–13	0–6	0–11
Noble[c]	40–138	17–64	0–23	0–18	4–29	0–20	0–8	0–13

[a] Seventy-three occupationally noise-exposed foundry workers.
[b] Thirty-six older people from the general low-income population.
[c] Twenty-three people attending an audiology clinic.

exposed. Men working in the moulding shops of small foundries would experience only a few noisy episodes in the normal working day; men working in the grinding and fettling departments of larger foundries would be continually exposed to very high noise levels.

It is also interesting to note that while the audiology clinic sample shows an average higher response to speech hearing (Section 1) and nonspeech detection (Section 2) than the older sample of McCartney et al., the opposite occurs in the case of localization and speech distortion (Sections 3 and 5). I interpret the latter reversal as a result of the different types of people making up the two samples. In the McCartney et al. group, discrimination problems were considerable in the majority of listeners, whereas in the clinic sample, discrimination difficulty was not necessarily the motivating influence to attend the clinic. Rather, dysfunctions like tinnitus and sheer loss of sensitivity were what brought most of these people to seek help. The diagnosis of sensorineural disorder was also marginal in some cases, for it is uncommon to find this as a pure disorder in people in the general non-noise-exposed population of that particular age. More typically it is in younger people and people of advanced age that a sensorineural disorder is the only problem.

With regard to the greater average spatial location problem in the older group in comparison with the clinic group, my earlier contention about a possible link between localization and discrimination difficulty may be invoked. If there is indeed a common underlying cause for these two functional disturbances, then it might be anticipated that increased discrimination difficulty would be associated with increased localization problems. Such a trend is not apparent within the occupational group (see Table 10.6), except insofar as spatial location and higher frequency threshold show some relationship, but it is observable *between* the occupational and clinic groups. Whereas mean speech hearing and nonspeech hearing scores in these two groups are 13 and 36 and 2 and 9, respectively, mean localization and speech distortion scores are 5 and 7 and 3 and 5, respectively. And whereas the maximum scores in the clinic sample, in the speech hearing and nonspeech hearing sections, exceed the occupational group's maximums, the contrary is the case, at least as far as spatial location is concerned. One should not push these results too far. It is a sufficient conclusion that data are not inconsistent with the earlier contention.

A final point to note is that the maximum Section 4 (emotional response) score in the occupational group exceeds the maximums in both the clinic and older-people samples. Three men in the occupational group had Section 4 scores above the clinic maximum. They turn out also to be the people who had the highest, second highest, and fourth highest total scores of the 73 men interviewed in that group. The total scores of all three exceeded the maximum total score (of 103) observed in the McCartney *et al.* group of older respondents. This can therefore explain the excess of their Section 4 scores over the Section 4 maximum score in the older group. However, the excess over the clinic group's Section 4 maximum cannot be explained in this way because all three of the occupational group respondents necessarily had total scale scores below the clinic maximum (of 138). The result from the occupational sample vis-à-vis the clinic sample suggests a real difference in extremity of emotional response between people in the two samples. Scrutiny of personal data regarding the high scorers from both occupational and clinic groups on this section of the questionnaire reveals no consistent factor, such as age, that might point the way to accounting for these findings.

One is left, on the basis of available data, with no solid basis for explanation. I can only speculate that men from a group of similarly noise-exposed peers who show an extreme effect on self-reported hearing difficulty—recall that the high scorers on Section 4 were high totalscale scorers—are witness to their greater plight in contrast to the majority of their colleagues, and knowing themselves to be so much worse off, they experience greater emotional disturbance as a result. The person attending a clinic but not of an age to be surrounded by peers with similar problems has not the same social signals that he or she is worse off than others suffering a similar disorder. Such people know they have difficulty in relation to the rest of their society, but they do not necessarily know that they are faring *so* poorly. They lack the constant comparison available to a person working alongside others exposed to the same damaging agent.

A supportive datum for this speculation lies in the fact that the high Section 4 scorers among the clinic sample were not necessarily the high total-scale scorers in that sample. The Section 4 and total scale scores plus the ranks of the total scale scores of the 5 highest Section 4 scorers from both the occupational and clinic groups are shown in Table 10.9 to illustrate this point. The 5 highest Section 4 scorers in the occupational sample are within the 7 highest total-scale scorers of the 73 persons in that group. By contrast, the rank positions of total-scale scores of the 5 highest Section 4 scorers in the clinic group are somewhat more dispersed throughout the range of total scale scores within that group ($N = 23$). This illustration is in a sense a more vivid way of saying that the correlation between Section 4 and total-scale scores in the clinic sample is probably lower than it is in the occupational sample. That turns out to be the case: $r_s = .624$ between Section 4 and total scale scores in the clinic sample as against .852 in the occupational sample.

If this speculation, with its item of supportive or at least suggestive evidence, can hold any weight, then it runs contrary to an hypothesis produced in Chapter 1 of this work. There it is stated that the handicap experienced by a person suffering occupational hearing disorder induced by noise may be less than the handicap experienced by one who suffers a hearing disorder in more "isolated" social circumstances (isolated in the sense of not necessarily being among others who have the same problem). This result, however, shows that the emotional disturbance felt by some people in the former situation may exceed that of people with equivalent or greater hearing difficulty in the latter situation.

We can substantiate this point by reference to the Section 4 scores of all possible pairs of people from both occupational and clinic groups who

TABLE 10.9

Scores on Section 4 (Emotional Response) of the Five Highest Scorers on That Section from the Occupational ($N = 73$) and Clinic ($N = 23$) Samples. Also Shown Are the Total Scale Scores and the Rank Position of These Total Scores (in Italics) of Each Group of Five Highest Section 4 Scorers

Section 4 score		Total scale score and rank position (r)	
Occupational sample	Clinic sample	Occupational sample	Clinic sample
39	29	127 *1*	138 *1*
36	28	124 *2*	118 *3*
32	25	113 *4*	70 *13*
27	25	75 *7*	71 *12*
25	24	95 *6*	110 *4*

can be matched on total scale scores. In Table 10.10, it is clearly shown that the Section 4 scores of the occupational group are fairly consistently higher than those of the clinic group. In other words, despite the *average* lower Section 4 scores of the occupational group (see Table 10.8), those with total scores in the clinic sample range show consistently higher Section 4 scores than matched respondents from the clinic sample. The reason for this more pronounced effect is unknown at the present time. My speculation about the fact of being able to compare oneself with others from a similar background and hence feel worse off in knowing that one *is* worse off (!), might hold a clue to explanation.

With this one presently inexplicable exception, results show that the Hearing Measurement Scale seems to provide a fairly consistent assessment across different samples of people. Where there are anomalies, results suggest that the scale may be exhibiting a sensitivity to consistent variations in the nature of hearing disturbance between people with different kinds of disorder. A more deliberate study would be required to substantiate this claim, but it is one that the author feels fairly confident in making. The Hearing Measurement Scale is obviously a sensitive instrument, as shown by the differential scores observed in different occupational groups (see Chapter 9, page 257). Its sensitivity to minor effects such as lip-reading skill will be demonstrated in Chapter 11. Given this sensitivity, it is not surprising that variations in hearing disturbance associated with even minor variations in type of disorder

TABLE 10.10

Pairs of Respondents from Occupational and Clinic Groups, Matched on Total Scale Scores, Showing the Generally Higher Section 4 (Emotional Response) Scores of the Former Compared with the Latter

	Total scores		Section 4 scores	
Pair	Occupational sample	Clinic sample	Occupational sample	Clinic sample
1	41	40	13	6
2	47	47	17	4
3	48	48	16	8
4	51	53	16	20
5	58	59	7	10
6	66	65	16	6
7	67	68	19	11
8	75	75	27	5
9	107	100	21	22
10	113	118	32	28
11	127	129	39	15
Means	72.7	72.9	20.3	12.3

should be revealed in the pattern of its measurement. Just as interesting, and equally important, is that the *context* of a disturbance, its social location and meaning, the factors identified in Chapter 1 as bearing upon experienced hearing handicap appear from the foregoing analysis to be detectable by the Hearing Measurement Scale.

COMPARISON ACROSS SCALES AND TESTS

Three performance measures were used in the McCartney *et al.* (1976) study: .5 to 2 kHz tonal threshold, SRT, and discrimination score for Campbell's (1965) W-22 half-lists. Discrimination was tested at the listener's comfortable listening level. In a prepublication draft (McCartney, personal communication), results were presented separately for both "better" and "poorer" ears—.5 to 2 kHz threshold average being the criterion. Correlations were made with Hearing Handicap and Hearing Measurement scale scores on a "better"–"poorer" ear basis. Table 10.11, adapted from McCartney *et al.* and from McCartney (personal communication), shows the correlation coefficients obtained between the two scales and between each scale and the various mechanical tests.

"Better" ear tonal threshold shows a fairly clear association with self-report, whereas "poorer" ear results on that test are barely related. SRT in either ear is at about the same low level of association with self-report. Discrimination score shows a pattern similar to tonal threshold but at lower correlation levels. The features of present interest are that results from both scales covary in their relations with performance and that this reflects their own significant interrelation. The Hearing Handicap Scale shows a closer degree of association with performance than the Hearing Measurement Scale, as would be anticipated from previous results and

TABLE 10.11

Correlations between Hearing Measurement Scale (HMS) and Hearing Handicap Scale (HHS) Scores and between Each and Various Performance Tests in 36 Older People[a]

	Test			
	.5 to 2 kHz tonal average	SRT	DS	HMS–HHS
"Better" ear				
HMS	.52*	.35	−.40	.67*
HHS	.62*	.40	−.44**	
"Poorer" ear				
HMS	.26	.25	−.20	
HHS	.36	.39	−.30	

* $p < .001$.
** $p < .01$.

[a] Adapted from McCartney *et al.*, 1976, and from McCartney (personal communication).

discussion about their respective content. The outcome shows that there are features of content common to the two scales, responsive to the same dimensions as functional tests. And the pattern of data suggests that the most significant feature common to both scales and performance is threshold sensitivity. This in turn suggests that discrimination score is not so vital in this kind of sample as a guide to everyday hearing difficulty, despite the fact that measured discrimination was a major problem for these people.

That result is at odds with that observed by Noble and Atherley (1970), in which discrimination figured to the same extent as SRT and both to a somewhat greater extent than tonal threshold in the noise-exposed group. The only potential source of explanation lies in the considerable difference in tonal threshold in the .5 to 2 kHz range between the above two groups. Listeners in the McCartney *et al.* study showed much higher average threshold levels in that range than those observed by Noble and Atherley. One is not arguing here for a restricted range effect. Noble and Atherley (1970) observed as wide, if not wider, a range of results but at a lower average level, than that observed by McCartney *et al.* It may be that threshold sensitivity in that audio-frequency range starts to become more important with regard to everyday hearing difficulty when levels approach those observed by McCartney *et al.* This cannot be taken as altogether satisfactory in explanation of these authors' result, because one would expect a concomitant relation between self-report and SRT if .5 to 2 kHz tonal threshold were the *causal* agent of difficulty (see Chapter 6). Intermediate influences must surely be at work, especially in view of the considerable discrimination impairment observed.

The explanation that suggests itself has to do with the SRT measurement. Noble (1969) observed that the discrimination problem in some men with occupational noise disorder was sufficiently gross to make measurement of SRT almost impossible. If an entire sample manifests this same problem, then perhaps SRT becomes merely a different way of assessing discrimination.

Until more extensive research into these kinds of samples is undertaken, no certain conclusions can be drawn regarding the interrelation between self-report and tested performance.

Study by Ward and Tudor

As mentioned in Chapter 2, a recent development within audiology is the attention being paid to rehabilitation in older people who acquire increasing partial deafness with advancing age. In the Netherlands and Scandinavia, programs designed with particular reference to this group have been under way for a number of years. Indeed, Ewertsen and Birk-Nielsen's (1973) questionnaire was produced within this sort of rehabilitation context.

A similar interest has quite rapidly surfaced recently in the United Kingdom and the United States. This has been brought especially to the present author's notice because of the increased amount of inquiry about the Hearing Measurement Scale in the past 2 years from research groups in these two countries whose particular concern is with older people and the rehabilitation procedures applicable in that population.

At the time of writing, preliminary results using the Hearing Measurement Scale are available from the work of Ward and Tudor (1976) at Exeter, England. Their concern has been to compare the pre- and post-treatment responses on the questionnaire and on speech tests of matched groups of older people participating in different kinds of training and rehabilitation procedures. It was the conclusion of these researchers, after reviewing available questionnaires, that the Hearing Measurement Scale was sufficiently all encompassing in its content, and particularly as regards emotional response to hearing difficulty, to commend its use in a program designed to improve both coping and listening skills. From the small amount of data available at present, it appears that following group and individual training sessions in the most effective use of a hearing aid substantial upward changes are observable in discrimination score (using the hearing aid) and that these changes are accompanied by equally substantial downward changes in scores on the speech sections (1 and 5) and emotional response section (4) of the Hearing Measurement Scale.

These results by themselves cannot be taken as meaningful. It will require results comparing different procedural treatment groups to find out whether consistent patterns of change emerge from this sort of application of the scale. But the result of telling significance is that as speech processing becomes easier (evidenced by both self-report and performance) emotional disturbance is reduced. This finding bears out the corollary observation that whenever a more than slight speech hearing problem exists an emotional disturbance is also observed. The result is promising, in more general terms, since it shows that a device like the Hearing Measurement Scale may find specialist application in people in whom it is often difficult to gauge by performance testing whether meliorative changes have indeed occurred.

Study by MacRae and Brigden

As part of the research study undertaken at the Australian National Acoustic Laboratories to find the tonal threshold averaging system that most effectively assessed everyday hearing handicap, MacRae and Brigden applied various questionnaires and performance tests to a large group of veterans. The aspect of this study that has publicly emerged is reported in MacRae and Brigden (1973) and discussed in Chapter 6. The performance test–questionnaire interrelations have not been and probably will not be published by these researchers, but the present author has been granted permission to present the results of that study in this work. While detailed results were not made available, for reasons of confidentiality of respondent's data, total scale scores and certain tonal threshold and speech test values were made available at the laboratory for transcription. The features of interest in these results are comparison once again of Hearing Measurement and Hearing Handicap scales, this time in a sample with noise-induced disorder, and comparison between each scale and various performance tests. Two additional features of considerable interest are (a) the relation between scale scores and the CID everyday sentence list scores in quiet and competing noise; and (b) comparison of scale scores with articulation index values calculated in the manner described in Chapter 6, Section III.F. The CID sentences have the most promising content as regards validity for assessment of everyday speech hearing ability, but they have not previously been subject to comparison against self-report measures.

Certain constraints attend analysis of MacRae and Brigden's data. As is mentioned in Chapter 6, these authors' (1973) results exhibit a fairly pronounced extremity effect, a large proportion of data points lying at the minimum and maximum ends of all the scaled measurements. This effect tends to provide very high correlational outcomes whose generalizability is uncertain. Restriction-of-range effects are so severe with regard to some performance test outcomes that correlation analysis is not worthwhile. A further constraint is that not all participants in the study were tested with each questionnaire, this being a somewhat secondary aspect of the whole program. Results from 99 of the 160 people involved in this aspect of the research can be used, however, as each of these was tested with both questionnaires and on all performance tests of present concern.

The resulting analyses are presented in Table 10.12. The strikingly high correlations, both between the scales and between each scale and the performance tests should not be relied upon too heavily for reasons mentioned above. The pattern of relationship within either scale–performance test data set is of prime interest as are the comparative outcomes for each scale.

It is evident that the articulation index provides the most powerful guide, based on tonal threshold, to everyday hearing difficulty in this sample of noise-deafened listeners. Furthermore, as compared with SRT, the everyday sentences are not so closely linked with everyday problems. The Hearing Handicap Scale is almost solely concerned with everyday speech hearing, and the fact that the differential outcome for SRT, as opposed to sentences, is maintained in that relational pattern strongly supports a conclusion that the effect is not caused simply by a confounding of scale score by nonspeech hearing content. Nor should one overlook the predictive power of .5 to 2 kHz tonal threshold in this

TABLE 10.12

Correlations between Hearing Measurement Scale (HMS) and Hearing Handicap Scale (HHS) Scores and between Each Scale and Various Performance Measures in the "Better" Ears of Listeners Tested by MacRae and Brigden at the Australian National Acoustic Laboratories ($N = 99$)

Test	HMS	rHHS, HMS .91	HHS
SRT	.846		.795
AI_{60}[a]	−.899		−.863
.5–2 kHz[b]	.880		.844
$CID_{60(Q)}$[c]	−.768		−.691
$CID_{60(N)}$[d]	−.762		−.735

[a] Articulation index for speech at 60 dB(A).
[b] "Better"-ear threshold average at .5 to 2 kHz ("better" ear = lower level at threshold at each tested frequency).
[c] CID everyday sentence list at 60 dB(A) in quiet listening.
[d] CID everyday sentence list at 60 dB(A) in background noise listening.

sample. That outcome is surprising, quite at odds with the result of Noble and Atherley (1970), but more akin to the (rather less reliable) result of Atherley and Noble (1971).

One should comment here on the use of "better" ear, for it might be assumed that use of this measure is the key to the difference in different studies. Noble (1967), however, correlated scores on the prototype questionnaire (Noble, 1968) with "both-ear" average thresholds at .5 to 6 kHz, .5 to 2 kHz, and 1 to 3 kHz in 32 men with various degrees of occupational noise disorder. Correlation was also made with "better" ears, "better" being defined in exactly the same way as MacRae and Brigden define it. In no case did the correlation differ significantly, nor was there a consistent change from use of the "better" ear rather than the "both-ear" average. Correlations in general were in the .37 to .48 range, the lowest value in fact being between scale score and "better" ear .5 to 2 kHz average. This result suggested that in the sample studied the "better"-ear approach was not fruitful. All the results considered so far, in fact, provide a confused picture of the .5 to 2 kHz–self-report interrelationship in people with noise-induced hearing disorder. Results are more consistent, however, as regards the role of frequencies higher than 2 kHz.

The other surprising outcome from analysis of MacRae and Brigden's study is the consistently closer association of performance with the Hearing Measurement Scale score than with the Hearing Handicap Scale score. This outcome is at odds with that of McCartney et al. (1976) though results are from different types of samples. Further study is obviously required and more detailed profiles of self-report, to unearth possible explanations for this outcome.

Overall, the data of MacRae and Brigden raise more questions than they answer, the only outcomes which conform at all with previous study in similar groups being the ascendant role of SRT and of the articulation index (hence of higher frequency threshold) in prediction of self-reported everyday hearing ability. The questions that remain with respect to the true role of .5 to 2 kHz threshold and of the CID everyday sentences clearly warrant further and detailed study, given the critical importance, actually and potentially, of both of these measures.

11

Advantages, Disadvantages, and Applications of Self-Report

ADVANTAGES OF SELF-REPORT

Theoretical

The three main theoretical advantages of self-report are that it can be a representative, meaningful, and nonassumptive method of hearing assessment. For it to gain these theoretical advantages over current mechanical testing, considerable developmental effort is required in the construction and scaling of a self-report inventory. The Hearing Measurement Scale is the only published instrument to date that emerged from this kind of detailed inquiry and development. That scale is by no means a full and final assessment tool in regard to hearing loss and handicap in the day-to-day world. There is ample scope for further developments, perhaps even radical changes not only to its format and content but by extension to the general field of self-reported hearing ability as well. I cannot at this stage conceive the ways in which change will occur, but I have no doubts that it will occur if audiology itself is to continue as a developing science.

As things stand at present, the representative quality of self-report is given in the Hearing Measurement Scale by the inclusion of items regarding aspects of everyday hearing experience and problems of impairment that partially deaf people themselves have identified in unstructured interviews. The distribution of items of different types and the different weights applying to scaled responses reflect the relative importance of various situations and problems for people who have difficulty in hearing. By contrast, the representativeness of a mechanical test springs from the theoretical orientation of the people devising that test, and the representativeness of assessment systems likewise expresses only what the systems' makers consider to be important qualities of hearing.

Meaningfulness is quite obviously attainable in self-report by ensuring that items really do refer to situations relevant and meaningful to the people being questioned. In this connection, of course, and in regard to representativeness, we have seen that some early efforts to devise self-report devices subverted these qualities so that the content of inventories merely reiterated the supposed content of mechanical tests. The questionnaire of Schein *et al.* (1970) is a good example of an instrument whose meaningfulness in the respondent's world is fairly low, whose content is obviously structured to ape the tonal threshold test.

But given a concern on the part of researchers to devise a scale that is not at odds with the "meaning world" of the people to be assessed, a great theoretical advantage is gained over tests whose meaning is obscure. Meaningfulness connotes the use of items that refer to recognizable and critical features of hearing in the world. A question such as one contained in the Hearing Measurement Scale referring to the respondent's pet domestic animal may appear slightly ludicrous and even trivial, but the unavoidable fact of the matter is that loss of audible contact with a domestic pet was a source of distress to those who experienced it. To ignore this fact would be to impose one's own terms of reference on what are and are not relevant and critical experiences for the partially deaf adult. Inclusion of such an item is not to provide a "Walt Disney" touch of sentimentality to the scale's content but simply to reflect what was observed in people's responses when questioned generally about their problems and their reactions to such problems.

This point relates to the quality of nonassumption that can be gained by careful use of the self-report method. There are two principal features of a nonassumptive framework in this connection, one in regard to meaning and relevance, the other in regard to scaling of responses. The second feature is also tied in with the interview style, about which more is said in the next section.

The first component of nonassumption lies in the putting of questions themselves. An assumptive approach would take it that the situations embodied in different questions are uniformly relevant to different people. Such an approach would further presume that the balance of items fairly represented the personal world of each respondent. Giolas (1970) has pointed out the error of such assumptions using the same sort of reason as given earlier here, namely, that different people engage in quite different activities. Communication is a vital feature of some people's lives; listening is the vital feature for others. Being able to detect various naturally occurring sounds is a source of pleasure and importance to some people; for others, extraneous sound is a source of distraction. A nonassumptive approach to an interview allows the definition of the person's daily existence to be filled out by that person. Items embodying situations in which a given person finds difficulty may at the same time not necessarily describe critical or typical circumstances for that person.

Negotiation over the meaning and relevance of a situation necessarily bears upon the particular scale score to be attached to the person's response. A nonassumptive approach to scoring shows quite free negotiation between interviewer and respondent over the degree of difficulty experienced by the respondent expressed in language preferred by the latter. A respondent might report that he always has trouble following group conversation outside the house but that he rarely encounters that circumstance because it is not a typical or important feature of his life. If it is established that such a circumstance has never figured prominently in that person's life and that nonexposure to that situation is not therefore the result of increasing difficulty within it, then scaling of response to that item must partly reflect the irrelevance of the situation to the respondent. What is more important, interviewer and respondent must agree that the negotiated scale point fairly reflects the degree of handicap the respondent feels and has expressed as a result of the difficulty within the given situation.

To be sure, such protracted conversation is only required now and again in a series of interviews. Because the great majority of items have a common meaning and relevance for the majority of respondents, most interviews using the Hearing Measurement Scale take about 10 to 15 minutes. But the exceptional cases need to be catered to, and in these circumstances interviews can last up to 30 to 60 minutes as the respondent with an unusual lifestyle negotiates with the interviewer the exact meaning for him or her of the circumstances mentioned in various items. But a nonassumptive framework of this kind pays off because both the interviewer and the person being interviewed come away from the encounter satisfied that a fair appraisal has been made of the hearing problems for that person, in that person's everyday world. This feature of interview is one that could be easily lost in a paper-and-pencil test.

The mechanical test, of course, has unmodifiable built-in assumptions about the lifestyle of the person being tested. With regard to speech tests, this framework is highly intrusive. Noble (1975b) pointed out that in the typical test of discrimination the assumption being made is that the dialect of the listener matches that of the speaker and assessor. It is well known that different dialects function using quite different phonemic clusters (Adler, 1972; Goodman, 1969; Willis, 1972). One cannot assume, therefore, when faced with a listener whose basilect (or natural dialect) is the one he uses more often and more readily than his acrolect (the dialectal form that approximates the standard form of the language in question), that the standard language discrimination test is any more valid for that person than it would be for someone who speaks a completely different language.

In self-reported assessment, the effect of dialect would be reflected straightforwardly in the degree of difficulty reported during the interview. Other intervening variables, such as lip-reading skill, are also reflected in degree of self-reported difficulty. This feature relates more to the practical advantage of self-report and is elaborated upon under that heading.

In sum, then, the theoretical advantages of self-report over currently used mechanical tests are considerable, provided the former type of scheme is constructed with an eye to these theoretical features. Nor would it be impossible, as I indicate earlier, to construct tests of function that also take account of these theoretical features. The time may come, then, when tests are sufficiently flexible and sophisticated to offer a truer guide to a person's hearing capability.

Practical

The most obvious practical advantage of interviewing is that no special equipment or elaborately controlled environment is needed to obtain the information being sought. Armed with questionnaire and tape recorder or with a blank inventory to be completed by the respondent, a researcher can gain a great deal of data in a short time. The utility of the test is very high. There is also a factor aiding this ease of administration. Among people with noise-induced disorder, functional tests must be conducted at least 12 hours, and preferably 36 hours, after the last noise exposure to avoid the variable effects of temporary threshold shift. An interview can be conducted at any time, however, because the circumstances being elicited are unrelated to a particular state of hearing that the person manifests at the time. In industrial surveys, typically very complex exercises to mount using traditional tests, the self-report aspect can be carried out with comparative ease, often in the person's own home at a time convenient to that person, and generally in a nonalien fashion.

Perhaps the most interesting kind of practical advantage shown in results using the Hearing Measurement Scale is the automatic way in which compensatory mechanisms are accounted for in the response profile. It has been shown by Sanders and Goodrich (1971) that lipreading is an involuntary compensating mechanism adopted even by hearing listeners in difficult listening conditions. A purely auditory test of hearing ability cannot take account of this compensatory skill. And given that visual acuity influences lip-reading skill, as Hardick, Oyer, and Irion (1970) showed, one can assume neither that its compensatory value will be constant across persons with similar hearing difficulty nor that its influence will automatically increase with increasing deafness. In point of fact, very few people who present themselves at audiology clinics are able to lip-read and one might even speculate that these may contain a self-selected group from the partially hearing population who for one reason or another have been unable to optimize use of this information source.

Noble (1974, 1975b, c) has pointed to a further variable that seems to affect critically the reliance on and use of lip-reading, namely, type of occupation. It has long been known that weavers have a particular aptitude at this skill. Kell *et al.* (1971) reported that 53% of the jute weavers in their sample relied upon lip-reading, and I have never encountered a weaver who did not have this ability to some extent. Barr (1884) makes the curious observation that women have a particular aptitude for lip reading, but I am not aware that this notion has ever been substantiated. It happens, however, that the industrial weaving trade is carried on mainly by women. I would speculate that Barr's observation may have sprung from the fact that in his day moustaches and beards were fashionable and of a kind that often partly concealed the male mouth. Barr himself, as is remarked and shown in Chapter 2, both sported this style and pointed out the difficulty it produces for partially deaf people. His observation about women's aptitude could thus be mistaken; it might rather have been that Victorian men had less labial and laryngeal information to go on.

Be that as it may, weavers report far greater reliance on lip-reading than either typical audiology clinic patients or even people from different yet equally noisy occupational backgrounds. Only 25% of the foundrymen I studied reported an ability to lipread. I have suggested that the nature of the working environment forces weavers to learn this skill in order to communicate with one another during working hours. Noise in a weaving shed is continuous; and the task, which is primarily that of repairing broken threads and restarting the machines, requires constant vigilance in a given spatial area, a performance that largely prevents face-to-face contact with other workers. One can therefore witness-lip reading in use across considerable distances among people working in weaving sheds.

By contrast, men in foundries by and large produce their own noise discontinuously when they themselves are working on a casting to trim it of spare metal using a pneumatic chisel or grinding the trimmed surface using an abrasive wheel. In addition, while they are working, they cannot attend to anything but the task before them. Furthermore, because of sparks and dust, goggles must be worn and sometimes face masks. All these features combine, first of all to *allow auditory* communication between bursts of noisy working activity and second, to *prevent visual* communication during noisy episodes. These constraints thus militate against acquisition of lip-reading skill, whereas the different occupational constraints in weaving positively demand its acquisition.

Now, the feature of interest is that these differences reveal themselves to some extent in the response patterns of the two groups to the Hearing Measurement Scale. In Table 11.1, mean scores are given on selected sections of the scale of three groups: 23 people attending at an audiology

TABLE 11.1

Mean Scores on the Speech Hearing Sections (1 and 5) and the Nonspeech Hearing Section (2) of the Hearing Measurement Scale of Three Groups of Respondents

Group	Section			N
	1	5	2	
Clinic sample	35.7	5.1	8.7	23
Foundrymen	19.4	4.2	1.9	14
Weavers	10.9	2.1	3.7	12

clinic, 14 grinders and trimmers from a foundry, and 12 weavers. It can be seen first of all that as one would expect the clinic sample shows very high scores on Section 1 (speech hearing) and Section 2 (nonspeech detection). The weavers' average score on Section 2 is twice as high as the average for the foundrymen but virtually half that of the foundrymen on Sections 1 and 5.

This outcome is taken from two heterogeneous groups showing widely and differently distributed scores, so not too much weight can be put on the result. However, it conforms with a similar comparison reported by Noble (1974) between the same group of weavers, a different group of foundrymen, and a group of drop-forge operators whose occupational circumstance is similar to that of the foundry workers.

The practical value of self-reported assessment is that it permits the variable influence of compensatory skill to mediate the response that a person will provide. A test that assesses only auditory function overlooks this sort of intermediate variable and thus does not truly reflect the difficulty experienced in everyday circumstances.

DISADVANTAGES OF SELF-REPORT

Theoretical

Among the theoretical disadvantages of self-report, probably the two most critical are variability in verbalizing phenomenal experience and change in cultural climate. Indeed, it could be said that the strengths of self-report are also its weaknesses. In gaining first-hand knowledge from the person about life experience, one is also buying into the troubled area of meaning and the translation of feeling into terms that may or may not precisely match that feeling and may or may not match across people, including the important dyad comprising respondent and interviewer. Similarly, in seeking to make the content of a self-report scale representative and relevant to the everyday world, one necessarily produces a scale with a quite closely defined spatiotemporal locus.

We take the second aspect first. Given that cultures vary both within and among themselves in time and space, the original location of a scale in that framework may become more and more part of the hinterland of a given culture. The situations referred to may become literally old-fashioned or, if not that, may alter in relevance and hence in meaning with passage of time in one culture or with transduction to other cultures. Two examples illustrate this point with regard to the Hearing Measurement Scale. First, there is the absence of reference to telephone use which occurred just because in the population in which the scale was developed telephones *at that time* (the mid 1960s) were a comparative rarity. The lifestyle of that same population has probably changed enough in 10 years to make the telephone a more common cultural item. As another instance, there is no reference in the scale to communication or listening in automobiles or transport generally, and again that occurred because mobility, car ownership indeed, was low in the test population. In Australia and the United States, and increasingly in the United Kingdom, automobile use is very much part of daily living. Were it the case that respondents happened to engage in extensive commuting to work, in company with others or in vehicles fitted with radio or stereo gear, then an important feature of daily life would not be touched on by the scale's present content.

This issue can be characterized as one of overlap between sets. One set is the life repertory of the typical respondent, the other is the ideal–typical life repertory represented by the scale. These are bound to be in phase during the development of a scale because its content is dictated by the repertory of typical respondents. Application to a new group is probably accompanied by a shift in the match-up between these two sets. Part of the scale's content will be outside the repertory of the new group; part of the new group's repertory will be outside that contained in the scale. The question becomes at what point the mismatch is sufficiently noticeable to require a restandardization, a bringing back into alignment of the two sets.

This sort of problem does not attend a test using tones: there being no meaning to start with, shifts of meaning cannot occur. The only way I can foresee of coping with the problem in self-report is in effect reenacting the original developmental steps in different cultures and within a given culture whenever in either of such contexts it is clear from responses to the open-ended questions in the scale that new cultural forms are emergent. I am referring here to the final questions in the Hearing Measurement Scale (see appendix to Chapter 9), in which respondents have opportunity first to describe issues not touched on in the interview and second to comment on questions they found hard to answer. These items are included so that recapitulation can occur if the respondent is uncertain about a given area of inquiry, and they also allow a fuller picture of the more idiosyncratic individual case. The point is that were an increasing proportion of people to identify an area not covered or to question the meaning of a specific area within the scale, these signs separately or together could be taken to indicate a shift in the match between sets and consequent need for a revision of content.

Nevertheless, despite this reparative possibility, this feature is a theoretical disadvantage of self-report that must be weighed against the advantages of the method.

The other main theoretical problem is one that cannot be so readily pinned down. Being a more purely methodological issue, this problem has philosophical implications. Put in straightforward terms, it is the ancient question of subjectivity. If I ask you to report your impression of some feature of your experience, how can I be sure that your appraisal is accurate? The answer, at first, is that I cannot; but the one-time reaction to that answer, namely, that subjective reports are worthless, is no longer satisfactory. The fact that I cannot be absolutely sure is no reason to reject such data. Rather, one must come at the problem in a different way.

The phenomenologists, particularly Schutz (1955), and more recently Berger and Luckmann (1967), have argued that experienced reality in everyday terms is a process of relationship between self and what is socially identified as the objective world. Any abstraction in regard to the world—and language is the most far-reaching abstraction confronting us—can no longer be identified as inherent in that world; it is, rather, a social object. Our descriptions of things are possible because we use an agreed-upon system of symbols, so that when I say "this book," you and I know what is being referred to. In the absence of a pure symbol system, we might resort to gesture—pointing, looking at, lifting, and so on. But for these actions to signify for you a reference to "this book," we both need to have previously agreed that such actions will have this signification. Without the prior social exchange to arrive at common meaning, gestures or words of mine can have no significance for anyone else. What this implies is that all meaningful action is *by definition* embedded in a social network.

What we mean, then, in using the term *subjective* is that the action, verbalization, or whatever performed by another has insufficient social basis to be meaningful. Equally, what we mean by *objective* is not that which is independent of our own social action—directly accessible and meaningful to each individual—but rather that which *does* have a relatively stable, agreed-upon significance.

It is usually at this point that philosophers become metaphorically violent and threaten the phenomenologists with an imaginary revolver. No fancy talk about intersubjective agreement is required, they say, to deal with the bald fact of one's demise following fatal gunshot wounds.

We will not meet this extreme form of opposition to the postulate in the present discourse because that would lead discussion astray.

In the more tranquil realms of everyday life, the intersubjectivity argument has considerable force. When I assert that a person's tonal audiogram shows that he cannot hear properly, I can only make that assertion within a previously agreed-upon background of what it means to use terms like "hear" and "hear properly" and, of course, "audiogram." This is not an objective fact I refer to in making the assertion but rather a fact within an objectivated world arrived at by prior consent between interested parties. What this book is trying to do, indeed, is undermine the very world in which assertions of the above sort are allowable as "objective fact."

Of course, worlds arrived at by scientific procedures are more enduring because better than the usual demonstrations are needed to obtain the consent of other parties to the enterprise about the significance of a given description. For instance, self-report as a methodology needs to struggle fairly hard to gain acceptance within the scientific community. That is a somewhat different issue, though obviously related, to the one of specific concern here. What we are centrally involved with is the "subjectivity" of self-reported assessment.

My method of dealing with this question, theoretically, is to argue that a scale whose content is first of all arrived at by negotiation with others and is continually renegotiated in any interview has moved from the position of pure "subjectivity" toward the "objective" end of the continuum. That argument only works, of course, if the prior argument about *subjective* and *objective* works; but by the term *works* I mean "gains the consent of interested parties." In other words, not only is there a point to be made about the social basis of the objective world, but there is also a point to be made about the social basis of *arguments* concerning the social basis of objective worlds.

To return once again to the original problem: I can increase certainty about self-report by undertaking to objectivate that report through negotiation with the other person. If I and the respondent agree about an assessment—if my reutterance of what the other person has reported gains that person's consent—then we have shifted his report from the subjective to the intersubjective and hence toward the objective. Let us not forget that we are using common language to arrive at this agreement. We do not have to devise a new symbol system and construct a reality from scratch; we are simply new players in an already established game. Furthermore, we have each separately played by the particular rules prior to engaging in this match because the interviewer has talked to others with similar problems and is practiced in the game and the respondent has witnessed his difficulty perpetually, verbalized about it, and had features of it confirmed in talking about it with others. The "subjectivity" of self-report cannot be characterized as an asocial subjectivity, for it has been objectivated long before any interview took place.

The only remaining problem, as I see it, concerns the access that the person has to his own experience. Here I think we can become somewhat more empirical. In regard to the Hearing Measurement Scale, the fairly high test–retest reliability after a 6-month interval supports a view that people are at least consistent in their appraisal of their own experiences. Furthermore, the fact that certain consistent reports were unrelated to overall opinion about state of hearing suggests that when a more evidently "subjective" response is demanded the individual may switch from a self-regarding posture to a more emotive, "subjective" attitude. I think it is quite feasible for people to adopt an "objective" view of themselves when the nature of the conversation invites them so to do. When the signal is given at the end of the interview to switch out of that role and provide a subjective opinion, the response may be at odds with the prior objective appraisal. Yet the latter, nonetheless, is consistent from one occasion of inquiry to another, however remote.

Notwithstanding the consistency of response overall, certain parts of the response pattern showed inconsistency, and this was especially marked in the initial questions about conversation. What this implies, however, is that there may be regions of experience which are variable rather than that the person is incapable of providing a verisimilar report. Conversational performance, at home and outside, with different people is presumably an occurrence of such variable successfulness that self-report may not be able to pin down a once-and-for-all appraisal.

Such a view is supported by data obtained in the initial study by Noble (1967). These data relate to a further important question of objectivity. One can reduce uncertainty about a self-report if it is corroborated by the report of others who know the respondent. This procedure was used by Noble (1967). While the person participating in the survey was interviewed by one researcher, his or her spouse or whomever he or she lived with was interviewed by another. A close association was observed between responses of both parties to items inquiring about more overt behavior—problems in detection of warning sounds, reduction of social contact, problems at public gatherings. But association was of only medium level between responses to items about difficulty in conversation. This lesser corroboration, plus the lower consistency on these items over time observed later in the reliability study (Noble, 1969), points to a real instability of self-reported appraisal in conversational speech hearing. More consistent responses were obtained on "listening" items (TV, radio), and this suggests that it is not speech hearing self-report per se that is inconsistent, only speech hearing in the more actually inconsistent conversational context.

In sum, the problem of a person's access to his or her own experience is a methodological debating point in regard to self-report. It may be wrong to classify this problem as a "disadvantage," rather it is a feature peculiar to the methodology and a probable source of inconsistency. That inconsistency, however, may or may not be intrinsic to the questionnaire itself; it may rather be inherent in certain referred-to instances of daily experience within the questionnaire's content.

Practical

The two major practical disadvantages of self-report are interviewer effects and fakability. Little needs to be said about either. It is evident that the different styles and skills of different interviewers, their inter- and intravariable willingness to negotiate with respondents about meaning and relevance, the social exchange whose character is bound to vary depending on the mutual regard of each party to the interview, all these must affect the responses and scores made. It is equally self-evident that respondents may fake an appraisal to give an impression of being worse off or better off than they know themselves actually to be. Neither problem is wholly beyond control. As regards the first, the use of tape recording allows later analysis of interviewing style so that different people may come to agree among themselves about sources of bias and ways of minimizing intrusion of the interviewer's world view on the respondent's world view. Tape recording also allows independent scoring of responses by someone other than the interviewer—an expedient adopted throughout the developmental stages of the Hearing Measurement Scale program.

As regards the second, it is my contention that faking will only occur when the respondent feels that the situation is not designed with his or her interest in mind. Faking in this test, as in others, is inseparable from the whole political context in which testing is carried out. At a practical level, faked responses may be detectable if the pattern of responding is quite at odds with typical patterns from similar people whose responses have been obtained in circumstances unlikely to produce faking. But the problem will not go away until the whole atmosphere of struggle and contest is replaced by one of mutual respect, and that can happen only with fundamental changes in social and political practice. I suggest that faking is less likely in a circumstance where responsibility is the business of all parties to the problem. The legislative structures in the Netherlands and in New Zealand mentioned in Chapter 3 may be conducive to this sort of atmosphere. I bring this point up again in the concluding chapter.

APPLICATIONS OF SELF-REPORT

In clinical practice and research, responses on a detailed questionnaire such as the Hearing Measurement Scale can provide significant data, bearing not only on the degree of everyday difficulty but also on the precise nature of that difficulty. A major research endeavor would be to investigate by factor analytic means the response patterns and profiles of different groups of people. A diagnostic or audiometric relation may well obtain within the fine structure of functional test response, type of disorder, and nature of self-reported disturbance. In the research described in Chapter 10, some indications of this possibility were noted, and more extensive study is certainly warranted. Whether a device like the Hearing Measurement Scale could have diagnostic usefulness cannot be foreseen at this stage, but it obviously has utility, by virtue of its standardized character, in rating the severity of disturbance. In any appraisal of the suitability of one or another program of treatment for different clients, self-report will have an increasing role.

The potential value of the method has already been realized in the rehabilitation context. Rating of change across time as a result of interventions of various sorts is a key feature of all such programs. Recently, Loeb, Cameron, Luz, Luz, and Vanderhei (1974) have used self-report to assess degrees of temporary injury and recovery paths.

The Hearing Measurement Scale was devised in the first place to assess handicap from persistent noise-induced disorder, and its capability in that context has been adequately demonstrated. There are several research studies of an industrial nature still to be done. One is to examine the feasibility of a paper-and-pencil form which will work in large-scale survey settings. That project is, as I mentioned, already under way. Of considerable importance would be a study along the lines of Burns and Robinson's (1970) paradigmatic investigation that would relate self-reported hearing loss and handicap to the degree of exposure to noise. Such a study would also demonstrate the extent to which features of different occupations influence experienced handicap, as suggested by the lip-reading effect described earlier.

Finally, in medicolegal settings, the Hearing Measurement Scale can obviously provide an assessment of experienced handicap, and its adoption by New Zealand as part of the assessment procedure in that country is evidence of such suitability. It is a simple empirical matter to discover whether and to what extent faking occurs in this sort of application. Data exist in plentiful supply from industrial samples in whom no likelihood of faking was involved. A comparison from matched samples of people claiming compensation would allow the robustness of the scale in that setting to be witnessed.

A final point to be mentioned in this connection is the issue of degrees of impairment and the low fence at which hearing handicap begins. I have always contended that an arbitrary limit of "normal" is inappropriate as a guide to evaluation. As is shown in Chapter 10 in discussion of the United States Public Health Service survey of 1935–1936, there appears to be a clearer lower boundary of impaired hearing at critical audio-frequencies, than an upper bound to normal hearing. A "low fence" is therefore better characterized as an obstacle to get under than one to get over. The criterion I have suggested (Noble, 1970) and attempted to defend (Noble, 1975c) is the lower limit or tenth centile score from an adequately representative sample of people with sensorineural disorder in the age range of compensation claimants, who present themselves at audiology clinics for treatment or hearing-aid fitting. Such a concept is in line with Davis's (1973) conception of the AAOO low fence as the "threshold level at which patients first *complain* of their handicap to a doctor rather than the threshold level at which they first *notice* difficulty [p. 1238]." Of course, Davis has no evidence that the AAOO fence is actually related to this behavior, but the point he puts is the same as mine. People who come to clinics for help are showing that their difficulty has reached a point that is no longer tolerable. This point will vary from person to person, and there will also be persons whose hearing is rapidly deteriorating because of disease, the effects of drugs, and so on. Within a clinic, a vast range of hearing difficulty is to be found—from the just noticeably intolerable to virtual deafness. The further suggestion I have made is that degree of handicap can be evaluated by locating an individual's self-report score on the distribution of clinic scores. If it is found that the individual score is at the nintieth centile of clinic scores, then it can be said he is 90% handicapped. Such a notion is perhaps arbitrary, but no more so than other rating systems and perhaps a touch more rational.

In conclusion, it is clear that there are opportunities for useful application of self-report in research, clinical, industrial, and medicolegal audiology. With increasing use and practice, the advantages and the limitations of the method will become clear. Eventually, self-report may give way to better tests of hearing function, but I suspect that occurrence is considerably in the future.

12

Future Trends

For reasons that have been given at various points, this book is partly a technical, partly a polemical treatise. From both points of view, the emphasis in this concluding phase is upon change. As stated earlier, science generally is both technical and radical. One reason some people persist in doing science is the hope to effect changes in "ways of seeing" certain problems. Dissatisfaction with current ways of seeing the particular topic area we have reviewed is what has sustained this author's interest in it. And a very powerful motive leading people to persist in the writing of books is undoubtedly the desire to affect the way others perceive problems and their solutions. A book is a more potent device for change than a journal article because it is larger, more far reaching, and (not least) repetitive. The monograph in our culture is a rhetorical device as well as a source of information. Although I have drawn attention to the rhetoric in this work, no monograph that is trying to be more than a technical manual is devoid of rhetoric. The foregoing sentences could not be written in a scientific journal because that kind of source deliberately inhibits them, but the book is one significant form in which such sentences are permitted.

In bringing this work to a close, I therefore want to make it clear that my purpose in undertaking the project has been to try to influence the course of events within the area of hearing assessment. The power of science, in my view, lies in the fact that the degree to which that endeavor may succeed rests in the evidence one can bring forward to support the case and not in the sentences which merely urge such change. One can, of course, select the evidence to provide this or that kind of picture, and I am not at all certain that selectivity of this kind is absent from the present work. But the game of selective representation cannot be consciously played with any lasting success. In any case, it was not mere caprice but rather evidence that brought this author to recognize the flaws in current practice in the first place.

Having said this much, I must add that evidence alone cannot change "ways of seeing." It requires, in addition, a wish or will for change that then permits evidence to be aligned in the preferred arrangement. This may seem to contradict what was just said, insofar as evidence cannot just be pushed around to satisfy a wish; but evidence can be restructured and presented in a new light. Unnoticed features can be emphasized, anomalies previously relegated to a footnote can be given center-stage treatment. This is an expression of science's radical role. The basic material, however, is still evidence.

I cannot precisely say what changes I would wish to take place. The prime concern is that consciousness regarding present practice be modified so that we see such practice as unsatisfactory. Beyond that, one may envision the unsatisfactory quality as arising from a political structure which will need to change before radical changes in this aspect of its social style can be brought about. Or one may see simply that as technical competencies improve adjustments must occur in the way problems are tackled. No revolution in thought or deed is needed; the process of evolution will engender new forms.

I think, first of all, that the prime mover in this particular segment of scientific inquiry, namely, impaired hearing caused by noise at work and at war, will diminish in importance over the next several decades. The war game may continue, but not on the grand scale of 1914–1918 or 1939–1945, or if on that scale, then using weaponry such that loss of hearing will not be a problem following it. Within industry, processes will just become quieter, simply because consciousness is radically changing about the safety and health of people at work. Workplaces are no longer regarded as special areas where higher risks are an inevitable part of the price of manufacture. That attitude is destined to vanish and be replaced by one that sees the industrial, mine, or farm process as simply another but not inferior sector of human performance in which injury resulting from the process is as lawfully punishable as criminal assault on Fifth Avenue. Occasional traumatic injuries from accidental events may still occur, but even these will diminish because such blast or sudden noise injuries result from generally unsafe processes. With improvement in safety engineering and radical alteration in industrial process, chances of accidental injury of this kind will be much reduced.

Along with this change in consciousness may emerge a new attitude to responsibility. On this score I cannot predict because it has to do with cultural movements, and one cannot easily foresee how these may develop. But signs now exist that the old employer–employee relationship is giving way to a contractual arrangement in which both management and shop floor are part of "labor" and the employer is increasingly, be it directly or indirectly, the state. In this latter arrangement, when I sue for damages, I am in a real way suing myself. Such a situation has been part of the older style of employer–employee interaction. The cost of injury being included in the cost of goods, as a consumer of these goods one pays part of that cost oneself. However, it is theoretically possible to avoid that cost by not consuming these goods. If the employer is the state, it is impossible to avoid that cost because it comes from state funds, and all pay taxes. If the state, as employer, takes responsibility for administering compensation, then the question of responsibility becomes more universal. In this sort of arrangement, one is one's own employer (as a taxpayer) as well as one's own employee. Of course, in practical terms, this arrangement is a myth because the state bureaucracy takes upon itself the role of "real" employer. But purely theoretically, the first description has a certain truth in it.

The purpose of this discussion is to attempt to get at the concept of responsibility, and what I am moving toward is a notion of universal responsibility within which, for example, the nature of legislation in the Netherlands and in New Zealand begins to make sense. In these countries, the state takes responsibility for all injury or disease arising from whatever cause. This move, in my view, if administered in a certain way, increases personal responsibility. Each person in the community can see how he or she has some responsibility, however slight, for the well-being and safety of all others. In compensation claims arising in industry, all that can presently be seen is the responsibility of the employer, and so the situation is necessarily one of conflict. The employer does not want all that responsibility exclusively, the employee wants none of it.

A changing climate of responsibility would, in my view, bring about change in the approach of all parties to compensation. The present atmosphere of conflict and the concomitant dishonest dealing on both sides—fraudulent claims, fraudulent assessment systems—would give way to a less impassioned and more rational approach. There would be no "sides" to align oneself with because all would be on the same "side." Eventually, too, compensation might be payable simply because one was "at risk," independent of any injury that might accrue from that risk. Under these conditions, assessment would be redundant as an evaluative ingredient in the claim and become simply a component of evidence along with more conventional testimony regarding the nature of the risk and the nature of one's exposure to it. This notion is perhaps too far fetched, however, to have meaning at present. The first notion, about changing responsibility, is not far fetched; it is becoming an increasing reality.

Notwithstanding the gradual disappearance of noise-induced hearing disorder from technological culture, assessment will remain important in other clinical circumstances. For while more widespread practices in medicine and community lifestyle persist, disease affecting hearing will also persist, and people will suffer congenital or adventitious disorder arising from the ill effects of drugs and the ill effects of technological life generally. The nature and severity of such effects will still need to be accurately gauged so that appropriate remediation can be provided.

The major change I foresee in the manner of that assessment relates to the changing social location of deaf and partially deaf people in the community. I would like to dwell a little on that theme; it is one we touched on in the opening chapter, and it is structurally fitting that it should be raised again at the close.

Despite many advances in popular and specialist thinking about deaf people, their liberation in society is a long way off. This is so because even "enlightened" deaf educators can see no future for deaf people except within the majority society. This attitude in itself is not unacceptable, but what is not seen as problematic is the nature and structure of that majority society. The problem for these educators lies in best means for inducting deaf children and adolescents into that society.

Deafness is still regarded by some so-called psychiatric experts as a problem condition in its own right which leads to personality disorder, psychosis, and the like (Mahapatra, 1974). Even though the evidence, as thoroughly reviewed for instance by Bonvillian, Charrow, and Nelson (1973), shows there to be no difference between deaf and hearing children with respect to cognitive competency, educators point to the social deprivation of deaf people as a supposedly critical problem for *them* (A. D. Evans, 1975; van Uden, 1975). What is not perceived through the psychiatric attitude and certainly not perceived through the attitude of some influential educators is that the problem of nonsocialization is a problem for the majority society, not a problem for deaf people. It certainly becomes a problem for the deaf when they discover that the social support system of their schools is withdrawn and they are suddenly faced with an alien world. And the problem for these people is, ironically, made worse precisely because their cognitive competency is equivalent to that of hearing people. Expectations about deaf people by hearing people will increase; the pressure will be on them all the more to demonstrate their equivalency.

But this can lead only to further problems so long as the majority society maintains its present structure. The liberation of oppressed groups is no longer seen solely in terms of integration with the power hierarchy of the society at large. Identification with majority society values is not the aim of pressure groups among women, blacks, homosexuals, delinquents, and the socially or mentally strange. The major aim of people in these groups seeking liberation is to be accommodated within society, not to be assimilated by society. And accommodation means that people who have power within the society must adjust practice and outlook. Minorities without power should not be required to do all the adjusting. In a very straightforward way as regards deaf people, this means that more hearing people need to learn their language and come to know their culture.

In schools, children are generally introduced to foreign cultures by learning languages other than their own. The utility of that practice for the majority of students is minimal. But I would predict that were signing to be offered in hearing children's schools, along with braille reading and other "secret" languages, the response would be immense. By this means, children would be given a code with which to circumvent the adult–teacher code, and in addition they would have ability to communicate with deaf or blind peers. For the latter feature to work, deaf children would certainly need to be taught along with hearing children, at least in the same institutions if not in the same classes. Cultural contact then would occur in two directions. In order to understand each other properly, both groups would have to develop certain faculties: signing on the hearing side and lip-reading on the deaf side. If the school system supported the development of these capabilities, the outcome would have a significant influence on both hearing and deaf children's perceptions of the world.

And this returns us to the starting point. Assessment by any system, but especially using self-report, requires that an understanding develop of the world view of the person being assessed. It perpetuates the oppression of deaf and partially deaf people if majority practice refuses to see the world in their terms. Only by understanding that world view can fair assessment be made, and this in turn means fair treatment of such people over and beyond the assessment context.

References

Adler, S. (1972). Dialectal differences and learning disorders. *Journal of Learning Disabilities, 5,* 344–350.
American Academy of Ophthalmology and Otolaryngology Committee on Conservation of Hearing (1959). Guide for the evaluation of hearing impairment. *Transactions of the American Academy of Ophthalmology and Otolaryngology, 63,* 236–238.
American Medical Association Council on Physical Therapy (1942). Tentative standard procedure for evaluating the percentage of useful hearing loss in medicolegal cases. *Journal of the American Medical Association, 119,* 1108–1109.
American Medical Association Council on Physical Medicine (1947). Tentative standard procedure for evaluating the percentage loss of hearing in medicolegal cases. *Journal of the American Medical Association, 133,* 396–397.
American Medical Association Council on Physical Medicine and Rehabilitation (1955). Principles for evaluating hearing loss. *Journal of the American Medical Association, 157,* 1408–1409.
American Medical Association Committee on Medical Rating of Physical Impairment (1961). Guide to the evaluation of permanent impairment; ear, nose, throat and related structures. *Journal of the American Medical Association, 177,* 489–501.
American National Standards Institute (1969). *American national standard specifications for audiometers,* ANSI S3.6–1969. New York: American National Standards Institute.
American Standards Association (1951). *American standard specification for audiometers for general diagnostic purposes,* Z24.5–1951. New York: American Standards Association.
Anastasi, A. (1961). *Psychological testing* (2nd ed.). New York: Macmillan.
Anderson, H., & Barr, B. (1966). Conductive recruitment. *Acta Oto-laryngologica, 62,* 171–184.
Atherley, G. R. C. (1967). Chronic acoustic trauma: A comparative study. Unpublished M.D. thesis, Univ. of Manchester.
Atherley, G. R. C., & Dingwall-Fordyce, I. (1963). The reliability of repeated auditory threshold determination. *British Journal of Industrial Medicine, 20,* 231–235.
Atherley, G. R. C., Hempstock, T. I., Lord, P., & Walker, J. G. (1967). Reliability of auditory threshold determinations using a circumaural-earphone assembly. *Journal of the Acoustical Society of America, 42,* 199–203.
Atherley, G. R. C., & Lord, P. (1965). A preliminary study of the effect of earphone position on the reliability of repeated auditory threshold determination. *International Audiology, 4,* 161–166.
Atherley, G. R. C., Lord, P., & Walker, J. G. (1966). Basis for the design of a circumaural earphone suitable for MAP determinations. *Journal of the Acoustical Society of America, 40,* 607–613.
Atherley, G. R. C., & Noble, W. G. (1967). Recent developments in audiometry. *Annals of Occupational Hygiene, 10,* 389–399.
Atherley, G. R. C., & Noble, W. G. (1969). Present hearing and past military gunfire experience. *Applied Acoustics, 2,* 199–205.
Atherley, G. R. C., & Noble, W. G. (1970). Effect of ear-defenders (ear-muffs) on the localization of sound. *British Journal of Industrial Medicine, 27,* 260–265.

References

Atherley, G. R. C., & Noble, W. G. (1971). Clinical picture of occupational hearing loss obtained with the hearing measurement scale. In D. W. Robinson (Ed.), *Occupational hearing loss*. London: Academic Press. Pp. 193–206.

Barr, T. (1884). *Manual of diseases of the ear*. Glasgow: Maclehose.

Barr, T. (1886). Enquiry into the effects of loud sounds upon the hearing of boilermakers and others who work amid noisy surroundings. *Proceedings of the Philosophical Society of Glasgow, 17*, 223–239.

Barr, T. (1889). The hearing of schoolchildren. *The Schoolmaster*, September 7.

Barr, T., & Barr, J. S. (1909). *Manual of diseases of the ear*. Glasgow: Maclehose.

Beasley, W. C. (1940a). Correlation between hearing loss measurements by air conduction on eight tones. *Journal of the Acoustical Society of America, 12*, 104–113.

Beasley, W. C. (1940b). Characteristics and distribution of impaired hearing in the population of the United States. *Journal of the Acoustical Society of America, 12*, 114–121.

Beasley, W. C. (1957). In H. Davis and J. R. Usher (Eds.), What is zero hearing loss? *Journal of Speech and Hearing Disorders, 22*, 662–690.

von Békésy, G. (1947). A new audiometer. *Acta Oto-laryngologica, 35*, 411–422.

von Békésy, G. (1970). Enlarged mechanical model of the cochlea with nerve supply. In J. V. Tobias (Ed.), *Foundations of modern auditory theory*. Vol. I. New York: Academic Press. Pp. 307–341.

Bench, J., Collyer, Y., Mentz, L., & Wilson, I. (1976). Studies in infant behavioural audiometry: III. Six-month-old infants. *Audiology, 15*, 384–394.

Bench, J., & Mentz, L. (1975). Stimulus complexity, state and infants' auditory behavioural responses. *British Journal of Disorders of Communication, 10*, 52–60.

Berger, P. L., & Luckmann, T. (1967). *The social construction of reality*. Harmondsworth, England: Penguin.

Bergman, M. (1966). Hearing in the Mabaans: A critical review of related literature. *Archives of Otolaryngology, 84*, 411–415.

Berkowitz, A. O., & Hochberg, I. (1971). Self-assessment of hearing handicap in the aged. *Archives of Otolaryngology, 93*, 25–28.

Bienvenue, G. R., & Siegenthaler, B. M. (1974). A clinical procedure for evaluating auditory localization. *Journal of Speech and Hearing Disorders, 39*, 469–477.

Binet, A., & Simon, T. (1905). Méthodes nouvelles pour le diagnostic du niveau intellectuel des anormaux. *Année Psychologique, 11*, 191–244.

Blumenfeld, V. G., Bergman, M., & Millner, E. (1969). Speech discrimination in an aging population. *Journal of Speech and Hearing Research, 12*, 210–217.

Bonvillian, J. D., Charrow, V. D., & Nelson, K. E. (1973). Psycholinguistic and educational implications of deafness. *Human Development, 16*, 321–345.

Brandy, W. T. (1966). Reliability of voice tests of speech discrimination. *Journal of Speech and Hearing Research, 9*, 461–465.

Bregman, A. S., & Campbell, J. (1971). Primary auditory stream segregation and perception of order in rapid sequences of tones. *Journal of Experimental Psychology, 89*, 244–249.

Bregman, A. S., & Dannenbring, G. L. (1973). The effect of continuity on auditory stream segregation. *Perception & Psychophysics, 13*, 308–312.

British Standards Institution (1954). *The normal threshold of hearing for pure tones by earphone listening:* BS 2497. London: British Standards Institution.

Broadbent, D. E. (1958). *Perception and communication*. Oxford, England: Pergamon.

Brown, R. E. C. (1948). Experimental studies on the reliability of audiometry. *The Journal of Laryngology and Otology, 62*, 487–524.

de Bruïne-Altes, J. C. (1946). *The symptom of regression in different kinds of deafness*. Groningen: J. B. Wolters.

Bryan, M. E., Parbrook, H. D., & Tempest, W. (1965a). A note on quiet threshold shift in the absence of noise. *Journal of Sound and Vibration, 2*, 147–149.

References

Bryan, M. E., Parbrook, H. D., & Tempest, W. (1965b). The variation of quiet thresholds with low level noise exposure. *Proceedings of the 5th International Congress on Acoustics*, Liège, September.

Bryan, M. E., & Tempest, W. (1971). Noise damage liability—evidence as to the state of knowledge. In D. W. Robinson (Ed.), *Occupational hearing loss*. London: Academic Press. Pp. 143–150.

Bunch, C. C. (1941). The development of the audiometer. *The Laryngoscope, 51*, 1100–1118.

Bunch, C. C. (1943). *Clinical audiometry*. St. Louis: C. V. Mosby.

Burk, K. W. (1958). Traditional and psychogalvanic skin response audiometry. *Journal of Speech and Hearing Research, 1*, 275–278.

Burns, W. (1971). The relation of temporary to permanent threshold shift in individuals. In D. W. Robinson (Ed.), *Occupational hearing loss*. London: Academic Press. Pp. 63–70.

Burns, W., & Robinson, D. W. (1970). *Hearing and noise in industry*. London: HMSO.

Campbell, R. A. (1965). Discrimination test word difficulty. *Journal of Speech and Hearing Research, 8*, 13–22.

Carhart, R. (1945). An improved method for classifying audiograms. *The Laryngoscope, 55*, 640–662.

Carhart, R. (1946a). Monitored live-voice as a test of auditory acuity. *Journal of the Acoustical Society of America, 17*, 339–349.

Carhart, R. (1946b). Speech reception in relation to pattern of pure tone loss. *Journal of Speech Disorders, 11*, 97–108.

Carhart, R. (1946c). Individual differences in hearing for speech. *Annals of Otology, Rhinology and Laryngology, 55*, 233–265.

Carhart, R. (1965). Problems in the measurement of speech discrimination. *Archives of Otolaryngology, 82*, 253–260.

Carhart, R., & Hayes, C. (1949). Clinical reliability of bone conduction audiometry. *The Laryngoscope, 59*, 1084–1101.

Carhart, R., & Jerger, J. F. (1959). Preferred method for clinical determination of pure-tone thresholds. *Journal of Speech and Hearing Disorders, 24*, 330–345.

Carhart, R., & Porter, L. S. (1971). Audiometric configuration and prediction of threshold for spondees. *Journal of Speech and Hearing Research, 14*, 486–495.

Castelo-Branco, A. (1971). Législation sur les troubles dus aux bruits dans différents pays. *Acta Oto-rhino-laryngologica Belgica, 25*, 131–138.

Cattell, J. McK. (1890). Mental tests and measurements. *Mind, 15*, 373–380.

Cawthorne, T., & Harvey, R. M. (1953). A comparison between hearing for pure tones and for speech. *Journal of Laryngology and Otology, 67*, 233–247.

Chaiklin, J. B., Ventry, I. M., & Barrett, L. S. (1961). Reliability of conditioned GSR pure-tone audiometry with adult males. *Journal of Speech and Hearing Research, 4*, 269–280.

Chalmers, A. F. (1976). *What is this thing called science?* St. Lucia: Univ. of Queensland Press.

Claass, A., & Jolivet, A. (1975). Réparation de la surdité et de l'hypoacusie professionnelles dans les différents pays de la communauté. In G. Rossi & M. Vigone (Eds.), *L'Uomo e il rumore*. Turin: Minerva Medica. Pp. 351–359.

Cole, R. A., & Scott, B. (1974). Toward a theory of speech perception. *Psychological Review, 81*, 348–374.

Coles, R. R. A. (1967). A noise-attenuating enclosure for audiometer earphones. *British Journal of Industrial Medicine, 24*, 41–51.

Coles, R. R. A. (1970). In discussion of Noble, W. G. A new concept of damage risk criterion. *Annals of Occupational Hygiene, 13*, 69–75.

Coles, R. R. A. (1975). Medico-legal aspects of noise hazards to hearing. *The Medico-Legal Journal, 43*, 3–19.

Collie, J. (1913). *Malingering and feigned sickness.* London: Arnold.
Committee on Compensation for Industrial Disease (1907). *Report of the Department Committee on Compensation for Industrial Disease.* London: HMSO.
Cordell, J. (1972). Noise legislation: A bibliography with abstracts. *Bibliographic Report No. 10.* Sydney: Commonwealth Acoustic Laboratories.
Corso, J. F. (1959). Age and sex differences in pure-tone thresholds. *Journal of the Acoustical Society of America, 31,* 498–507.
Corso, J. F. (1963). Age and sex differences in pure-tone thresholds. *Archives of Otolaryngology, 77,* 53–73.
Corso, J. F. (1976). Presbycusis as a complicating factor in evaluating noise-induced hearing loss. In D. Henderson, R. P. Hamernik, D. S. Dosanjh, & J. H. Mills (Eds.), *Effects of noise on hearing.* New York: Raven Press. Pp. 497–524.
Corso, J. F., & Cohen, A. (1958). Methodological aspects of auditory threshold measurements. *Journal of Experimental Psychology, 55,* 8–12.
Corso, J. F., Wright, H. N., & Valerio, M. (1976). Auditory temporal summation in presbycusis and noise exposure. *Journal of Gerontology, 31,* 58–63.
Cronbach, L. J., Rajaratnam, N., & Gleser, G. C. (1963). Theory of generalizability: A liberalization of reliability theory. *British Journal of Statistical Psychology, 16,* 137–163.
Curry, E. T. (1949). A study of the relationship between speech thresholds and audiometric results in perception deafness. *Journal of Speech and Hearing Disorders, 14,* 104–110.
Cutting, J. E., & Rosner, B. S. (1974). Categories and boundaries in speech and music. *Perception & Psychophysics, 16,* 564–570.
Dadson, R. S., & King, J. H. (1952). A determination of the normal threshold of hearing and its relation to the standardization of audiometers. *Journal of Laryngology and Otology, 66,* 366–378.
Dallos, P., Billone, M. C., Durrant, J. D., Wang, C.-y., & Raynor, S. (1972). Cochlear inner and outer hair cells: Functional differences. *Science, 177,* 356–358.
Danloux-Dumesnils, M. (1969). *The metric system.* London: Athlone Press.
Davis, H. (1948). The articulation area and the social adequacy index for hearing. *The Laryngoscope, 58,* 761–778.
Davis, H. (1960). Military standards and medicolegal rules. In H. Davis & S. R. Silverman (Eds.), *Hearing and deafness* (2nd ed.). New York: Holt. Pp. 242–264.
Davis, H. (1965). Slow cortical responses evoked by acoustic stimuli. *Acta Oto-laryngologica, 59,* 179–185.
Davis, H. (1970a). Anatomy and physiology of the auditory system. In H. Davis & S. R. Silverman (Eds.), *Hearing and deafness* (3rd ed.). New York: Holt. Pp. 47–82.
Davis, H. (1970b). Hearing handicap, standards for hearing, and medicolegal rules. In H. Davis & S. R. Silverman (Eds.), *Hearing and deafness* (3rd ed.). New York: Holt. Pp. 253–279.
Davis, H. (1970c). Audiometry: Pure tone and simple speech tests. In H. Davis & S. R. Silverman (Eds.), *Hearing and deafness* (3rd ed.). New York: Holt. Pp. 179–220.
Davis, H. (1971). A historical introduction. In D. W. Robinson (Ed.), *Occupational hearing loss.* London: Academic Press. Pp. 7–12.
Davis, H. (1973). Some comments on "Impairment to hearing from exposure to noise" by K. D. Kryter. *Journal of the Acoustical Society of America, 53,* 1237–1239.
Davis, H., & Kranz, F. W. (1964). The international standard reference zero for pure-tone audiometers and its relation to the evaluation of impairment of hearing. *Journal of Speech and Hearing Research, 7,* 7–16.
Davis, H., Morgan, C. T., Hawkins, J. E., Galambos, R., & Smith, F. W. (1950). Temporary deafness following exposure to loud tones and noise. *Acta Oto-laryngologica,* Supplement 88.
Davis, H., & Silverman, S. R. (1970). Appendix. In H. Davis & S. R. Silverman (Eds), *Hearing and deafness* (3rd ed.). New York: Holt. Pp. 481–495.

Davis, H., Stevens, S. S., Nichols, R. H., Jr., Hudgins, C. V., Marquis, R. J., Peterson, G. E., & Ross, D. A. (1947). *Hearing aids: An experimental study of design objectives.* Cambridge, Massachusetts: Harvard Univ. Press.
Davis, H., & Usher, J. R. (1957). In H. Davis & J. R. Usher (Eds.), What is zero hearing loss? *Journal of Speech and Hearing Disorders, 22,* 662–690.
Delaney, M. E. (1971). Some sources of variance in the determination of hearing level. In D. W. Robinson (Ed.), *Occupational hearing loss.* London: Academic Press. Pp. 97–108.
Delaney, M. E., & Whittle, L. S. (1967). Reference equivalent threshold sound pressure levels for audiometry. *Acustica, 18,* 227–231.
Dewey, G. (1923). *Relative frequency of English speech sounds.* Cambridge, Massachusetts: Harvard Univ. Press.
Dix, M. R., Hallpike, C. S., & Hood, J. D. (1948). Observations upon the loudness recruitment phenomenon, with especial reference to the differential diagnosis of disorders of the internal ear and VIII nerve. *Proceedings of the Royal Society of Medicine, 41,* 516–526.
Dix, M. R., Hallpike, C. S., & Hood, J. D. (1949). "Nerve" deafness: Its clinical criteria, old and new. *Proceedings of the Royal Society of Medicine, 42,* 527–536.
Doerfler, L. G., & McClure, C. T. (1954). The measurement of hearing loss in adults by galvanic skin response. *Journal of Speech and Hearing Disorders, 19,* 184–189.
Duncan, S., Jr. (1975). On the structure of speaker–auditor interaction during speaking turns. *Language in Society, 2,* 161–180.
Eby, L. G., & Williams, H. L. (1951). Recruitment of loudness in the differential diagnosis of end-organ and nerve fibre deafness. *The Laryngoscope, 61,* 400–414.
Egan, J. P. (1948). Articulation testing methods. *The Laryngoscope, 58,* 955–991.
Elliott, L. L. (1963). Prediction of speech discrimination scores from other test information. *Journal of Auditory Research, 3,* 35–45.
Elliott, L. L. (1964). Note on predicting speech-discrimination scores. *Journal of the Acoustical Society of America, 36,* 1961–1962.
Elpern, B. S. (1960). Differences in difficulty among the CID W-22 auditory tests. *The Laryngoscope, 70,* 1560–1565.
Elpern, B. S. (1961). The relative stability of half-list and full-list discrimination tests. *The Laryngoscope, 71,* 30–36.
Engelberg, M. (1965). Relationship of pure tones to speech reception threshold. *Annals of Otology, Rhinology and Laryngology, 74,* 234–240.
Engelberg, M. (1968). Test–retest variability in speech discrimination testing. *The Laryngoscope, 78,* 1582–1589.
Evans, A. D. (1975). Experiential deprivation: Unresolved factor in the impoverished socialization of deaf school children in residence. *American Annals of the Deaf, 120,* 545–552.
Evans, E. F. (1975). The sharpening of cochlear frequency selectivity in the normal and abnormal cochlea. *Audiology, 14,* 419–442.
Ewertsen, H. W., & Birk-Nielsen, H. (1973). Social hearing handicap index. *Audiology, 12,* 180–187.
Eysenck, H. J. (1953). *The structure of human personality.* London: Methuen.
Eysenck, H. J. (1967). *The biological basis of personality.* Springfield, Illinois: Thomas.
Fairbanks, G. (1958). Test of phonemic differentiation: The rhyme test. *Journal of the Acoustical Society of America, 30,* 596–600.
Falconer, G. A., & Davis, H. (1947). The intelligibility of connected discourse as a test for the "threshold for speech." *The Laryngoscope, 57,* 581–595.
Fletcher, H. (1929). *Speech and hearing.* New York: Van Nostrand.
Fletcher, H. (1950). A method of calculating hearing loss for speech from an audiogram. *Journal of the Acoustical Society of America, 22,* 1–5.
Fletcher, H. (1953). *Speech and hearing in communication.* New York: Van Nostrand.

Fletcher, H., & Munson, W. A. (1933). Loudness, its definition, measurement and calculation. *Journal of the Acoustical Society of America, 5,* 82–108.

Fletcher, H., & Steinberg, J. C. (1929). Articulation testing methods. *Bell System Technical Journal, 8,* 806–854.

Flodgren, E., & Kylin, B. (1961). Sex differences in hearing in relation to noise exposure. *Acta Oto-laryngologica, 52,* 358–366.

Fowler, E. P. (1936). A method for the early detection of otosclerosis. *Archives of Oto-laryngology, 24,* 731–741.

Fowler, E. P. (1937). Measuring the sensation of loudness. *Archives of Otolaryngology, 26,* 514–521.

Fowler, E. P. (1941). Hearing standards for acceptance, disability rating and discharge in the military services and in industry. *The Laryngoscope, 51,* 937–956.

Fowler, E. P. (1942). A method for measuring the percentage of capacity for hearing speech. *Journal of the Acoustical Society of America, 13,* 373–382.

Fowler, E. P. (1947). The percentage of capacity to hear speech, and related disabilities. *The Laryngoscope, 57,* 103–113.

Fox, M. S. (1957). In discussion of Glorig, A. Some medical implications of the 1954 Wisconsin state fair hearing survey. *Transactions of the American Academy of Ophthalmology and Otolaryngology, 61,* 160–171.

Fox, M. S. (1965). Comparative provisions for occupational hearing loss. *Archives of Otolaryngology, 81,* 257–260.

French, N. R., Carter, C. W., & Koenig, W. (1930). The words and sounds of telephone conversations. *Bell System Technical Journal, 9,* 290–324.

French, N. R., & Steinberg, J. C. (1947). Factors governing the intelligibility of speech sounds. *Journal of the Acoustical Society of America, 19,* 90–119.

Fry, D. B. (1961). Word and sentence tests for use in speech audiometry. *The Lancet,* July 22, 197–199.

Galbraith, J. K. (1974). *Economics and the public purpose.* London: Deutsch.

Gengel, R. W. (1973). On the reliability of discrimination-performance in persons with sensorineural hearing-impairment using a closed-set test. *Journal of Auditory Research, 13,* 97–100.

Gibson, J. J. (1950). *The Perception of the Visual World.* Boston: Houghton.

Gibson, J. J. (1966). *The senses considered as perceptual systems.* Boston: Houghton.

Giolas, T. G. (1970). The measurement of hearing handicap: A point of view. *Maico Audiological Library Series, 8,* 20–23.

Giolas, T. G., & Duffy, J. R. (1973). Equivalency of CID and revised CID sentence lists. *Journal of Speech and Hearing Research, 16,* 549–555.

Gjaevenes, K. (1969). Estimating speech reception threshold from pure tone hearing loss. *Journal of Auditory Research, 9,* 139–144.

Glass, D. C., & Singer, J. E. (1972). *Urban stress: Experiments on noise and social stressors.* New York: Academic Press.

Glorig, A. (1954). Malingering. *Annals of Otology, Rhinology and Laryngology, 63,* 802–815.

Glorig, A. (1958). A report of two normal hearing studies. *Annals of Otology, Rhinology and Laryngology, 67,* 93–111.

Glorig, A. (1971). In discussion of papers. In D. W. Robinson (Ed.), *Occupational hearing loss.* London: Academic Press. P. 83.

Glorig, A., & Davis, H. (1961). Age, noise and hearing loss. *Annals of Otology, Rhinology and Laryngology, 70,* 556–571.

Glorig, A., & Nixon, J. (1960). Distribution of hearing loss in various populations. *Annals of Otology, Rhinology and Laryngology, 69,* 497–516.

Glorig, A., & Nixon, J. (1962). Hearing loss as a function of age. *The Laryngoscope, 72,* 1596–1610.

Glorig, A., Quiggle, R., Wheeler, D. E., & Grings, W. (1956). Determination of the normal hearing reference zero. *Journal of the Acoustical Society of America, 28,* 1110–1113.

Glorig, A., Ward, W. D., & Nixon, J. (1961). Damage risk criteria and noise-induced hearing loss. *Archives of Otolaryngology, 74,* 413–423.

Goffman, E. (1961). On the characteristics of total institutions. In D. R. Cressey (Ed.), *The prison: Studies in institutional organization and change.* New York: Holt. Pp. 15–106.

Goldman, J. L. (1944). A comparative study of whisper tests and audiograms. *The Laryngoscope, 54,* 559–572.

Goodman, K. S. (1969). Dialect barriers to reading comprehension. In J. Baratz & R. Shuy (Eds.), *Teaching black children to read.* Washington: Center for Applied Linguistics. Pp. 14–28.

Goodnow, J. J. (1976). The nature of intelligent behavior: Questions raised by cross-cultural studies. In L. Resnick (Ed.), *The nature of intelligence.* New York: Erlbaum. Pp. 169–188.

Graham, J. T. (1960). Evaluation of methods for predicting speech reception threshold. *Archives of Otolaryngology, 72,* 347–350.

Green, D. M. (1960). Psychoacoustics and detection theory. *Journal of the Acoustical Society of America, 32,* 1189–1203.

Green, S. (1975). Variation of vocal pattern with social situation in the Japanese monkey (*Macaca fuscata*): A field study. In L. A. Rosenblum (Ed.), *Primate behavior: Developments in field and laboratory research.* Vol. IV. New York: Academic Press. Pp. 1–102.

Gregory, R. L., & Wallace, J. G. (1963). Recovery from early blindness: A case study. *Monographs of the Experimental Psychology Society,* No. 2, Cambridge, England.

Greven, A. J., & Oosterveld, W. J. (1975). The contralateral ear in Ménière disease. *Archives of Otolaryngology, 101,* 608–612.

Grime, R. P. (1975). *The law of noise-induced hearing loss and its compensation.* Southampton, England: Wolfson Unit for Noise and Vibration Control.

Grubb, P. (1963a). A phonemic analysis of half-list speech discrimination tests. *Journal of Speech and Hearing Research, 6,* 271–275.

Grubb, P. (1963b). Some considerations in the use of half-list speech discrimination tests. *Journal of Speech and Hearing Research, 6,* 294–297.

Guttman, L. (1944). A basis for scaling qualitative data. *American Sociological Review, 9,* 139–150.

Hallpike, C. S. (1967). The loudness recruitment phenomenon: A clinical contribution to the neurology of hearing. In A. B. Graham (Ed.), *Sensorineural hearing processes and disorders.* London: Churchill. Pp. 489–499.

Hallpike, C. S., & Hood, J. D. (1951). Some recent work on auditory adaptation and its relationship to the loudness recruitment phenomenon. *Journal of the Acoustical Society of America, 23,* 270–274.

Hallpike, C. S., & Hood, J. D. (1959). Observations upon the neurological mechanism of the loudness recruitment phenomenon. *Acta Oto-laryngologica, 50,* 472–486.

Hardick, E. J., Oyer, H. J., & Irion, P. E. (1970). Lipreading performance as related to measurements of vision. *Journal of Speech and Hearing Research, 13,* 92–100.

Harris, J. D. (1946). Free voice and pure tone audiometer for routine testing of auditory acuity. *Archives of Otolaryngology, 44,* 452–467.

Harris, J. D. (1953). A brief critical review of loudness recruitment. *Psychological Bulletin, 50,* 190–203.

Harris, J. D. (1954). Normal hearing and its relation to audiometry. *The Laryngoscope, 64,* 928–957.

Harris, J. D. (1960). Combinations of distortion in speech. *Archives of Otolaryngology, 72,* 227–232.

Harris, J. D. (1965). Pure-tone acuity and the intelligibility of everyday speech. *Journal of the Acoustical Society of America, 37,* 824–830.

Harris, J. D., Haines, H. L., & Myers, C. K. (1952). Loudness perception for pure tones and speech. *Archives of Otolaryngology, 55,* 107–133.

Harris, J. D., Haines, H. L., & Myers, C. K. (1956). A new formula for using the audiogram to predict speech hearing loss. *Archives of Otolaryngology, 63,* 158–176.

Harris, J. D., Haines, H. L., & Myers, C. K. (1960). The importance of hearing at 3 kc for understanding speeded speech. *The Laryngoscope, 70,* 131–146.

Harris, J. D., Haines, H. L., Kelsey, P. A., & Clack, T. D. (1961). The relation between speech intelligibility and the electroacoustic characteristics of low fidelity circuitry. *Journal of Auditory Research, 1,* 357–381.

Hartley, B. P. R., Howell, R. W., Sinclair, A., & Slattery, D. A. D. (1973). Subject variability in short-term audiometric recording. *British Journal of Industrial Medicine, 30,* 271–275.

Hawkins, J. E. (1971). The role of vasoconstriction in noise-induced hearing loss. *Annals of Otology, Rhinology and Laryngology, 80,* 903–913.

Heaton, J. M. (1968). *The eye: Phenomenology and psychology of function and disorder.* London: Tavistock.

Hempstock, T. I., & Atherley, G. R. C. (1971). Tinnitus and noise-induced tinnitus. In D. W. Robinson (Ed.), *Occupational hearing loss.* London: Academic Press. Pp. 207–216.

Hempstock, T. I., Bryan, M. E., & Tempest, W. (1965). Normal operating conditions for free-field automatic audiometry. *Proceedings of the 5th International Congress on Acoustics,* Liège, September.

Hempstock, T. I., Bryan, M. E., & Webster, J. B. C. (1966). Free-field threshold variance. *Journal of Sound and Vibration, 4,* 33–44.

Hickling, S. (1966). Studies on the reliability of auditory threshold values. *Journal of Auditory Research, 6,* 39–46.

High, W. S., Fairbanks, G., & Glorig, A. (1964). Scale for self-assessment of hearing handicap. *Journal of Speech and Hearing Disorders, 29,* 215–230.

High, W. S., & Gallo, R. P. (1963). Audiometric reliability in an industrial hearing conservation program. *Journal of Auditory Research, 3,* 15–34.

High, W. S., & Glorig, A. (1962). The reliability of industrial audiometry. *Journal of Auditory Research, 2,* 56–65.

High, W. S., Glorig, A., & Nixon, J. (1961). Estimating the reliability of auditory threshold measurements. *Journal of Auditory Research, 1,* 247–262.

Hinchcliffe, D., & Hinchcliffe, R. (1974). Administrative and legal control of noise and its effects (part II). *British Journal of Audiology, 8,* 101–108.

Hinchcliffe, R. (1959). The threshold of hearing as a function of age. *Acustica, 9,* 303–308.

Hirsh, I. J. (1952). *The measurement of hearing.* New York: McGraw-Hill.

Hirsh, I. J., Davis, H., Silverman, S. R., Reynolds, E. G., Eldert, E., & Benson, R. W. (1952). Development of materials for speech audiometry. *Journal of Speech and Hearing Disorders, 17,* 321–337.

Hodgson, K. W. (1953). *The deaf and their problems.* London: Watts.

Holt, E. E. (1882). Boiler-maker's deafness and hearing in a noise. *Transactions of the American Otological Society, 3,* 34–44.

Hood, J. D. (1950). Studies in auditory fatigue and adaptation. *Acta Oto-laryngologica,* Supplement 92.

Hood, J. D. (1960). A comparative study of loudness recruitment in cases of deafness due to Ménière's disease, head injury and acoustic trauma. *Acta oto-rhino-laryngologica Belgica, 14,* 224–233.

Hood, J. D. (1968). Speech discrimination and its relationship to disorders of the loudness function. *International Audiology, 7,* 232–238.

Hood, J. D., & Poole, J. P. (1971). Speech audiometry in conductive and sensorineural hearing loss. *Sound (British Journal of Audiology), 5,* 30–38.

References

House, A. S., Williams, C. E., Hecker, M. H. L., & Kryter, K. D. (1965). Articulation-testing methods: Consonantal differentiation with a closed-response set. *Journal of the Acoustical Society of America, 37,* 158–166.

Hudgins, C. V., Hawkins, J. E., Karlin, J. E., & Stevens, S. S. (1947). The development of recorded auditory tests for measuring hearing loss for speech. *The Laryngoscope, 57,* 57–89.

Hughson, W., & Thompson, E. (1942). Correlation of hearing acuity for speech with discrete frequency audiograms. *Archives of Otolaryngology, 36,* 526–540.

Huizing, H. C. (1949). The symptom of recruitment and speech intelligibility. *Acta Otolaryngologica, 36,* 346–355.

Huizing, H. C., & Reyntjes, J. A. (1952). Recruitment and speech discrimination loss. *The Laryngoscope, 62,* 521–527.

International Association of Industrial Accident Boards and Commissions (1961). Report of administration and procedure committee on compensation for impairment of hearing. Honolulu, Hawaii, mimeograph.

International Organization for Standardization (1964). *Standard reference zero for the calibration of pure-tone audiometers, ISO recommendation R389.* Geneva: ISO.

Jackson, J. E., Fassett, D. W., Riley, E. C., & Sutton, W. L. (1962). Evaluation of the variability in audiometric procedures. *Journal of the Acoustical Society of America, 34,* 218–222.

Jerger, J. (1960). Bekesy audiometry in analysis of auditory disorders. *Journal of Speech and Hearing Research, 3,* 275–287.

Jerger, J. (1961). Recruitment and allied phenomena in differential diagnosis. *Journal of Auditory Research, 1,* 145–151.

Jerger, J. (1962). Comparative evaluation of some auditory measures. *Journal of Speech and Hearing Research, 5,* 3–17.

Jerger, J. F., Shedd, J. L., & Harford, E. (1959). On the detection of extremely small changes in sound intensity. *Archives of Otolaryngology, 69,* 200–211.

Jerger, J., Speaks, C., & Trammell, J. L. (1968). A new approach to speech audiometry. *Journal of Speech and Hearing Disorders, 33,* 318–328.

Johnson, K. O. (1957). Veterans compensations for hearing loss. *Journal of Speech and Hearing Disorders, 22,* 731–733.

Jung, C. G. (1923). *Psychological types.* London: International Library of Psychology, Philosophy and Scientific Method.

Keck, R. C. (1955). Legal aspects of noise. *Noise Control, 1*(3), 35–38, 58, 60.

Kell, R. L., Pearson, J. C. G., Acton, W. I., & Taylor, W. (1971). Social effects of hearing loss due to weaving noise. In D. W. Robinson (Ed.), *Occupational hearing loss.* London: Academic Press. Pp. 179–191.

Kesey, K. (1962). *One flew over the cuckoo's nest.* London: Methuen.

Kiang, N. Y. S., Moxon, E. C., & Levine, R. A. (1970). Auditory-nerve activity in cats with normal and abnormal cochleas. In G. E. W. Wolstenholme & J. Knight (Eds.), *Sensorineural hearing loss.* London: Churchill. Pp. 241–273.

Kreul, E. J., Bell, D. W., & Nixon, J. C. (1969). Factors affecting speech discrimination test difficulty. *Journal of Speech and Hearing Research, 12,* 281–287.

Kreul, E. J., Nixon, J. C., Kryter, K. D., Bell, D. W., Lang, J. S., & Schubert, E. D. (1968). A proposed clinical test of speech discrimination. *Journal of Speech and Hearing Research, 11,* 536–552.

Kryter, K. D. (1962). Methods for the calculation and use of the articulation index. *Journal of the Acoustical Society of America, 34,* 1689–1697.

Kryter, K. D. (1970). *The effects of noise on man.* New York: Academic Press.

Kryter, K. D. (1973). Impairment to hearing from exposure to noise. *Journal of the Acoustical Society of America, 53,* 1211–1234.

Kryter, K. D., Williams, C., & Green, D. M. (1962). Auditory acuity and the perception of speech. *Journal of the Acoustical Society of America, 34,* 1217–1223.

Kuhn, T. S. (1962). The structure of scientific revolutions. *International Encyclopedia of Unified Science, 2*(2). Chicago: Chicago Univ. Press.

Kylin, B. (1960). Temporary threshold shift and auditory trauma following exposure to steady-state noise. *Acta Oto-laryngologica,* Supplement 152.

Lakatos, I. (1970). Falsification and the methodology of scientific research programmes. In I. Lakatos & A. Musgrave (Eds.), *Criticism and the growth of knowledge.* Cambridge, England: Cambridge Univ. Press. Pp. 91–196.

Lamb, L. E., & Peterson, J. L. (1967). Middle ear reflex measurements in pseudohypacusis. *Journal of Speech and Hearing Disorders, 32,* 46–51.

Lansberg, M. P. (1954). Modern aspects of the recruitment phenomenon. *Archives of Otolaryngology, 60,* 712–730.

Lebo, C. P., & Reddell, R. C. (1972). The presbycusis component in occupational hearing loss. *The Laryngoscope, 82,* 1399–1409.

Liberman, A. M., Delattre, P., & Cooper, F. S. (1952). The role of selected stimulus-variables in the perception of the unvoiced stop consonants. *American Journal of Psychology, 65,* 497–516.

Liberman, A. M., Cooper, F. S., Shankweiler, D. P., & Studdert-Kennedy, M. (1967). Perception of the speech code. *Psychological Review, 74,* 431–461.

Licklider, J. C. R., & Pollack, I. (1948). Effects of differentiation, integration and infinite peak clipping upon the intelligibility of speech. *Journal of the Acoustical Society of America, 20,* 42–51.

Lindeman, H. E. (1969). Results of speech intelligibility survey in cases of noise traumata. *International Audiology, 8,* 626–632.

Loeb, M., Cameron, P. D., Luz, G. A., Luz, S., & Vanderhei, S. L. (1974). Hearing levels in U.S. Army basic training: Relationship to questionnaire responses. *Journal of Auditory Research, 14,* 247–257.

The Machinist (1975). State benefits for loss of hearing. *The Machinist, 30*(16), August.

MacRae, J. H. (1975–76). A procedure for classifying degree of hearing loss. *Journal of the Oto-Laryngological Society of Australia, 4,* 26–35.

MacRae, J. H. (1977). The effect of random variability of hearing levels on AMA (1971) and NAL (1974) percentage hearing loss values. *Informal Report 44.* Sydney: National Acoustic Laboratories.

MacRae, J. H., & Brigden, D. N. (1973). Auditory threshold impairment and everyday speech reception. *Audiology, 12,* 272–290.

Mahapatra, S. B. (1974). Deafness and mental health: Psychiatric and psychosomatic illness in the deaf. *Acta Psychiatrica Scandinavica, 50,* 596–611.

Martin, M. C. (1974). Critical bands in sensori-neural hearing loss. *Scandinavian Audiology, 3,* 133–140.

Massaro, D. W. (1974). Perceptual units in speech recognition. *Journal of Experimental Psychology, 102,* 199–208.

Maxwell, G. (1963). *Ring of bright water.* London: Longmans.

Mazzella di Bosco, M. (1975). Tutela della sordità professionale in Italia. In G. Rossi & M. Vigone (Eds.), *L'Uomo e il rumore.* Turin: Minerva Medica. Pp. 340–350.

McCandless, G. A., & Lentz, W. E. (1968). Evoked response (EEG) audiometry in nonorganic hearing loss. *Archives of Otolaryngology, 87,* 123–128.

McCartney, J. H., Maurer, J. F., & Sorenson, F. D. (1976). A comparison of the hearing handicap scale and the hearing measurement scale with standard audiometric measures on a geriatric population. *Journal of Auditory Research, 16,* 51–58.

McClelland, D. C., Atkinson, J. W., Clark, R. A., & Lowell, E. L. (1953). *The achievement motive.* New York: Appleton.

McFarlan, D. (1940). Speech hearing and speech interpretation testing. *Archives of Otolaryngology, 31,* 517–528.

Merrell, H. B., & Atkinson, C. J. (1965). The effect of selected variables upon discrimination scores. *Journal of Auditory Research, 5,* 285–292.

Meyer zum Gottesberge, A., & Plath, P. (1967). Statistical investigation on speech discrimination in noise induced hearing loss. *International Audiology, 6,* 15–17.

Miller, G. A., Heise, G. A., & Lichten, W. (1951). The intelligibility of speech as a function of the context of the test materials. *Journal of Experimental Psychology, 41,* 329–335.

Miller, G. A., & Nicely, P. E. (1955). An analysis of perceptual confusions among some English consonants. *Journal of the Acoustical Society of America, 27,* 338–352.

Mills, A. W. (1972). Auditory localization. In J. V. Tobias (Ed.), *Foundations of modern auditory theory.* Vol. II. New York: Academic Press. Pp. 303–348.

Mullins, C. J., & Bangs, J. L. (1957). Relationships between speech discrimination and other audiometric data. *Acta Oto-laryngologica, 47,* 149–157.

Nabokov, V. (1964). Notes on prosody. In *Eugene Onegin,* by Aleksandr Pushkin. Translated by V. Nabokov, with a commentary. New York: Bollingen Foundation. Vol. III, Appendix 2.

National Acoustic Laboratories (1974). Procedure for determining percentage loss of hearing. Sydney: National Acoustic Laboratories.

Nelson, H. A. (1957). Legal liability for loss of hearing. In C. M. Harris (Ed.), *Handbook of noise control.* New York: McGraw-Hill. Ch. 38.

Niemeyer, W. (1967). Speech discrimination in noise-induced deafness. *International Audiology, 6,* 42–47.

Niemeyer, W., & Sesterhenn, G. (1974). Calculating the hearing threshold from the stapedius reflex threshold for different sound stimuli. *Audiology, 13,* 421–427.

Nixon, J., Glorig, A., & High, S. W. (1962). Changes in air and bone conduction thresholds as a function of age. *Journal of Laryngology and Otology, 76,* 288–298.

Noble, W. G. (1967). The assessment of disability from chronic acoustic trauma. Unpublished M.A. thesis, Univ. of Manchester.

Noble, W. G. (1968). The assessment of disability from chronic acoustic trauma. *International Audiology, 7,* 353–359.

Noble, W. G. (1969). A scale for the measurement of hearing loss and disability. Unpublished Ph.D. thesis, Univ. of Manchester.

Noble, W. G. (1970). A new concept of damage risk criterion. *Annals of Occupational Hygiene, 13,* 69–75.

Noble, W. G. (1971). *Test manual for the hearing measurement scale.* Armidale, Australia: Univ. of New England, Department of Psychology.

Noble, W. G. (1973). Pure tone acuity, speech-hearing ability and deafness in acoustic trauma: A review of the literature. *Audiology, 12,* 291–315.

Noble, W. G. (1974). Critical factors in the assessment of deafness due to noise. *Maico Audiological Library Series, 11,* 32–34.

Noble, W. G. (1975a). Auditory localization and its impairment. *Maico Audiological Library Series, 14*(1).

Noble, W. G. (1975b). What are speech tests a measure of? *Proceedings of the First Conference of the Audiological Society of Australia.* Sydney: Audiological Society of Australia. Pp. 5–12.

Noble, W. G. (1975c). Assessment of hearing handicap: Comment on the "Kryter series." *Journal of the Acoustical Society of America, 57,* 750–752.

Noble, W. G., & Atherley, G. R. C. (1970). The hearing measurement scale: A questionnaire for the assessment of auditory disability. *Journal of Auditory Research, 10,* 229–250.

Noble, W. G., & Russell, G. (1972). Theoretical and practical implications of the effects of hearing protection devices on localization ability. *Acta Oto-laryngologica, 74,* 29–36.

Palva, T. (1952). Finnish speech audiometry: Methods and clinical applications. *Acta Oto-laryngologica*, Supplement *101*.

Palva, T. (1955). Studies of hearing for pure tones and speech in noise. *Acta Oto-laryngologica*, *45*, 231–243.

Palva, T. (1957). Self-recording threshold audiometry and recruitment. *Archives of Otolaryngology*, *65*, 591–602.

Pearson, J. C. G., Kell, R. L., & Taylor, W. (1973). An index of hearing impairment derived from the pure-tone audiogram. In W. Taylor (Ed.), *Disorders of auditory function*. London: Academic Press. Pp. 129–150.

Portmann, M., Aran, J.-M., & Lagourgue, P. (1973). Testing for "recruitment" by electrocochleography. *Annals of Otology, Rhinology and Laryngology*, *82*, 36–43.

Pugh, J. E., Horwitz, M. R., & Anderson, D. J. (1974). Cochlear electrical activity in noise-induced hearing loss. *Archives of Otolaryngology*, *100*, 36–40.

Quiggle, R. R., Glorig, A., Delk, J. H., & Summerfield, A. B. (1957). Predicting hearing loss for speech from pure tone audiograms. *The Laryngoscope*, *67*, 1–15.

Quist-Hanssen, S., & Steen, E. (1960). Observed and calculated hearing loss for speech in noise-induced deafness. *Acta Oto-laryngologica*, Supplement *158*, 277–281.

Reed, M. (1970). Deaf and partially hearing children. In P. Mittler (Ed.), *The psychological assessment of mental and physical handicaps*. London: Methuen. Pp. 403–441.

Resnick, D. M. (1962). Reliability of the twenty-five word phonetically balanced lists. *Journal of Auditory Research*, *2*, 5–12.

Riegel, K. F. (1973). An epitaph for a paradigm: Introduction for a symposium. In K. F. Riegel (Ed.), *Intelligence: Alternative views of a paradigm*. Basel: Karger. Pp. 1–7. Originally published as *Human Development*, 1973, *16*(1–2).

Robinson, D. W., Shipton, M. S., & Whittle, L. S. (1975). Audiometry in industrial hearing conservation–I. NPL Acoustics Report Ac 64. Teddington, England: National Physical Laboratory.

Robinson, D. W., Shipton, M. S., & Whittle, L. S. (1975). Audiometry in industrial hearing conservation–II. NPL Acoustics Report Ac 71. Teddington, England: National Physical Laboratory.

Robinson, D. W., & Whittle, L. S. (1973). A comparison of self-recording and manual audiometry: Some systematic effects shown by unpractised subjects. *Journal of Sound and Vibration*, *26*, 41–62.

Roeser, R. J., & Rose, D. E. (1968). Electroencephalographic audiometry and the determination of cochlear pathology. *Journal of Auditory Research*, *8*, 135–141.

Rose, D. E., Keating, L. W., Hedgecock, L. D., Schreurs, K. K., & Miller, K. E. (1971). Aspects of acoustically evoked responses: Inter-judge and intra-judge reliability. *Archives of Otolaryngology*, *94*, 347–350.

Rose, D. E., Keating, L. W., Hedgecock, L. D., Miller, K. E., & Schreurs, K. K. (1972). A comparison of evoked response audiometry and routine clinical audiometry. *Audiology*, *11*, 238–243.

Rosen, S. (1969). Epidemiology of hearing loss. *International Audiology*, *8*, 260–277.

Rosen, S., Bergman, M., Plester, D., El-Mofty, A., & Satti, M. H. (1962). Presbycusis study of a relatively noise-free population in the Sudan. *Annals of Otology, Rhinology and Laryngology*, *71*, 727–743.

Rosen, S., Preobrajensky, N., Khechinashvili, S., Glazunov, I., Kipshidze, N., & Rosen, H. V. (1970). Epidemiologic hearing studies in the USSR. *Archives of Otolaryngology*, *91*, 424–428.

Ross, M., & Huntington, D. A. (1962). Concerning the reliability and equivalency of the CID W-22 auditory tests. *Journal of Auditory Research*, *2*, 220–228.

Ross, M., Huntington, D. A., Newby, H. A., & Dixon, R. F. (1965). Speech discrimination of hearing-impaired individuals in noise. *Journal of Auditory Research*, *5*, 47–72.

Russell, G. (1975). Effects of earplugs and earmuffs on horizontal plane sound localization. Unpublished Ph.D. thesis, Univ. of New England.

Sabine, P. E. (1942). On estimating the percentage loss of useful hearing. *Transactions of the American Academy of Ophthalmology and Oto-laryngology, 46,* 179-196.

Sanders, D. A., & Goodrich, S. J. (1971). The relative contributions of visual and auditory components of speech to speech intelligibility as a function of three conditions of frequency distortion. *Journal of Speech and Hearing Research, 14,* 154-159.

Schein, J. D., Gentile, A., & Haase, K. W. (1970). Development and evaluation of an expanded hearing loss scale questionnaire. National Center for Health Statistics, Series 2, No. 37. Rockville, Maryland: U.S. Dept. of Health, Education and Welfare.

Schmidt, P. H. (1967). Presbycusis. *International Audiology,* Supplement no. 1.

Schuknecht, H. F. (1953). Lesions of the organ of Corti. *Transactions of the American Academy of Ophthalmology and Otolaryngology, 57,* 366-383.

Schuknecht, H. F. (1970). Functional manifestations of lesions of the sensorineural structures. In J. V. Tobias (Ed.), *Foundations of modern auditory theory.* Vol. I. New York: Academic Press. Pp. 383-404.

Schutz, A. (1955). Symbol reality and society. In L. Bryson, L. Finkelstein, H. Hoagland, & R. M. McIver (Eds.), *Symbols and society.* New York: Harper. Reprinted in *Alfred Schutz Collected Papers* 1 (M. Natanson, Ed.). The Hague: Martinus Nijhoff, 1973, Pp. 287-356.

Seligman, M. E. P. (1975). *Helplessness.* San Francisco: W. H. Freeman.

Sesterhenn, G., & Breuninger, H. (1977). Determination of hearing threshold for single frequencies from the acoustic reflex. *Audiology, 16,* 201-214.

Sharrah, J. S. (1966). Compensation for hearing loss. *Industrial Medicine and Surgery, 35,* 275-277.

Sher, A., & Owens, E. (1974). Consonant confusions associated with hearing loss above 2000 Hz. *Journal of Speech and Hearing Research, 17,* 669-681.

Siegel, S. (1956). *Nonparametric statistics for the behavioral sciences.* New York: McGraw-Hill.

Siegenthaler, B. M. (1949). A study of the relationship between measured hearing loss and intelligibility of selected words. *Journal of Speech and Hearing Disorders, 14,* 111-118.

Siegenthaler, B. M., & Strand, R. (1964). Audiogram-average methods and SRT scores. *Journal of the Acoustical Society of America, 36,* 589-593.

Silverman, S. R., & Hirsh, I. J. (1955). Problems related to the use of speech in clinical audiometry. *Annals of Otology, Rhinology and Laryngology, 64,* 1234-1244.

Silverman, S. R., Thurlow, W. R., Walsh, T. E., & Davis, H. (1948). Improvement in the social adequacy of hearing following the fenestration operation. *The Laryngoscope, 58,* 607-631.

Simmons, F. B. (1970). Monaural processing. In J. V. Tobias (Ed.), *Foundations of modern auditory theory.* Vol. I. New York: Academic Press. Pp. 345-379.

Simonton, K. M., & Hedgecock, L. D. (1953). A laboratory assessment of hearing acuity for voice signals against a background of noise. *Annals of Otology, Rhinology and Laryngology, 62,* 735-747.

Speaks, C., & Jerger, J. (1965). Method for measurement of speech identification. *Journal of Speech and Hearing Research, 8,* 185-194.

Speaks, C., Jerger, J., & Trammell, J. (1970). Measurement of hearing handicap. *Journal of Speech and Hearing Research, 13,* 768-776.

Spoendlin, H. (1972). Innervation densities of the cochlea. *Acta Oto-laryngologica, 73,* 235-248.

Spoor, A. (1967). Presbycusis values in relation to noise induced hearing loss. *International Audiology, 6,* 48-57.

Steinberg, J. C., & Gardner, M. B. (1937). The dependence of hearing impairment on sound intensity. *Journal of the Acoustical Society of America, 9*, 11–23.

Steinberg, J. C., & Gardner, M. B. (1940). On the auditory significance of the term hearing loss. *Journal of the Acoustical Society of America, 11*, 270–277.

Steinberg, J. C., Montgomery, H. C., & Gardner, M. B. (1940). Results of the world's fair hearing tests. *Journal of the Acoustical Society of America, 12*, 291–301.

Stephens, S. D. G. (1969). Auditory threshold variance, signal detection theory and personality. *International Audiology, 8*, 131–137.

Stephens, S. D. G. (1971). Some individual factors influencing audiometric performance. In D. W. Robinson (Ed.), *Occupational hearing loss*. London: Academic Press. Pp. 109–120.

Stephens, S. D. G. (1976). The input for a damaged cochlea—a brief review. *British Journal of Audiology, 10*, 97–101.

Sunderman, F. W., & Boerner, F. (1950). *Normal values in clinical medicine*. Philadelphia: Saunders.

Suter, A., & von Gierke, H. E. (1975). Evaluation and compensation of occupational hearing loss in the United States. In G. Rossi & M. Vigone (Eds.), *L'Uomo e il rumore*. Turin: Minerva Medica. Pp. 359–366.

Swets, J. A. (1961). Is there a sensory threshold? *Science, 134*, 168–177.

Swets, J. A., Tanner, W. P., Jr., & Birdsall, T. G. (1961). Decision processes in perception. *Psychological Review, 68*, 301–340.

Symons, N. S. (1955). Legal and legislative developments in New York state. *Noise Control, 1*(1), 72–74.

Symons, N. S. (1958). Workmen's compensation benefits for occupational hearing loss. *Noise Control, 4*, 300–304, 332.

Szasz, T. S. (1956). Malingering: "Diagnosis" or social condemnation? *Archives of Neurology and Psychiatry, 76*, 432–443.

Szasz, T. S. (1971). *The manufacture of madness*. London: Routledge & Kegan Paul.

Taylor, W., Pearson, J. C. G., Kell, R., & Mair, A. (1967). A pilot study of hearing loss and social handicap in female jute weavers. *Proceedings of the Royal Society of Medicine, 60*, 1117–1121.

Taylor, W., Pearson, J., Mair, A., & Burns, W. (1965). Study of noise and hearing in jute weaving. *Journal of the Acoustical Society of America, 38*, 113–120.

Thompson, G., & Hoel, R. (1962). "Flat" sensorineural hearing loss and PB scores. *Journal of Speech and Hearing Disorders, 27*, 284–285.

Thorndike, E. L. (1932). *A teacher's word book of the twenty thousand words found most frequently and widely in general reading for children and young people* (rev. ed.). New York: Columbia Univ. Press.

Tonning, F.-M. (1975). Auditory localization and its clinical applications. *Audiology, 14*, 368–380.

Trier, T. R., & Levy, R. (1965). Social and psychological characteristics of veterans with functional hearing loss. *Journal of Auditory Research, 5*, 241–256.

van Uden, A. (1975). The place of manual communication in the education of deaf children seen from the viewpoint of a fully oral education-philosophy. Presented at the Seminar on, "The place of manual communication in the education of deaf children". London, April.

United States Public Health Service (1938). Preliminary analysis of audiometric data in relation to clinical history of impaired hearing. *The National Health Survey, Hearing Study Series*, Bulletin No. 2. Washington, D.C.: U.S. Public Health Service.

Vargo, S. W. (1974). Compression amplification and hearing aids. *Maico Audiological Library Series, 12*, 5–8.

Ventry, I. M. (1976). Pure tone–spondee threshold relationships in functional hearing loss: A hypothesis. *Journal of Speech and Hearing Disorders, 41,* 16–22.

Ventry, I. M., & Chaiklin, J. B. (1962). Functional hearing loss: A problem in terminology. *Asha, 4,* 251–254.

Ventry, I. M., & Chaiklin, J. B., Eds. (1965a). Multidiscipline study of functional hearing loss. *Journal of Auditory Research, 5,* 179–272.

Ventry, I. M., & Chaiklin, J. B. (1965b). The efficiency of audiometric measures used to identify functional hearing loss. *Journal of Auditory Research, 5,* 196–211.

Ventry, I. M., Trier, T. R., & Chaiklin, J. B. (1965). Factors related to persistence and resolution of functional hearing loss. *Journal of Auditory Research, 5,* 231–240.

Walsh, T. E., & Silverman, S. R. (1946). Diagnosis and evaluation of fenestration. *The Laryngoscope, 56,* 536–555.

Ward, P. R., & Tudor, C. (1976). Project to evaluate follow up services for adults issued with hearing aids: Progress report 2. Univ. of Exeter, Institute of Biometry and Community Medicine.

Ward, W. D. (1970). Musical perception. In J. V. Tobias (Ed.), *Foundations of modern auditory theory.* Vol. I. New York: Academic Press. Pp. 405–447.

Ward, W. D. (1971). Presbycusis, sociocusis and occupational noise-induced hearing loss. *Proceedings of the Royal Society of Medicine, 64,* 200–203.

Ward, W. D., Fleer, R. E., & Glorig, A. (1961). Characteristics of hearing losses produced by gunfire and by steady noise. *Journal of Auditory Research, 1,* 325–356.

Ward, W. D., Glorig, A., & Sklar, D. L. (1959). Susceptibility and sex. *Journal of the Acoustical Society of America, 31,* 1138.

Watson, L. A., & Tolan, T. (1949). *Hearing tests and hearing instruments.* Baltimore: Williams & Wilkins.

Webster, J. C. (1964). Important frequencies in noise-masked speech. *Archives of Otolaryngology, 80,* 494–504.

Weissler, P. G. (1968). International standard reference zero for audiometers. *Journal of the Acoustical Society of America, 44,* 264–275.

Wells, H. G. (1904). The country of the blind. *Strand Magazine,* April. Reprinted in *H. G. Wells: Selected short stories.* Harmondsworth, England: Penguin, 1958. Pp. 123–146.

Westerman, S. T. (1975). Noise pollution: Practical aspects concerning workers worldwide. *Eye, Ear, Nose and Throat Monthly, 54,* 387–393.

Wever, E. G., & Lawrence, M. (1954). *Physiological acoustics.* Princeton, New Jersey: Princeton Univ. Press.

Wheeler, L. J., & Dickson, E. D. D. (1952). The determination of the threshold of hearing. *Journal of Laryngology and Otology, 66,* 379–395.

Wiggins, J. S. (1973). *Personality and prediction: Principles of personality assessment.* Reading, Massachusetts: Addison-Wesley.

Williams, C. R. (1957). Medico-legal aspects. In J. Sataloff (Ed.), *Industrial deafness.* New York: McGraw-Hill. Pp. 52–60.

Willis, C. (1972). Perception of vowel phonemes in Fort Erie, Ontario, Canada, and Buffalo, New York: An application of synthetic vowel categorization tests to dialectology. *Journal of Speech and Hearing Research, 15,* 246–255.

Witting, E. G., & Hughson, W. (1940). Inherent accuracy of a series of repeated clinical audiograms. *The Laryngoscope, 50,* 259–269.

Worden, F. G., & Galambos, R., Eds. (1972). Auditory processing of biologically significant sounds. *Neurosciences Research Program Bulletin, 10,* No. 1.

Yamamoto, T. (1971). Occupational deafness. In *Encyclopedia of health and occupational safety.* Geneva: ILO. Pp. 368–370.

Young, M. A., & Gibbons, E. W. (1962). Speech discrimination scores and threshold measurements in a non-normal hearing population. *Journal of Auditory Research, 2,* 21–33.

Zwislocki, J. J. (1975). Phase opposition between inner and outer hair cells and auditory sound analysis. *Audiology, 14,* 443–455.
Zwislocki, J., Maire, F., Feldman, A. S., & Rubin, H. (1958). On the effect of practice and motivation on the threshold of audibility. *Journal of the Acoustical Society of America, 30,* 254–262.
Zwislocki, J. J., & Sokolich, W. G. (1973). Velocity and displacement responses in auditory-nerve fibers. *Science, 182,* 64–66.

Index

A

Adaptation of tonal threshold, 90–96
Amplitude modulation, 11–13
  in discrimination of nonspeech sound, 11
  in spatial location, 12–13
  in theory of speech perception, 11
Articulation function, 141–142
Articulation index, 142
  applied to tonal threshold–speech discrimination relationship, 167–168
  correlation with self-report measures, 303–305
Assessment of hearing, *see also* Assessment systems, and specific hearing tests
  concept of, 25–26
  for compensation, 29–30, 39, 46–57, 323
  in conservation of hearing programs, 29
  in evaluation of treatment programs, 28–29
  historical origin, 26, 27
  outline for change in, 239–240
  in rehabilitation programs for old people, 29
  scientist's role in, 30–31, 51–52
  in young children, 28
Assessment systems, 41–46, 129–130
  AAOO–AMA, 44–46, 50–51, 53, 57, 162–163
  average of .5, 1, and 2 kHz ("three average"), 120–121, 124, 125, 127–128, 130, 131, 132, 133, 134, 136, 137, 138
  in countries other than the United States, 54–57
  Fowler (1941), 41–42, 115–116
  Fowler (1942), 42, 116, 130
  Fowler-Sabine (AMA, 1942), 43, 119
  Fowler-Sabine (AMA, 1947), 43–44, 53, 124–125, 135
  Fletcher's ".8 rule," 41, 112–113
  Kryter's and Harris's recommendations, 46, 162, 165
  multiple regression, 129, 130, 131–133, 135, 138–139
  Sabine (1942), 42–43
  "two average," 124, 129, 134–135, 137–138
Audiogram, *see* Tonal audiogram shape
Audiometric zero, 173–174, 176–179, 181–184, *see also* National standards
Auditory perception, *see also* Hearing
  classical theory of, 3–4, 11–12
Auditory world, 4–7, 12
Average Evoked Response Audiometry, 226–227

B

Békésy audiogram types, 210, 211–212

C

Communication, 6–10
  in frogs and monkeys, 8–9
  versus listening, 6–7, 261–263, 289–290
  man–animal and man–machine, 7
  sign language, 14
  speaking–listening process, 6
  vocalized language, 7–10
Compression–amplification hearing aids, 217
Conductive disorder, description, 19
Consistency, *see also* Reliability, and specific hearing tests, 62, 64–65, 75

D

Deafness
  "realization" and liberation, 15–16, 324–325
  social and phenomenal world of, 13–16
"Disability," 40
Disorder (as against disturbance) of hearing, 33, 40, 118
Disyllable ("spondee") word lists
  Central Institute for the Deaf (CID), revision of PAL lists by, 36–37
  Psycho-Acoustic Laboratory (PAL) lists, 35–36, 120

343

Index

E

Epidemiology, 174, 185–186

F

Fakability, see "Functional hearing loss"
Familiarization, see Adaptation of tonal threshold; Learning
"Filter" hypothesis, 155–156, 157–159, 165
Frequency modulation, 8, 9, 10, 11, 12–13
   in monkeys' language, 8, 9
   as spectral change in spatial location, 12–13
   in theory of speech perception, 9, 10, 11
"Functional hearing loss," 218–231
   alleged contaminating effect in listener samples, 135
   categorical error of the concept, 228–229
   definition, 219–220
   fakability concept as alternative to, 229–231
   logical problems in identification, 122–123, 137
   multidisciplinary study of, 221–224, 227–228
   speech-tone threshold relations in, 227–228

G

Galvanic Skin Response (GSR) audiometry, 223, 224–225
Generalizability, 71–73
Gibsonian theory, 4–6, 7
   acoustic specification of sources, 5–6
   "ecological acoustics," 4, 5, 8
   nature of information in, 4–5, 7

H

Handicap, 13, 14–15, 20, 28, see also Hearing handicap
   of deafness due to powerlessness, 14–15
   deafness viewed as, 13, 28
   in sensorineural as against conductive disorder, 20
Hearing, see also Normal hearing
   auditory act, 3, 236
   in the everyday world, 236–242
   as handicap in deaf culture, 15
   versus listening, 5–6

Hearing conservation and tonal threshold test reliability, 82–85
Hearing handicap, 40, 111
Hearing Handicap Scale, 248–250
   correlation with Hearing Measurement Scale, 300–301, 303–304
   correlation with performance test results, 278–282, 300, 303–304
"Hearing impairment," 40
"Hearing loss," 39, 40, 69–70
Hearing Measurement Scale, 257–258
   background development, 252–255, 307, 313
   comparative results from different samples, 295–300
   correlation with performance test results, 283–295, 300–305
   facsimile, 264–268
   and lip-reading, 311–312
   reliability and sensitivity of, 255–257
   validity and operational characteristics of, 258–263
Higher Frequency Threshold, see Tonal audiogram shape
Hörmesser (standardized mechanical noisemaker), 32
Human speech, see also Frequency modulation; Communication
   critical features and boundaries, 9, 10
   place of articulation, 9–10
   syllables, 10
   vowel and consonant energy, 34

I

Impaired hearing, see individual types (sensorineural, conductive, etc.)
Intelligibility, see also Sensorineural disorder; Speech discrimination testing
   and cue-reduction, 155–159
   effect of lexical population size on, 35, 36

L

Learning, see also Adaptation of tonal threshold; Speech perception
   as familiarization in tonal threshold tests, 75, 90–92, 93
   of spatial invariants, 12
Lip-reading, 310–312
   occupation as mediating factor in acquisition of, 311–312

Index

Localization, *see* Spatial location
"Low fence," 195–198, 318–319

M

"Malingering," 220–221, *see also* "Functional hearing loss"
  transformation into "Functional hearing loss," 221
Ménière's disease
  abnormal loudness adaptation in, 144–145
  and tonal threshold test reliability, 81–82
Modulation, *see* Frequency modulation; Amplitude modulation
Monosyllable word lists, 34–37, 104–107
  Bell Telephone Lists, 34–35
  Bell Telephone numerals, 35, 113
  Central Institute for the Deaf (CID), revision of PAL lists by, 36–37, 104–107
  Psycho-Acoustic Laboratory (PAL) lists, 36, 104–105

N

National standards, 176–178, 184, *see also* Normal hearing
  current United States zero (ANSI, 1969), 178
  former British zero (BSI, 1954), 178
  former United States zero (ASA, 1951), 176–178
  International Organization for Standardization zero (ISO, R 389), 178, 184
  and threshold test reliability, 87
Noise-induced hearing disorder, 21, 26–27, 170–171
  Barr's epidemiological study of (1886), 26–27, 174–175
  characteristic audiogram shape, 119
  effect of remote history of noise exposure, 192
  effect on spatial location, 21
  reasons for discrimination impairment in, 170–171
  self-report study of, 254–263, 296–300
  and tonal threshold–speech discrimination relationship, 143–146, 149–155, 159–162, 163–165, 166–168, 169–170
  and tonal threshold–speech reception threshold relationship, 122, 124–125, 131, 136, 139
Normal hearing, 173
  as "best available" and "best expectable" hearing, 175, 183–184, 198
  controversy about the former Anglo-American mismatch, 179–184
  "Limits of normal," 195–198
Normal hearing as an age-related variable, 185–195
  male–female difference, 190–193
  studies in people unexposed to ordinary noise, 186–189, 190
Normal threshold of hearing, *see* Normal hearing; National standards
Numerals, 112–115, *see also* Monosyllable word lists
Numerals testing, *see also* Intelligibility
  as mere detection of speech, 114–115

P

Partial deafness, 13, 16–19, 308–310
  acquired in adulthood, 17–19
  akin to being part-black, 16–17
  social–phenomenal world of, 13, 16–19, 308–310
Partial hearing, *see* Partial deafness
Phenomenology, 314–316
Phonetic balancing, 36, 37
"Primary auditory stream segregation," 10–11
Presbycusis, 185, 189, *see also* Normal hearing as an age-related variable

Q

"Quiet threshold shift," 93–96
  threshold variability and individual differences in, 95–96

R

Recruitment, 200–216
  attacked as a concept, 210–212
  as diagnostic device, 201–203, 211–212
  explanatory hypotheses of, 203–208
  Fowler's original studies of, 201
  measurement by alternate loudness balancing, 201, 202, 208–210, 211–212
  in Ménière's disease, 203, 209, 214–216
  in noncochlear pathology, 203, 211

and speech discrimination in sensorineural disorder, 146–147, 148, 155–156, 163, 212–213, 216–217, 290
theory of effect on speech discrimination, 213–216
Reliability, 61–64, 86–87, *see also* Generalizability; Variability of threshold, individual hearing tests
  distinct from variability of threshold, 86–87, 92
  models for measurement of, 64–66
  statistics used to express, 76–77
Rhyme tests, 37, 107–108

S

Sampling, 118–119, 186–189
  as an issue in age-related hearing research, 186–189, 193–195
  selection by diagnosis versus audiogram shape, 118–119
Science, as technical and as radical activity, 30, 321–322
Screening tests, 32, 66–67
Self-report, 242–243, 252–254, 307–319, *see also* Self-report inventories; Self-report and tonal threshold
  applicability in clinical assessment, 317–318
  applicability in noisy industry, 310, 318
  distinction between scaled and nonscaled questionnaires, 243–244
  dubious reaction to, 25
  interviewer bias and faking in, 317
  interviewing versus paper-and-pencil testing, 252–254
  meaningful quality of, 307–308
  nonassumptive quality of, 308–309
  of normal hearing, 181, 182, 183–184
  and problem of accessibility of experience, 316–317
  and problem of subjectivity, 314–316
  representative quality of, 307
  as social science technique, 242–243
  and speech discrimination score, 278, 279, 280, 281, 287–288, 300–301, 302, 303–305
  and speech reception threshold, 278, 282–283, 287–288, 300–301, 303–305
  stability of content across time and space, 312–314

temporal versus intensitive scaling, 253–254
  used in assessment for compensation, 55, 318–319
  utility of, 109, 310
Self-report inventories, *see also* Hearing Handicap Scale; Hearing Measurement Scale
  Dundee scale (Taylor *et al.*), 243–244, 247–248
  Lindeman's questionnaire, 247
  revision of 1960–1963 USPHS survey scale, 246–247
  Social Hearing Handicap Index, 250–252
  St. Louis scale, 245–246
  USPHS survey scale of 1935–1936, 244–245
Self-report and tonal threshold
  "Dundee Index," 282
  results using the Hearing Handicap Scale, 278, 280, 281–282, 300, 303–304
  results using the Hearing Measurement Scale, 287–289, 292–293, 294–295, 300–301, 303–305
  USPHS survey of 1935–1936, 270–276
Sensitivity of a test, 63
Sensorineural disorder, 19–20, 170–171, 217–218
  effect on speech discrimination, 20, 142, 145–146
  reasons for discrimination impairment in, 170–171, 217–218
  tonal threshold–speech discrimination relationship in, 145–146, 163
  tonal threshold–SRT relationship in, 127–129, 131
Sentence lists, 34–35, 36, 38
  Bell Telephone, 34–35, 117
  CID everyday, 38, 108, 303–305
  Psycho-Acoustic Laboratory, 36
Signing, as a natural language, 14, 17
SISI test, 210, 211
Social Adequacy Index, 45–46, 245–246
Sociocusis, 193–195
Spatial location, 11–13, 20–22
  comparison of self-report and performance in, 291–292
  effect of unilateral disorder on, 21
  implications of disruption for speech perception, 21–22, 260–261, 263
  role of pinna(e), 12
  self-reports of ability in, 21

Speech detection threshold, 75
  reliability, 100–101
Speech discrimination testing, 75, 102, 140–141
  as analog of everyday hearing, 237
  assumption about dialect in, 309
  at fixed acoustic level, 161
  interlist consistency and, 104–108
  intralist stability and, 106
  response mode and reliability of, 103–104
  talker effect on reliability of, 102–103
Speech perception, *see also* Human speech; Communication
  Cole and Scott's Theoretical Model of, 9, 10–11
  emotional disturbance accompanying breakdown of, 258, 259, 302
  improvement with specific practice, 136, 149, 155
Speech reception threshold, 35–36, 75, 140
  as analog of everyday hearing, 237, 290
  reliability, 100–101
Speech tests, *see* Tests of hearing, and specific types of lists
Speeded speech, 156–157, 163–164, *see also* Tonal audiogram shape
Stability, 62, 65–66, 75, *see also* Reliability and specific hearing tests
Stapedius Reflex Threshold Audiometry, 225–226

T

Tests of hearing, *see also* Assessment systems, and specific hearing tests
  for assessment as against diagnosis, 31–32
  consonant-confusion test, 149
  distinct from assessment systems, 31
  nonstandardized speech tests, 34
  short forms of speech test lists, 109
  watch-tick test, 32, 33, 174–175
"The Country of the Blind," 15
Thomas Barr (otologist), biographical note, 26
Threshold concepts, 91–92, *see also* specific hearing tests
Tinnitus, 22–23
  as imposed stimulus, 22
Tonal audiogram shape

Carhart's classifications, 119–122, 137, 138–139
  as critical auditory variable, 118–121
  "flat" versus "unsymmetrical" distinction, 117, 123, 125, 127–128, 129–130, 142–143
  high frequency threshold elevation and speech hearing, 142–143, 144, 148, 153–154, 155–157
Tonal threshold tests, 32–34
  basic features, 32–33
  bone conduction reliability, 81–82
  earphone placement and reliability of, 89–90
  limited informativeness of, 33–34
  operator-effect and reliability of, 78–79, 80
  reliability in clinical–industrial samples, 77–86
  signal type and consistency in, 88–89
  test conditions and reliability of, 79
  testing technique and reliability of, 79–80, 82, 87–89
Transitions, *see* Frequency modulation; Amplitude modulation
Tuning curves, 206–208

U

United States Public Health Service
  Hearing Survey of 1935–1936 self-report scale, 244–245
  National Hearing Survey (1935–1936), 176–177, 179–183, 195–196, 198, 270–276
  revision of 1960–1963 Hearing Survey self-report scale, 246–247
Utility, 66–67, 108–109, *see also* Screening tests

V

Validity, 67–71, *see also* Generalizability
  definitions of concurrent and predictive, 68
  definitions of theoretical construct and content, 69–71
Validity of Discrimination Score for estimating hearing handicap, 169, 237–238

Validity of Speech Reception Threshold for estimating hearing handicap, 169, 237–238
Validity of tonal threshold
for estimating speech detection threshold, 113–116
for estimating speech discrimination score, 112, 140–171
for estimating speech reception threshold, 112, 116–117, 119–140
Variability of threshold, 90–99, *see also* Threshold concepts
and different states of hearing, 96–97
and motivational–personality variables, 97–99
Veterans Administration, 52–53, 53–54, 99, 119, 222, 223

W

Wisconsin State Fair hearing surveys, 50, 132, 186, 187
Workmen's compensation, 47–50